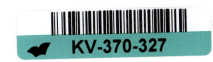

RECENT ADVANCES IN
MULTIPLE SCLEROSIS THERAPY

RECENT ADVANCES IN MULTIPLE SCLEROSIS THERAPY

Proceedings of the Vth Congress of the European Committee for Treatment and Research in Multiple Sclerosis (ECTRIMS), Brussels, 16–18 March 1989

Hosted by the CHARCOT FOUNDATION of the Belgian Research Group for Multiple Sclerosis.

Editors:

R.E. GONSETTE
P. DELMOTTE
Belgian National Center for Multiple Sclerosis
Melsbroek, Belgium.

 1989

EXCERPTA MEDICA, AMSTERDAM - NEW YORK - OXFORD

International Congress Series No. 863
ISBN 0 444 81111 7

This book is printed on acid-free paper.

Published by:
Elsevier Science Publishers B.V.
(Biomedical Division)
P.O. Box 211
1000 AE Amsterdam
The Netherlands

Sole distributors for the USA and Canada:
Elsevier Science Publishing Company Inc.
655 Avenue of the Americas
New York, NY 10010
USA

Printed in The Netherlands

FOREWORD

The Organizing Committee of the Vth ECTRIMS Congress was particularly delighted to welcome participants coming from nearly all over Europe and even from the five continents.

We were hesitant, maybe even reluctant to some point, to determine the treatment of Multiple Sclerosis (MS) as the main theme of this Vth ECTRIMS meeting. It was indeed the first time in Europe that a congress of this importance was mainly dedicated to MS therapy, which is always regarded suspisciously within the scientific world.

As the first immunosuppressive treatments go back to about the years 60, we thought that it could be possible to draw some conclusions either positive or negative, from the numerous clinical trials made in nearly all European countries since more than 25 years. Shortly after taking this decision, we heard that 2 meetings were programmed with the same theme in the United States at the end of 88 and beginning 89, which gave us confidence. It was most natural in these conditions for European searchers to sum up their experience and also to confront it with that of their American colleagues and we wish to thank them for coming and sharing their experience with us.

All those who have been facing MS treatment for decades will understand how exceptional it is that 3 main meetings are dedicated within a few months to MS therapy. Indeed for many years, MS treatment seemed such an impossible aim for an objection which is more an excuse than a good reason. We often hear, and this suits the public opinion, that as long that no cause is known for a disease, mastering it remains impossible. However, we have learnt from the past that we can act on a disease long before knowing its real cause. The most important point is indeed to know what are the pathophysiological mechanisms responsible of signs and symptoms.

It is true that in this field MS has remained a mystery until some years ago. We are now able to classify it with certainty within the group of immune diseases, even if we cannot yet determine the actual cause of these immune disorders. European searchers have been suspecting the role of immunity in MS for many years now, and let us not forget that immunosuppressive treatments in MS have been used for the first time in Europe.

MS has the advantage of fascinating immunologists all over the world. It is now common practice, when a new immunologic parameter is discovered to investigate it in MS. Undoubtedly the major discoveries in this field during these last few years, will have an utmost influence in solving the problem of MS. Basic research allows us to understand better each day some of the immune pathological mechanisms involved in the development of the disease. At the same time, techniques modifying immunity have increased tremendously and it was logical to check what happened in MS when modifying these mechanisms.

Unfortunately, MS brings up specific problems as far as effects of treatments are concerned. Firstly, we know that animals are not susceptible to get MS and we do not yet have a perfect experimental animal model. Secondly, the fluctuating evolution of the disease makes it difficult to evaluate the effects of our experimental treatments. Thirdly, we know from recent MRI longitudinal studies that there is no strict correlation between the evolution of the lesions inside the brain and clinical symptoms.

Early European clinical studies have, for these reasons, been imperfect, which sometimes leads to criticism from our American colleagues. They had however the advantage of bringing two important contributions in our way of conceiving MS treatment: 1. immunotherapy is feasible in MS; 2. intense and prolonged immunosuppression can be effective in some patients.

Hence the numerous trials of immune techniques since a decade, not to actually eradicate MS, but in the hope of halting the progression. The ECTRIMS executive committee therefore felt that now was the most appropriate time to evaluate current results and define future perspectives.

The first part of the Congress was devoted to clinical and paraclinical parameters which ought to be used to objectively assess disease activity. As everybody knows we do not yet have the perfect functional and/or neurological scale but it would however be of the utmost importance to know which of the existing ones are the most reliable, and to define changes accepted by all as reflecting a true disease progression.

During these last years some new neurophysiological and mainly neuroradiological techniques have allowed us to better analyze the hidden face of the disease in such a way that they have even sometimes modified some of our concepts. We have good reasons to believe that MRI will unable us, in certain conditions not yet defined, to evaluate the effects of treatments faster and with more objectivity.

We wish to thank Prof. Hommes for accepting to draw concluding remarks from the presented papers and to define the best criteria to objectively assess both disease activity and effects of treatments.

As a matter of fact, on the second day treatments was dealt with. Too much time and money have been wasted in endless clinical trials, the inefficiency of which is however obvious. The role of ECTRIMS is to take a firm and clear position, independently of pharmaceutical companies and medical schools, concerning the usefulness or not to pursue such clinical trials. It should also be possible to define what trials ought to be developed in well trained centers and which should further be conducted in multicenter studies. Could the combination of two or more immune techniques bring better results like in cancer treatment for instance.

All these treatments, we must stress, only concern a small number of patients, those with a rapidly progressing disease and for whom it is anyway the last hope.

But we are every day confronted with the large number of patients whose disease is slowly but inexorably progressing. We know that within 25 years most of them will be severely handicapped and no effective help can to day be given. Several low risks immune techniques to reduce on the long term the relapse rate as well as the progression in those young patients have been recently suggested.

One of them, the COP I seems to have been quite seriously tested. If the positive effects on relapses seemed attractive there were some contradictions in the presentation of the results in progressive forms on successive meetings. It is furthermore unfortunate that red tape, political and financial problems prevent us from confirming or invalidating COP I effects in large multicenter studies.

Obviously we cannot yet take position concerning the efficiency of low risks treatments possibly suggested in young patients. It is therefore our duty to organize clinical studies able to answer firmly to the question: is such or such low risk treatment useful in early stages of the disease. Even more that the fact of following this types of treatment often implies high costs for the patients.

Prof. Mertin had to face the difficult task to suggest guidelines in these various fields. We thank him for doing so.

A last session was dedicated to another important problem: that of gathering and collecting clinical and paraclinical data in order to yet better understand the disease and mainly to make the most of our experience in therapeutic trials. The only way in this field is databasing.

For the first time, American and European computerized clinical files were presented and compared. Even if there was little chance of taking definite decisions, this round table will hopefully enable us in a near future to put together a computerized file which will serve as a common denominator to exchange and exploit MS data accumulated all over the world. This initiative shows once more the need of exchanging basic and clinical data in MS on an international level. Prof. Confravreux who has a wide experience in this field since years had accepted to be the chairman of this round table. He has reported about an European proposal for computerization of MS patients data, recently accepted by the ECTRIMS' executive committee.

Finally, it is very encouraging, with the United States of Europe in view, to hear that since December 88 MS research is officially part of the IVth Medical and Health Research programme of the CEC. Prof. Hommes, general secretary of ECTRIMS, is the keystone of this project.

This Vth ECTRIMS Congress dealt with three well defined objectives in the frame of MS treatment. The presentations and discussions were of high standard of quality and once again, we would like to thank all the participants for their contribution to the success of this meeting.

R.E. GONSETTE, MD
President Vth ECTRIMS Congress

ACKNOWLEDGEMENTS

We are grateful to: Commission of the European Communities, Ministerie van de Vlaamse Gemeenschap, Fonds National de la Recherche Scientifique – Nationaal Fonds voor Wetenschappelijk Onderzoek, Société Belge de Neurologie – Belgische Vereniging voor Neurologie, American National Multiple Sclerosis Society, Ligue Belge de la Sclérose en Plaques, Communauté Française, for sponsoring this congress.

The Organizing Committee acknowledges gratefully the generous support of: SANDOZ Brussels and SANDOZ Basel, CODALI Brussels, Laboratoires André GUERBET Paris, Lab. DELALANDE Brussels, UPJOHN Brussels.

CONTENTS

Neurophysiological techniques

Biological markers

Concluding remarks

TREATMENTS: RESULTS AND FUTURE PROSPECTS

Corticotherapy

Interferons

Cyclosporine A

Azathioprine

Cyclophosphamide

Other immunosuppressive treatments

Symptomatic treatments

FREE COMMUNICATIONS

POSTERS

ASSESSMENT OF DISEASE ACTIVITY

NATURAL HISTORY, CLINICAL ASSESSMENT, PROGNOSTIC FACTORS

© 1989 Elsevier Science Publishers B.V. (Biomedical Division)
Recent advances in multiple sclerosis therapy.
R.E. Gonsette, P. Delmotte, editors.

INTER-RATER VARIABILITY ON MULTIPLE SCLEROSIS DISABILITY SCALES IN A BLINDED, PROSPECTIVE CLINICAL TRIAL

J.H. NOSEWORTHY, M.K. VANDERVOORT, C. WONG, LONDON, ONTARIO, AND THE CANADIAN COOPERATIVE MULTIPLE SCLEROSIS STUDY GROUP, VANCOUVER, CALGARY, SASKATOON, WINNIPEG, LONDON, HAMILTON, TORONTO, OTTAWA, AND MONTREAL, CANADA.
Department of Clinical Neurological Sciences, University Hospital, 339 Windermere Road, London, Ontario, Canada N6A 5A5

INTRODUCTION

Although early evidence suggests that it may be possible to use serial MRI studies to follow the course of multiple sclerosis (MS) (1,2), there is no universally available, verified method of measuring objectively responses to therapeutic intervention. Of the four scales considered to be part of the Minimum Record of Disability by the International Federation of Multiple Sclerosis Societies (Expanded Disability Status Scale, Functional Systems, Incapacity Status Scale, and Environmental Status Scale), only the Expanded Disability Status Scale (EDSS; 3) and Functional Systems (FS; 4) are appropriate for use in therapeutic trials. The Functional Systems record the neurological abnormalities resulting from MS. Each FS score can be compared over time with itself to measure the changes within that anatomical system during the period of observation. The Expanded Disability Status Scale, an updated version of the Disability Status Scale (5), uses the scores from the FS to define the lower range of the scale. The EDSS is largely derived from the results of an observed neurological examination, symptoms are discarded and only deficits due to MS are considered in deriving this final score.

The degree of inter-rater and intra-rater reliability in the use of these scales has been tested by several investigators. Kuzma and colleagues (5 examiners in total; 6) repeatedly examined 10 patients on 2 occasions within a week and found that the FS and DSS (as well as the standard neurologic examination) provided reliable and reproducible information with no significant differences between the five examiners on the majority of the examination items. Amato and colleagues reported on the inter-observer and intra-observer reliability in the Kurtzke scoring systems in MS (7). Forty MS patients were examined by one neurologist in the presence of three others, and each physician independently assigned FS and EDSS scores. Patients were brought back one month later to assess intra-rater reliability. Using a weighted Kappa index (which takes into account the relative levels of disagreement between any two observers) the degree of inter-rater and intra-rater agreement was found to be very high (weighted Kappa values greater than 80%) for the EDSS, for the pyramidal, bladder and bowel, and sensory functions of the FS. Lower scores were observed in the cerebellar,

4

Table: Percent agreement and Kappa statistics.

	PERFECT AGREEMENT		$\geq$ 1 STEP AGREEMENT	
	%	K	%	K
EDSS	69.7	.62	94.5	.89
FS				
Pyramidal	69.4	.47	98.2	.88
Cerebellar	46.5	.32	82.1	.58
Brainstem	58.2	.45	96.6	.90
Sensory	48.5	.31	85.9	.60
Bowel & Bladder	57.9	.43	94.9	.82
Visual	69.6	.59	92.0	.81
Cerebral	70.2	.47	96.5	.76

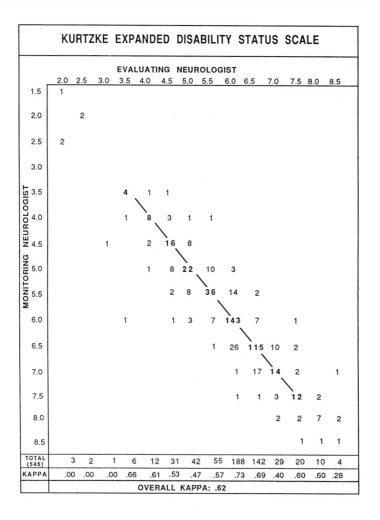

brainstem, and mental subsections of the FS. Finally, in 1988, Amato and colleagues (4 examiners) working in pairs examined a total of 24 patients (8). Using the Kappa index, inter-observer agreement ranged from 30-50% with the largest degree of disagreement being found in the sensory and mental functions of the FS. Agreement within one point on these scales was seen in greater than 85% of the cases, however. These investigators concluded that a two-unit difference on each of these scales probably indicated a reliable index of clinical change.

MATERIAL AND METHODS

This report describes the degree of inter-rater variability in the use of the EDSS and FS in the 9 centre randomized, blinded, and placebo-controlled Canadian Cooperative Study of Cyclophosphamide and Plasma Exchange in Patients with Progressive MS. These disability scales are being used to measure whether these treatments are beneficial for patients whose illness has been steadily progressive (decline of EDSS by greater than or equal to 1.0 within the preceding twelve months in patients with an EDSS of between 4.0 and 6.5). Each of the 168 enrolled patients is seen consecutively by two neurologists at entry and, thereafter, at six-monthly intervals. The two physicians are not permitted to discuss their findings nor consult with their prior records. To measure the degree of inter-rater agreement in excess of that expected by chance, the Kappa statistic was calculated using a "perfect" agreement vs. "imperfect" agreement paradigm. It was not possible with this study design to assess the degree of intra-rater variability.

RESULTS AND DISCUSSION

The EDSS scores from the 545 paired examinations in 168 patients is shown in the figure. If there were perfect agreement between the two examiners on the assignment of the EDSS at each of the 545 examinations all the results would fall on the highlighted diagonal line. In fact, perfect agreement is seen in 69.7% of the cases. Agreement within one step (a difference of 0.5 points on the EDSS), however, is seen in almost 95% of the examinations. There are a sufficient number of observations between 4.5 and 7.5 on the EDSS scale to suggest that the degree of variability is similar within this range. Similar results were found for the pyramidal score of the FS. In 545 paired examinations, perfect agreement was seen in 69.4% of the cases. Agreement within one step (a full 1.0 point on the FS) was seen in greater than 98% of the examinations. The Kappa statistic for each step between 0 and 5 on the pyramidal scale suggests that there is a similar degree of concordance between examiners throughout most of the range of the scale. Concordance was less satisfactory for the cerebellar and sensory FS scales. Perfect agreement is seen in only 46.5 and 48.5% of these cases respectively, with agreement within one step in approximately 82-86% of the cases. Again, the Kappa statistics suggest that between 0 and 4 on the cerebellar and sensory scales there is a similar degree of inter-rater variability.

The table summarizes the degree of perfect agreement and agreement within one step in these 545 paired examinations. The Kappa statistic is given for each parameter. Perfect agreement in the range of 69% was seen for the EDSS, pyramidal, visual, and cerebral scores of the FS. Perfect agreement was less than 50%, however, for the cerebellar and sensory scores. Inter-rater reliability improved markedly for concordance within one step, being greater than 80% in all cases, and greater than 94% in the EDSS, pyramidal, brainstem, bowel/bladder, and cerebral scores. In most cases, the Kappa values for perfect agreement all fell within the .4 -.75 range, values which would rate a "moderate to substantial" degree of inter-rater agreement according to Landis and Koch (9). If one permits a one step error between examiners, the Kappa statistic improves markedly, and with the exception of the cerebellar, cerebral, and sensory FS scales, is in the "almost perfect" range (9).

We have sufficient observations to calculate Kappa statistics for perfect agreement for the first five grades of each of the Functional Systems. These data (not shown) suggest that there is no single grade on any of the Functional Systems on which the raters' performance differ significantly from the overall Kappa for that particular Functional System scale.

Our experience suggests that although there is a considerable degree of concordance between neurologists using these ordinal disability scales, there remains a modest degree of disagreement in the assignment of each measure of disability. We would conclude from this study that two experienced neurologists agree within one step on the degree of disability in at least 94% of cases on the EDSS and pyramidal, brainstem, and cerebral FS scores but disagree by two or more steps in 15-18% of cases on the cerebellar and sensory scores (FS). The degree of inter-rater variability between examiners is similar throughout the range of most of the FS scales and from 4.0 - 7.5 on the EDSS. Inter-rater variability and momentary changes in patient performance may account for changes of a single step in the FS and EDSS scales. A change of greater than one step is needed to infer an important change in clinical status.

REFERENCES
1. Isaac C, Li DKB, Genton M, et al (1988). Neurology 38:1511-1515.
2. Willoughby EW, Grochowski E, Li DKB, et al (1989). Ann Neurol 25:43-49.
3. Kurtzke JF (1983). Neurology 33:1444-1452.
4. Kurtzke JF (1961). Neurology 11:686-694.
5. Kurtzke JF (1955). Neurology 5:580-583.
6. Kuzma JW, Namerow NS, Tourtellotte WW, et al (1969). J Chron Dis 21:803-814.
7. Amato MP, Groppi C, Siracusa GF, Fratiglioni L (1987). Ital J Neurol Sci, Suppl 6:129-132.
8. Amato MP, Fratiglioni L, Groppi C, et al (1988). Arch Neurol 45:746-748.
9. Landis JR, Koch GG (1977). Biometrics 33:159-174.

The Canadian Cooperative Multiple Sclerosis Study Group

This study group consists of the following investigators, committees, and participating centres (members of the executive committee are indicated by an asterisk): Central Coordinating Centre (University of Western Ontario), London, Ont.: principal investigator J.H. Noseworthy*; study coordinator M.K. Vandervoort*; safety committee: R. Roberts, chairman, Hamilton, Ont., J.P. Antel, Montreal, P.Q., J.F. Kurtzke, Washington, D.C.

Participating centres (in order of number of eligible patients entered): University of Western Ontario, London, Ont.: J.H. Noseworthy*, M.K. Vandervoort*, W.P. Mcinnis, G.C. Ebers*, G.P.A. Rice, B.G. Weinschenker, D. Hollomby, N. Muirhead. The University of Calgary, Calgary, Alta., T.P. Seland, co-director*, O. Suchowersky, C. Harris, J. Klassen. University of Manitoba, Winnipeg, Man.: A. Auty, J.M. Del Campo, J. Todd, H. Rayner. University of British Columbia, Vancouver, B.C.: D. Paty, S. Hashimoto, R. Farquhar, K. Eisen, W.B. Benny. University of Toronto, Toronto, Ont.: T. Gray, G. Sawa, K.H. Shumak*, A. Royal, E. McBride, J.J. Freedman. University of Saskatchewan, Saskatoon, Sask.: D.J. MacFadyen, W. Hader, E. Ashenhurst, M. Schmaltz, D. Sheridan, R. Card. University of Montreal, Montreal, P.Q.: P. Duquettte, L. Roy, J. Pleines, Y. Lapointe. McMaster University, Hamilton, Ont.: J.E. Paulseth, R. Lo, M. Gent*, D.W. Taylor*, B. Neufeld, J.A. McBride. University of Ottawa, Ottawa, Ont.: R. Nelson, D. Preston, G. Rock, L. Huebsch.

© 1989 Elsevier Science Publishers B.V. (Biomedical Division)
Recent advances in multiple sclerosis therapy.
R.E. Gonsette, P. Delmotte, editors.

INTERRATER RELIABILITY IN THE USE OF THE KURTZKE SCALE FOR MULTIPLE SCLEROSIS: CLUES TO THE VALIDATION OF CLINICAL DATA FROM COOPERATIVE STUDIES.

MARIA PIA AMATO, LAURA FRATIGLIONI, LUIGI AMADUCCI, GIANFRANCO SIRACUSA, CINZIA GROPPI

Institute of Neurology - University of Florence

INTRODUCTION

Despite the growing use in clinical trials and prognostic studies on Multiple Sclerosis (MS) of quantitative methods for assessing neurological status, there has been rather little information on the reliability of such methods. This is an essential requirement of any measuring device and provides the foundation for applying research results to clinical practice (1). This report deals with a detailed analysis of the inter-rater reliability of the Kurtzke Functional Systems (FS) and Expanded Disability Status Scale (EDSS) (2).

MATERIALS AND METHODS

Our sample consisted of the 24 patients with definite MS according to Poser's criteria (3), who were referred, during the month of June 1986, to the Institute of Neurology of the University of Florence. The experiment was conducted by four neurologists with comparable experience, arranged into six pairs. Each pair examined four patients in turn, with each member of the pair serving as the first examiner for two patients and as the second examiner for the remaining two. Each neurologist of the pair examined and scored patients independently. The extent of inter-rater agreement was determined by means of the Fleiss's generalization of the kappa index which measures agreement among multiple raters (4,5). The numerical values of kappa were judged according to Landis and Koch (6).

RESULTS

The raw data for each pair of raters in scoring EDSS are shown in Table 1. Two trends emerge from these raw data: disagreements were evenly distributed among the six pairs of observers and in most cases raters differed by no more than 0.5 or 1.0 score units. The same trends were evident from FS scoring, too. From the raw data we calculated three different kappa indexes (Table 2): kappa 1 when raters had to assign exactly the same score to be considered in agreement; kappa 2 when raters who differed by no more than one point were considered to agree and, finally, kappa 3 when raters who differed by at most two points were considered as agreeing. In terms of the kappa 1 index, we found rather low levels of inter-rater agreement. In particular only in Cerebellar, Brain-stem and Bowel and Bladder functions and for EDSS did the kappa coefficients reach 50%, which is regarded as a moderate level of agreement. Mental, Sensory, and, surprisingly, Pyramidal functions, too, showed the lowest levels of kappa 1 values. When raters who differed by no more than one point were said to agree , as expressed by the kappa 2 values, inter-examiner agreement was always greater than 85%, which represents close to perfect agreement. Agreement was just about perfect among raters differing by at most 2 points, as the kappa 3 column shows. Finally, we analyzed the kappa values for the first and the second half of the EDSS, taking a score of 5 as a cutoff. Agreement was 32% for EDSS scores between 1 and 4 (9 patients) and 59% for scores between 5 and 8.5 (15 patients).

TABLE 1 : POINT-DIFFERENCES AMONG EACH PAIR OF RATERS IN EDSS SCORES

		EDSS scores				
Observer	N patients	0	0.5	1.0	1.5	2
A/B	4	2	2	0	0	0
A/C	4	3	0	1	0	0
A/D	4	1	1	2	0	0
B/C	4	2	1	1	0	0
B/D	4	1	2	0	1	0
C/D	4	3	0	1	0	0

Table 2: INTER-RATER RELIABILITY ON KURTZKE FS AND EDSS

KURTZKE SCALE	K1	K2	K3
FS			
Pyramidal	0.28	0.95	1.0
Cerebellar	0.56	0.87	0.87
Brainstem	0.50	0.93	1.0
Bladder-bowel	0.50	1.0	1.0
Sensory	0.32	0.93	1.0
Mental	0.32	0.87	0.94
EDSS	0.49	0.94	1.0

12

DISCUSSION

In the present study we found fair to moderate inter-rater agreement in scoring MS patients on the Kurtzke scale. Mental, Sensory and, surprisingly, Pyramidal Functions proved to be the most variable. Furthermore, a fair degree of agreement was found on the first half of the EDSS (scores <5) , where the evaluation depends entirely on the FS scores. Almost perfect inter-rater agreement could be obtained when a one-point difference was the criterion for agreement. When numerical scores form the basis for clinical judgements a point difference of only one unit on the Kurtzke disability scale is generally taken as a sufficient index of clinical change. Our data suggest that a one point difference might simply reflect variability inherent in the neurological examination itself , rather than a real modification in the disease . Therefore we feel that a difference of at least two score points on the EDSS would constitute a more reliable indicator of clinical change, expecially in long-term multicenter studies. Training programs for raters and periodic control of inter-rater variability seem highly advisable to increase the quality of data obtained in clinical research.

REFERENCES

1. Koran LM (1975): The reliability of clinical methods, data and judgements : N England J Med 293:695-701.

2. Kurtzke JF (1983): Rating neurological impairment in multiple sclerosis. An expanded disability status scale (EDSS) . Neurology 33:1444-1452.

3. Poser Cm, Paty DW, Scheinberg L, et al (1983): New diagnostic criteria for multiple sclerosis:guidelines for research protocols. Ann Neurol 13:227-231.

4. Feinstein AR (1985): Statistical indexes of association, in Feinstein AR (ed):Clinical epidemiology:The architecture of clinical research . Philadelphia, WB Saunders Co, pp 184-185.

5. Fleiss JL (1971): Measuring nominal scale agreement among many raters. Psychol Bull 76:378-382.

6. Landis JR, Koch GG (1977): The measurement of observer agreement for categorical data. Biometrics 33:159-173.

© 1989 Elsevier Science Publishers B.V. (Biomedical Division)
Recent advances in multiple sclerosis therapy.
R.E. Gonsette, P. Delmotte, editors.

HLA, Gm AND Km ALLOTYPES: INFLUENCE UPON MULTIPLE SCLEROSIS SUSCEPTIBILITY, COURSE AND PROGNOSIS.

Christian CONFAVREUX*, Thibault MOREAU*, Hervé BETUEL**,
Lucette GEBUHRER**, Jean-Philippe SALIER***, Jean-Jacques VENTRE*, PHilippe
MESSY****, Albert BIRON**** and Gilbert AIMARD*.
* Hôpital Neurologique, **Centre de Transfusion Sanguine and
**** Département Informatique des Hospices Civils de Lyon, Lyon.
*** INSERM U 295, Saint-Etienne du Rouvray, FRANCE.

There are, presently, very convincing lines of evidence demonstrating genetic background influence upon Multiple Sclerosis (MS) susceptibility. By contrast, genetic background influence upon MS severity is still a matter of discussion. For instance, the rare monozygotic twins concordant for MS may, indeed, show very discordant courses of their disease. Anyway, there is an urgent need for predictive tools in MS, available, if possible, from the onset of the disease. This was the rationale for this genetic study.

MATERIAL AND METHODS

Among the 1150 MS patients who have entered the Lyon MS database since 1976 (1), there are presently 355 patients who have been typed for HLA-A and -B antigens, 141 for HLA-C and -DR, 126 for HLA-DQ and 118 for G1m, K1m and Bf antigens. The number of tested antigens was 14 for HLA-A, 20 for HLA-B, 7 for HLA-C, 12 for HLA-DR and 1 for HLA-DQ (DQW1).

For assessing genetic influence, if any, on MS susceptibility, the prevalence of the given antigens was compared in our MS population and a group of regional blood donors.

For any single antigen and the more prevalent antigen combinations, clinical characteristics of the disease were compared between positive and negative patients. In particular, disease onset parameters (age, symptoms and signs, remittent or progressive mode of onset), disease course parameters (intervals from disease onset to second relapse, progression onset or "second event"; "cumulative" symptoms and signs) and disease severity (intervals from disease onset to moderate or severe disability assessed by means ± standard deviations, medians and distributions or actuarial curves; M / D ratio, i.e. quotient of MacAlpine's disability level and disease duration; MS severity index (1); S/B ratio, i.e. severe to benign cases ratio). I t must be emphasized that we considered as significantly influencing MS severity, only single antigens or antigens combinations for which we found several concordant and statistically significant results from the analysis of clinical parameters. Antigens associated with only a single significant result were considered as not significantly influencing MS severity, owing to the number of tested antigens.

Chi-square, Fisher's and Student's tests were used where appropriate. The level of significance was chosen at 0,05.

RESULTS

Genetic influence upon MS susceptibility

After correction of p according to the number of tested antigens, we found a significant excess of A30, DR2, G1m(1), G1m(23), BfF and BfS antigens or the B7DR2 antigens combination when the MS population was compared to the control group, whereas A31 and C6 antigens were significantly decreased.

Genetic influence upon MS onset or course parameters

No significant result was observed at this level whatever the single antigens or the antigens combinations which were tested.

Genetic influence upon MS severity

When single antigens were tested, significant results were obtained only for A10, B12, DR11 and Km1. The presence of A10 or DR11 antigens was associated with a more severe course of the disease while B12 or Km1 antigens indicated a more benign prognosis.

Among the various tested antigens combinations, a trend for a more rapid course of the disease was found in association with A2+Km1-, A2+Gm3+ or A2+BfS+. The only significant result concerned the B7+Gm1+Gm3+ combination which was an indicator of a poor outcome. However, this combination was encountered in 12 out of 118 patients only.

DISCUSSION

Our results about the influence of the HLA system upon MS susceptibility are in good agreement with whose published for caucasian MS patients (2, 3). However, by contrast with the scottish study (3), we found a similar frequency for DQW1 in MS patients and controls.

17

Concerning genetic influence upon clinical characteristics or severity in MS, published results are rather discordant. For instance, presence of DR2 antigen would be associated with a better prognosis (4) or a worse prognosis (5) or would have no significant prognostic value (6,7,8). In our material, we encountered three situations:
- antigens affecting MS susceptibilty in our series or in other series from MS caucasian patients do not affect MS severity. This was particularly true for A3, B7, DR2 and DQW1.
- among antigens not affecting MS susceptibility, there were some affecting MS severity: A10 and DR11 were associated with a poor outcome whereas, for B12 and Km1, it was with a more benign course. Consequently, there appeared to exist an independance in the influence, if any, of HLA, Gm, Km or Bf antigens upon susceptibility to and severity of MS in our series. The reasons for such a phenomena is intriguying.
- combinations of antigens may show an effect upon MS severity when constitutive single antigens do not. The HLA, Gm, Km and Bf genes code for molecules directly involved in the immune response. Some alleles enhance immune response when others slow down it. Moreover, it may be anticipated that antigens combinations may exert additive effects in one direction or the opposite.

At the concrete level of the individual patient, influence of some antigens on MS severity, although significant it may be, is not sufficient to be considered as a decisive predictive tool. Discrepancies between results from various series must be emphasized, the more recent concerning Km1. By contrast to our observations, Berr et al (9) found that presence of this antigen was associated with a more severe MS outcome.

CONCLUSION

The influence of some HLA and Gm antigens upon MS susceptibility is confirmed in the present series. Anyway, the absolute linkage, if it does exist, between MS and a given allele is still to be discovered. We are far from the situation which prevails in narcolepsy with DR2 (10). Otherwise, genetic studies in MS have not yet succeeded so far in providing an objective and reliable predictive tool of the outcome.

ACKNOWLEDGEMENTS

The support of the "Association pour la Recherche sur la Sclérose En Plaques" (ARSEP) is acknowledged.

18

REFERENCES

1. Confavreux C, Aimard G, Devic M (1980) Brain 103: 281-300

2. Batchelor JR (1985) In: Matthews WB, Acheson ED, Batchelor JR, Weller RO (eds) McAlpine's Multiple Sclerosis. Churchill Livingstone, Edinburgh, London, Melbourne and New-York, pp 281-300

3. Francis DA, Batchelor JR, McDonald WI, Hing SN, Dodi IA, Fielder AHL, Hern JEC, Downie AW (1987) Brain 110: 181-196

4. Madigand M, Oger JJF, Fauchet R, Sabouraud O, Genetet B (1982) J Neurol Sci 53: 519-529

5. Jersild C, Fog T, Hansen GS, Thomsen M, Svejgaard A, Dupont B (1973) Lancet ii: 1221-1225

6. Poser S, Ritter G, Bauer HJ, Grosse-Wilde H, Kuwert EK, Raun NE (1981) J Neurol 225: 219-221

7. Dejaegher L, De Bruyere M, Ketelaer P, Carton H (1983) J Neurol 29: 167-174

8. Govaerts A, Gony J, Martin-Mondiere C, Poirier JC, Schmid M, Schuller E, Degos JD, Dausset J (1985) Tissue Antigens 25: 187-199

9. Berr C, Dugoujon JM, Clanet M, Cambon-Thomsen A, Alperovitch A (1989) N Eng J Med 320: 467

10. Confavreux C, Gebuhrer L, Betuel H, Freidel C, Bastuji H, Aimard G, Devic M, Jouvet M (1987) J Neurol Neurosurg Psychiat 50: 635-636

© 1989 Elsevier Science Publishers B.V. (Biomedical Division)
Recent advances in multiple sclerosis therapy.
R.E. Gonsette, P. Delmotte, editors.

THE OCULAR-SENSITIVE FORM OF MULTIPLE SCLEROSIS

E. ROULLET, P. AMARENCO, R. MARTEAU

Service de Neurologie, Hôpital Saint-Antoine, 184, Rue du Faubourg St-Antoine,
75571 PARIS cédex 12 - FRANCE.

INTRODUCTION

The prognosis of Multiple Sclerosis (MS) is highly variable and benign and severe forms have been described according to variable criteria (1, 2, 3, 4). However, factors predicting benign outcome cannot reliably be used as prognostic tools in clinical practice, and some are controversial. The localization of plaques in very benign cases has not been assessed, as these patients do not usually come to autopsy. Plaques are not evenly distributed (5, 6) and the topographic presentation of MS may be genetically determined (7). It is our clinical experience that most patients with a benign outcome have a special clinical form of MS, mainly with ocular and sensitive symptoms (OS). We studied the clinical and MRI characteristics of OS MS patients followed at our clinic.

METHODS

Patients. The clinical evolution and disability of all patients followed at our clinic are prospectively assessed according to well-established criteria : attacks and progression are categorized following Brown's criteria (8) and disability scored using Kurtzke Disability Status Scale (9). In early 1988, we entered clinical and paraclinical data in a specially designed computer program. The data of patients rated as OS were reanalyzed. We only considered definite MS patients (10) who had an exclusive history of visual and/or sensory symptoms and/or signs : optic neuritis, diplopia, oscillopsia on one hand, paresthesias, useless hand, proprioceptive ataxia, Lhermitte's sign on the other. The main clinical data were tabulated and compared to those of our whole population with definite MS (350 patients at that time).

Paraclinical data. Cerebrospinal fluid (CSF) was considered as positive (i.e. suggestive of MS) if it contained more than 10 cells per mm3 or oligoclonal banding on cellulose acetate electrophoresis. MRI was done at 3 different facilities in 10 patients. The number and localization of high signal zones (HSZ) visible on T2-weighted slices were compared to those of 13 non-OS unselected patients with intermediate disability (Kurtzke score : 3 to 6, mean 4.78 ± 1.83) and same duration of MS (9.28 ± 6.24 vs 9.36 ± 4.83 years). MRI assessment was carried out blind to clinical data.

RESULTS

Thirty-six patients were initially rated as OS. Eleven were rejected. In 9, careful analysis of history showed the presence of motor, cognitive and/or vestibular symptoms or signs : in 1, the diagnosis was not definite and in 1, clinical data were considered too inaccurate for analysis.

The main clinical and paraclinical data are presented in Table 1 :

TABLE 1

Clinical data

	Ocular-sensitive MS (n = 25)	Whole MS population (n = 350)	
Male/female	4/21	115/235	NS
Remittent forms	25/25	168/347	
Age at onset	27.8 ± 10.4	29.2 ± 8.7	NS
Age (years)	43.1 ± 17.2	43.2 ± 12.1	NS
Duration of follow-up	14.0 ± 8.8	14.1 ± 9.7	NS
Disability (Kurtzke)	1.8 ± 1.0	4.5 ± 2.0	$p < 0.01$
R1 R2 (months)	31.5	35.5	NS
Auto-immune diseases	3/25	9/317	$p < 0.02$
CSF (positive)	12/18	166/234	NS

All OS patients had exacerbating-remitting MS ; 14 (out of 15) could be classified as benign forms (Kurtzke grade 3 or less after 10 years of illness). Age at onset, duration of MS and follow-up and interval between the first two relapses were not different from those of our whole MS population. Auto-immune diseases were associated with MS in 3 patients (auto-immune thrombocytopenia and diabetes : 1 patient ; uveitis : 1 patient ; diabetes : 1 patient).

MRI data showed a tendency for less MS burden in the OS group. There were more patients with confluent lesions and more patients with more than 5 lesions on MRI in the 'classic MS' group than in the OS group, but these results did not reach statistical significance. Patients with no brainstem and/or cerebellar lesions were less numerous in the OS group (table 2).

TABLE 2

MRI data

	OS MS (n = 10)	Classic MS (n = 13)	
Number of lesions			
< 5	6	4	NS
≥ 5	4	9	
Confluent lesions			
absence	7	7	NS
presence	3	6	
Brainstem/cerebellar lesions (presence)	2/10	8/13	p<0.05

DISCUSSION

In a horizontal survey of 350 MS patients, 25 (7 %) presented with exclusive ocular and sensitive symptoms and signs. Age, age at onset and duration of illness were similar to those of our whole MS population. Most where females and all where remittent forms. Disability was lower and auto-immune diseases were more frequent than in the control group. MRI quantification of lesions showed a tendency for less burden in ocular-sensitive patients, with slight overlapping of the two groups. These data are in agreement with earlier studies concerning 'benign MS' (1, 3, 4) ; they show female preponderance and exclusively remitting forms in this group. Although obtained with a smaller population, MRI data are similar to those of Koopmans and al (5) and show that clinico-imaging correlations can be obtained in some sub-groups of patients. Auto-immune diseases associated with MS have been recently reviewed (11, 12) and this association is considered nothing more than chance ; however, our data indicate that such an association may be restricted to a sub-group of patients. These results are consistent with the hypothesis of a particular genetic background of some benign MS patients.

ACKNOWLEDGEMENTS

This study was in part granted by ARSEP (Association pour la Recherche sur la Sclérose en Plaques). Isabelle Mège typed the manuscript.

22

REFERENCES

1   - Mc Alpine D, Compston ND, Lumsden CE. Multiple Sclerosis. Edinburgh and London. E and &S Livingstone Ltd, 1955.

2   - Confavreux C, Aimard G, Devic M. Course and prognosis of Multiple Sclerosis assessed by the computerized data processing of 349 patients. Brain, 1980,103:281-300.

3   - Thompson AJ, Hutchinson N, Brazil J, Feighery C, Martin EA. A clinical and laboratory study of benign Multiple Sclerosis. QJ Med, 1986, 225 : 69-80.

4   - Bonduelle M, Bouygues P, Degos CF, Gauthier C. Les formes bénignes de la sclérose en plaques. Réévaluation. Rev. Neurol., 1979, 135 : 593-604.

5   - Koopmans RA, Li DKB, Grochowski E, Cutler PJ, Paty DW. Benign versus chronic progressive multiple sclerosis : magnetic resonance imaging features. Ann. Neurol., 1989, 25 : 74-81.

6   - Ikuta F, Zimmerman HM. Distribution of plaques in seventy autopsy cases of Multiple Sclerosis in the United States. Neurology, 1976, 26 (part 2) : 26-28.

7   - Shibasaki H, Kuroda Y, Kuroiwa Y. Clinical studies of Multiple Sclerosis in Japan : classical Multiple Sclerosis and Devic's disease. J. Neurol. Sci., 1974, 23 : 215-222.

8   - Poser CM, Paty DW, Scheinberg K et al. New diagnostic criteria for Multiple Sclerosis. Guidelines for research protocols. Ann. Neurol. 1983, 13 : 227-231.

9   - Kurtzke JF. Further notes on disability evaluation in Multiple Sclerosis with scale modifications. Neurology, 1965, 15 : 654-661.

10 - Brown JR, Beebe GW, Kurtzke JF et al. The design of clinical studies to assess therapeutic efficacy in MS. Neurology, 1979, 18 (part 2) : 1-23.

11 - Aisen ML, Aisen PS, La Rocca NG, esser BS, Scheinberg L. Features of connective tissue disease in unselected Multiple Sclerosis patients. Ann. Neurol., 1987, 22 : 151.

12 - De Keyser J. Auto-immunity in Multiple Sclerosis. Neurology, 1988, 38 : 371-374.

PROGNOSTIC FACTORS IN A MULTIPLE SCLEROSIS INCIDENCE MATERIAL AT A 25 YEAR FOLLOW-UP

B. Runmarker, O. Andersen
Dep. of Neurology, Sahlgren Hospital, S-413 45 Göteborg, Sweden

INTRODUCTION

The long-term prognosis in MS is considered to be difficult or even impossible to predict. Some clinical factors like bout frequency were found to be important by some authors, but not by others. A possibility to perform an unbiased study of the long-term prognosis was provided by the Göteborg incidence material, which was recently reinvestigated.

MATERIAL AND METHODS

Material. 306 MS patients with onset of disease from January 1 1950 until December 31, 1964 were followed in the department of Neurology, and clinical data concerning these patients have been published earlier (Ref.1). The material was updated, and most of the patients were personally examined by the authors, so that a follow-up time of at least 25 years was reached in virtually all living patients. Only 5 patients were completely lost to follow-up. Furthermore, we have revised the diagnosis of all patients according to the Poser criteria. There was a total of 236 definite MS patients. 49 of these were autopsy verified, 165 were clinical definite and 22 lab-supported definite. 17 had clinical probable MS. 53 cases of possible MS were excluded, leaving 253 patients to be included in the statistical analysis.

Statistical methods. The life-table method was used, and as the critical, absorbing event we used the start of chronic progression of the disease. Patients lost to follow-up and patients dying from other causes than MS were censored from the calculations from that year.

RESULTS

Of the whole material, 15 % had a progressive course from onset. The chance to be in a non-progressive course is decreasing with a longer follow-up time, and after 25 years this chance was 22% (95% conf. limits : $\pm$ 5%)(Fig. 1).

Influence of sex. There were 152 females and 101 males, giving a sex ratio of 1.50:1. There was a significant difference in prognosis between the sexes, with a higher risk of developing a progressive course for men (Fig. 2).

Influence of age at onset. The age at onset influences prognosis, the higher the age at onset, the worse the prognosis (Fig. 3).

24

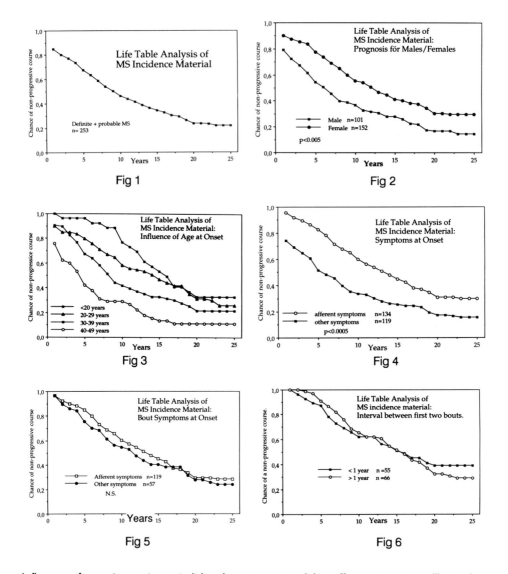

Fig 1

Fig 2

Fig 3

Fig 4

Fig 5

Fig 6

<u>Influence of symptoms at onset.</u> It has been suggested that afferent symptoms like optic neuritis and sensibility symptoms might give a better prognosis. The material was divided according to the type of symptoms at onset. Patients with mainly afferent symptoms were compared to the remainder (having mainly efferent or combined symptoms). The group with mainly afferent symptoms had a significantly better prognosis (Fig 4).

However, there is a confounding factor. There is a strong interdependence between motor symptoms and chronic progression. After excluding patients not having a distinct bout onset, there was no longer any clear difference between the groups (Fig 5).

Similarly, patients with optic neuritis had a better prognosis than the remainder, but there was no significant difference when only patients with bout onset were included.

Initial symptoms from other regions, the brain stem, the spinal cord and the cerebral hemispheres did not significantly differ in prognosis from the rest.

Influence of length of remission. The frequency of relapses during the first years has been stated to influence prognosis. The material was divided in two groups according to the length of the first remission ; that is,more than one year, or less. There was no significant difference between the groups. Patients having a progressive course before the second relapse were excluded. (Fig. 6).

To evaluate the efficacy of these parameters as compared to simple extrapolation of the course during the first years, the material was divided into two groups according to their neurological deficit score 5 years after onset, one with high score and one with low. As expected, the prognosis was significantly better for the latter group, but still in this group the chance for a non- progressive course was only 37%. (Fig. 7)

We tried to define a group with a more benign course than this, and with less risk for progression. To do this, we combined different factors associated with a good prognosis. So far, we have not been able to find a really benign group. For example, the group of females with onset before 30 years of age, and only afferent symptoms at onset, still have only 40% chance to avoid a progressive course.

Influence of pregnancy. It has been shown that pregnancy influences the rate of relapses before and after delivery (Ref 2,3,4). Most authors agree that there is a trend towards a lower relapse rate during the pregnancy, and a higher rate post-partum. In fact, in an earlier study on this material there seemed to be an overall beneficial effect on the relapse rate, the analysis made on onset bouts only (Ref 5). Therefore we wanted to study if there was any long-term effect of pregnancy.

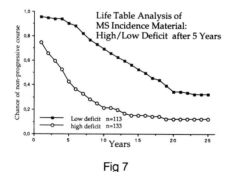

Fig 7

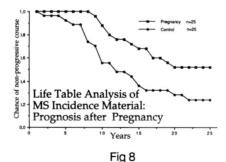

Fig 8

The disease course was compared between two groups: 25 women who became pregnant after onset of the disease, and a group of women without any pregnancy. In a case-control study the pregnant females and the controls were matched according to their neurological deficit score at the time of pregnancy.

With this method, there was a significantly better prognosis after pregnancy (Fig. 8). The data suggest that pregnancy protects from the progressive course. Each year, the risk of entering a state of progression was more than three times higher for the non-pregnant women (95% confidence limits: 1.11, 11.4). Even though there are considerable changes in the immune system during pregnancy, the explanation for this possible long-term effect is unclear.

CONCLUSIONS

1. The present study confirms that a progressive course, higher age at onset, male sex and motor symptoms predict an unfavourable course.

2. In the long run, the course of the disease seems rather homogenous in a large group of patients. The chance to escape a progressive course shows only a limited variation between prognostic subgroups, i.e. between 10-40%.

3. There are a number of factors that influence prognosis. However, they tend to be strongly interdependent, and so far it has been difficult to find a predictor more efficient than simply using the neurological deficit score 5 years after onset.

4. Preliminary, there seems to be a long-term beneficial effect of pregnancy, the reason for which is unclear.

5. Clinical prognostic factors should be paid attention to when studying lab predictors , in order to avoid confounding factors.

REFERENCES
1. Broman T, Andersen O, Bergmann L: Clinical studies on Multiple sclerosis. Acta Neurol Scand 1981;63:6-33
2. Korn-Lubetzki I, Kahana E, Cooper G, et al: Activity of multiple sclerosis during pregnancy and puerperium. Ann Neurol 1984;16:229-231.
3. Poser S, Poser W: Multiple sclerosis and gestation. Neurology 1983;33:1422-1427
4. Ghezzi A, Caputo D: Pregnacy: A factor influencing multiple sclerosis? Eur Neurol 1981;20:517-519
5. Andersen O: Reduced risk of MS onset during pregnancy. Acta Neurol Scand Suppl No 98,1984;69:370-71

© 1989 Elsevier Science Publishers B.V. (Biomedical Division)
Recent advances in multiple sclerosis therapy.
R.E. Gonsette, P. Delmotte, editors.

COURSE OF MULTIPLE SCLEROSIS: EARLY PROGNOSTIC FACTORS.
RESULTS AFTER A FOLLOW-UP OF THREE YEARS.

Coordinating center: Istituto Neurologico "C. Besta", Milan — Filippini G,
Solari A, Paggetta C. Participating centers: Osp. di Rovereto — Neurology
Div., Rossi G; Osp. di Niguarda, Milan — Neurology Div., Bevilacqua L; Ist.
S. Raffaele, Milan — Neurology Dept. IV, Comi GC, Martinelli V; Pavia
University Neurology Dept. — Cosi V, Citterio A, Bergamaschi R; Ferrara
University Neurology Dept. — Altobelli A, Casetta I; Florence University
Neurology Dept. — Amato MP; Pisa University Neurology Dept. — Meucci G; Bari
University Neurology Dept. — Logroscino GC; Palermo University Neurology
Dept. — Savettieri G, Marchesi G.

INTRODUCTION

This paper reports on first results from a long-term prospective
study carried out in 9 neurology departments, the Italian
Multicenter Prognostic Study on Multiple Sclerosis (IMPS-MS).
The prognosis of 35 patients with isolated optic neuritis (ON)
who entered the study is also considered.

MATERIAL AND METHODS

The series consisted of 313 newly-diagnosed patients recruited
between 1984 and 1987 in 9 neurology departments and residents
in the same province as the centers. The other inclusion criteria
were first symptoms occurring within three years prior to diagnosis
and cerebrospinal fluid (CSF) examination available at diagnosis.
The degree of diagnostic certainty, according to the McDonald-
Halliday classification, was verified by a clinical commission (1).
The diagnosis of ON was made using clinical criteria.
Reduction in visual acuity together with a defect in the central
visual field, a negative neurological history and a normal
neurological examination had to be present.
Neurological assessment at diagnosis and at each clinical follow-up
was recorded by the Minimal Record of Disability for MS (2).

Each patient has been reexamined every six months and during exacerbations.

TABLE I

MEAN AGE AT ONSET (YEARS) ($\pm$ STANDARD DEVIATION) IN MALES AND FEMALES BY DIAGNOSTIC LEVEL IN 313 PATIENTS.

2 - way ANOVA (Optic Neuritis Excluded): sex p=0.19; diagnostic level p < 0.001

Diagnostic level	Age at onset		
	Males	Females	All
Definite	30.3 (9.3)	28.5 (10.5)	29.1 (10.1)
Early Probable	28.6 (8.1)	28.6 (9.4)	28.6 (8.9)
Progressive Probable	36.9 (8.9)	35.5 (9.3)	36.1 (9.0)
Progressive Possible	35.5(11.3)	36.2 (7.2)	35.9 (9.3)
Suspected	28.5 (8.6)	27.7 (8.9)	28.0 (8.7)
Optic Neuritis	29.7(11.4)	26.7 (8.9)	27.7 (9.7)

RESULTS AND DISCUSSION

Three hundred and twenty-four patients were initially recruited. Two hundred and seventy-eight had MS according to the McDonald-Halliday criteria; for 35 patients the diagnosis was ON, and 11 were misdiagnosed.

As regards the MS patients, 104 were male and 174 female. The mean age at onset was 30 years for males, and 28 years for females. The cases which were progressive from the start (progressive possible and progressive probable MS), had a significantly higher age at onset (Table 1).

The most common symptom at onset was motor pareses, referred by 112 patients. One hundred patients had disturbances of sensation, 85 had problems in coordination or equilibrium, 44 started with diplopia, 32 had visual disturbances, 16 had disturbances of the fifth and 14 of the seventh cranial nerve respectively.

After a mean follow-up of two years, 17 MS patients, that is 6%, entered the progressive phase of the disease.

Of the 35 patients with ON, 9 (26%) developed MS.

In 5 cases the interval from ON to MS diagnosis was less than one year and they, therefore, were diagnosed as early probable MS.

The male-female ratio for those ON patients who developed MS was .26 and .73 for those patients who did not develop the disease, the difference being not statistically significant. This suggests a higher conversion rate for women than for men as reported in other studies (3,4).

The positive predictive value of CSF oligoclonal bands respect to the development of MS in the 35 patients with ON was 30%; their negative predictive value was 90% (Table 2). The specificity and sensitivity of oligoclonal bands were respectively 30% and 60%.

The data presented here, relative to a three years follow-up, obviously need re-evaluation over time, since some of them will change-and others need confirmation.

TABLE II

PREDICTIVE VALUES, SPECIFICITY AND SENSITIVITY OF C.S.F. OLIGOCLONAL BANDING ANALYSIS FOR THE DEVELOPMENT OF M.S. IN 35 UNCOMPLICATED OPTIC NEURITIS AFTER A MEAN FOLLOW-UP OF TWO YEARS.

Positive predictive value = 30%
Negative predictive value = 90%
Specificity = 30%
Sensibility = 90%

	MS Present	MS Absent	Total
Oligoclonal bands present	8	18	26
Oligoclonal bands absent	1	8	9
Total	9	26	35

30

REFERENCES

REFERENCES

1. McDonald WI, Halliday AM. Diagnosis and classification of multiple sclerosis. Br Med Bull 1977; 33: 611-617.

2. Minimal Record of Disability for Multiple Sclerosis. International Federation of Multiple Sclerosis, National Multiple Sclerosis Society.

3. Kinnunen E. The incidence of optic neuritis and its prognosis for multiple sclerosis. Acta Neurol Scand 1983; 68: 371-377

4. Rizzo JF, Lessell S. Risk of developing multiple sclerosis after uncomplicated optic neuritis: a long-term prospective study.

COGNITIVE FUNCTIONS

© 1989 Elsevier Science Publishers B.V. (Biomedical Division)
Recent advances in multiple sclerosis therapy.
R.E. Gonsette, P. Delmotte, editors.

AN OVERVIEW OF CLINICAL AND RESEARCH ISSUES REGARDING COGNITIVE IMPAIRMENT
AMONG MS PATIENTS

RANDOLPH B. SCHIFFER, M.D., and ERIC D. CAINE, M.D.
Departments of Neurology and Psychiatry; Strong Memorial Hospital, Rochester,
New York 14642, U.S.A.

Multiple studies since the Second World War have confirmed a high frequency
of cognitive deficits among MS patients (for a review see reference 1). A
summary prevalence estimate of such deficits among MS patients would be that
50% of all patients, regardless of neurologic disease severity, have
demonstrable cognitive deterioration. A curious fact about the dementia
associated with MS is that not only are the patients often unaware of its
presence, but so are the doctors (2).

Physicians and patients tend to overlook the dementia of MS because in most
instances it is not glaringly obvious, as are the cognitive deficits of
patients with syndromes such as Alzheimer's or Huntington's Disease. Many
aspects of language remain intact in MS, as (typically) does global personality
function, orientation and navigational skills, praxis, and prosody. Most
commonly the MS patients demonstrate a generalized slowing of cognitive
processing. It is not known whether this is related to the fatigue which is so
common, or to a primary disturbance of attention. Verbal and visual memory
functions are affected, in which typically repetition and recognition memory
for word lists is intact, with impaired active retrieval of information from
storage. With regard to the visuoconstructive and visuoperceptive difficulties
of these patients, we do not yet know whether they experience a primary
impairment of visuospatial learning and manipulative skills, or whether the
difficulties emanate from underlying sensorimotor deficits. MS patients also
tend to demonstrate abnormalities on tests involving conceptual thinking and
abstract reasoning, and verbal fluency may be decreased.

We are most interested in the potential neuroimmunologic substrate of this
cognitive disturbance, but unfortunately, most of our present evidence bears
only indirectly on this issue. We do know several curious things about the
cognitive disturbance. Despite what one might expect, there is but a weak
correlation between cognitive deficits and general neurologic deficits as
measured by Kurtzke's Expanded Disability Status Scale (3-5). It seems that
the cognitive deficits are present within some patients, whether the disease is
newly diagnosed or longstanding, and whether general neurologic disability is
mild or severe (6). There does seem to be a connection between clinical
disease pattern and the presence of cognitive deficits. Patients who have

entered the chronic progressive phase of the illness are more likely to be demented than are those in the relapsing-remitting phase of the disease (7).

Cognition in MS may be strangely independent of clinically defined neurologic exacerbations of the disease (8,9). This issue has not been the specific focus of either of the clinical studies cited, but is mentioned by these authors. To clarify these issues, we will need prospective studies of cognition in MS patients, and at the present time these are few, and the results are conflicting. In the older literature, Canter (10) performed sequential assessments at six-month intervals on 47 MS patients using the Wechsler-Bellevue Scale. He found a pattern of deterioration upon 9 of the 11 subtests over this relatively brief period of time. We found similar evidence that cognitive deterioration can occur over a six-month period in 11 MS patients selected for the presence of depression (unpublished). We assessed these 11 patients using a neuropsychological test battery while they were depressed, and repeated the assessment six months later after successful treatment of the depression. We were looking for evidence of "pseudodepression," or cognitive deficits associated with depression, which might improve after resolution of the affective disorder. To our surprise, we found suggestive evidence that cognition actually deteriorated across several language and verbal-fluency related cognitive tests. This deterioration seemed to be evident despite the mitigating factors of practice effects, the relatively short test-retest interval, and the clinical improvement in depression. This pattern of test performance is presented graphically in Figure I, in which the 50th percentile line on the ordinate has been determined by the performance of eight matched MS control patients without affective disorder.

Two other relatively small prospective studies have failed to find progression in cognitive deficits among MS patients. In 1966, Fink and Houser reported sequential testing of 44 severely impaired MS patients using the Wechsler Adult Intelligence Scale (11). They did not find significant change after a one-year interval. And at a recent European Congress, Medaer and colleagues reported no cognitive deterioration in 85 MS clinic attenders in a test-retest study with mean follow-up interval of 24 months (12). This present lack of concensus in the literature will have to be resolved by future studies.

An additional intriguing aspect of this cognitive performance problem among MS patients is that magnetic resonance imaging seems to be sensitive to the underlying pathophysiology. In four recent studies using various ways of objectifying MR results, all found positive correlations between measures of lesion severity by MR and cognitive deficits (13-16). This finding is of particular interest to neuroimmunologists since it is known that MR lesions may "come and go" in MS patients, without overt change in their clinical status.

It is possible that the MR technology is picking up a dimension of the disease process which is also picked up by neuropsychological test batteries.

MS PILOT STUDY

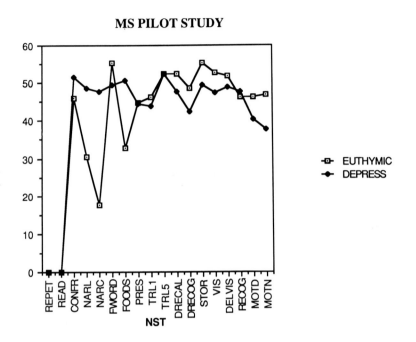

Figure 1

Since we understand multiple sclerosis as at least in part an autoimmune disease characterized by abnormal function within both T cell and B cell systems, what we would really like to know is whether cognitive performance among these patients has direct neuroimmunologic significance. This is a difficult question to approach experimentally, and no studies are available which directly examine relationships between cognitive performance and neuro-immunologic parameters. We have attempted to develop at least some preliminary data concerning cognition and B cell abnormalities in the 11 MS patients whose cognitive performance is depicted in Figure I above. Free kappa light chains (i.e., light chains not covalently bound to functional immunoglobulin molecules) have been demonstrated in the CSF of MS patients both by immuno-assays and by immunoelectrophoresis (17-20). Our group at the University of Rochester has previously presented data indicating that elevated CSF free kappa chains are relatively specific for MS, although this parameter is not known to

36

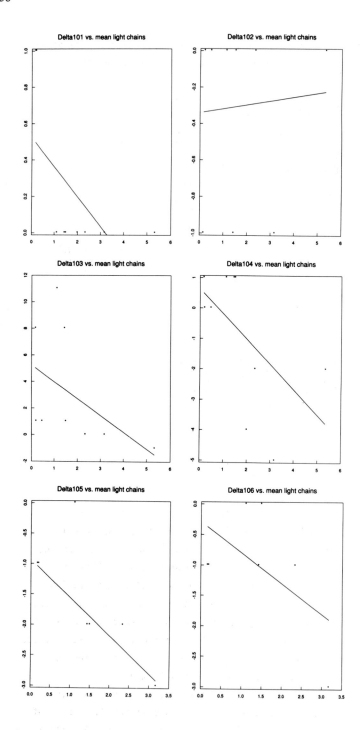

Figure 2

vary with fluctuations in disease activity (21,22). We have made a preliminary attempt to relate these CSF free kappa chain levels to the observed cognitive decrements in language-related functions among the patients depicted in Figure I. In Figure II we present individual graphs depicting line plots for each of the six language subtests which seemed to "pick up" the cognitive deterioration observed in those patients over a six-month interval. The absolute deterioration in cognition is plotted on the ordinate in the units of each test, versus the mean of two separate CSF free kappa chain determinations on the abscissa.

Although the numbers of patients are few, and these data remain quite preliminary, one can see a trend in five of these variables for cognitive deterioration to be relatively greater as the absolute level of free CSF kappa chains rises. We would hope that future research concerning cognition in MS would attempt to relate behavioral changes in an imaginative way to underlying measures of T and B cell function.

REFERENCES

1. Rao SM (1986) Neuropsychology of Multiple Sclerosis: A Critical Review. J Clin Exp Neuropsychology 8:503-542.
2. Peyser JM, Edwards KR, Poser CM, Filskov SB (1980) Cognitive Function in Patients with Multiple Sclerosis. Arch Neurol 37:577-579.
3. Rao SM, Glatt S, Hammeke TA, McQuillen MP, Khatri BO, Rhodes AM, Pollard S (1985) Chronic Progressive Multiple Sclerosis: Relationship Between Cerebral Ventricular Size and Neuropsychological Impairment. Arch Neurol 42:678-682.
4. Lyon-Caen O, Jouvent R, Hauser S, Chaunu MP, Benoit N, Widlocher D, Lhermitte F (1986) Cognitive Function in Recent Onset Demyelinating Diseases. Arch Neurol 43:1138-1141.
5. Van Den Burg W, Van Zomeren AH, Minderhoud JM, Prange AJA, Meijer NSA (1987) Cognitive Impairment in Early Stages of Multiple Sclerosis. Arch Neurol 44:494-501.
6. Ivnik RJ (1978) Neuropsychological Test Performance as a Function of the Duration of MS Related Symptomatology. J Clin Psychol 39:304-312.
7. Heaton RK, Nelson LM, Thompson DS, Burks JS, Franklin GM (1985) Neuro-psychological Findings in Relapsing-Remitting and Chronic-Progressive Mutliple Sclerosis. J Consult and Clin Psychology 53:103-110.
8. Harrower MR, Kraus J (1951) Psychological Studies on Patients with Multiple Sclerosis. Arch Neurol 66:44-51.
9. Grant I, McDonald WI, Trimble MR, Smith E, Reed R (1984) Deficient Learning and Memory in Early and Middle Phases of Multiple Sclerosis. J Neurol Neurosurg Psychiatry 47:250-255.
10. Canter AH (1951) Direct and Indirect Measures of Psychological Deficit in Multiple Sclerosis. Parts I and II. J Gen Psychology 44:3-25, 27-50.
11. Schiffer RB, Caine EC (1989) The Interaction Between Cognition and Affective Disorder in Multiple Sclerosis. Excerpta Medica, in press.

12. Fink SL, Houser HB (1966) An Investigation of Physical and Intellectual Changes in Multiple Sclerosis. Arch Phys Med and Rehab, 56-61

13. Medaer R, Hellebuyck H, Swerts M, Caes P (1989) A Prospective Survey on Cognitive Function in MS. Presented at the 5th ECTRIMS Congress, Brussels, March 16-18.

14. Huber SJ, Paulson GW, Shuttleworth EC, et al. (1987) Magnetic Resonance Imaging Correlates of Dementia in Multiple Sclerosis. Arch Neurol 44:732-736.

15. Franklin GM, Heaton RK, Nelson LM, et al. (1988) Correlation of Neuro-psychological and MRI Findings in Chronic/Progressive Multiple Sclerosis. Neurology 38:1826-1829.

16. Reischies FM, Baum K, Breu H, et al. (1988) Cerebral Magnetic Resonance Imaging Findings in Multiple Sclerosis. Arch Neurol 45:1114-1116.

17. Rao SM, Leo GJ, Haughton VM, et al. (1989) Correlation of Magnetic Resonance Imaging with Neuropsychological Testing in Multiple Sclerosis. Neurology 39:161-166.

18. Bollengier F, Rabinovitch N, Lowenthal A (1978) Oligoclonal Immuno-globulins, Light Chain Ratios, and Free Light Chains in Cerebrospinal Fluid and Serum from Patients Affected with Various Neurological Diseases. J Clin Chem Clin Biochem 16:165-173.

19. Mattson DH, Roos RP, Hopper JE, Arnason BGW (1982) Light Chain Composition of CSF Oligoclonal IgG Bands in Multiple Sclerosis and Subacute Sclerosing Panencephalitis. J Neuroimmunol 3:63-76.

20. Vandvik B (1977) Oligoclonal IgG and Free Light Chains in the Cerebro-spinal Fluid of Patients with Multiple Sclerosis and Infectious Diseases of the Central Nervous System. Scand J Immunol 6:913-922.

21. Laurenzi MA, Marra M, Kam-Hansen S, Link H (1980) Oligoclonal IgG and Free Light Chains in Multiple Sclerosis Demonstrated by Thin-Layer Polyacrylamide Gel Isoelectric Focusing and Immunofixation. Ann Neurol 8:241-247.

22. Rudick RA, Pallant A, Bidlack JM, Herndon RM (1986) Free Kappa Chains in Multiple Sclerosis Spinal Fluid. Ann Neurol 20:63-69.

23. Rudick RA, Peter DM, Bidlack JM, Knutson DW (1985) Free Light Chains in Cerebrospinal Fluid. Neurology 35:1443-1449.

© 1989 Elsevier Science Publishers B.V. (Biomedical Division)
Recent advances in multiple sclerosis therapy.
R.E. Gonsette, P. Delmotte, editors.

A PROSPECTIVE SURVEY ON COGNITIVE FUNCTIONING IN M.S.

R. MEDAER, M. SWERTS, P. CAES, H. HELLEBUYCK

M.S. and Rehab. Centre - 3583 Overpelt - Belgium

In 1984, at the M.S. and Rehab. centre of Overpelt, we began to submit M.S. patients to a standardised battery of neuro-psychological tests. From a total of 104 patients with a well documented diagnosis of M.S., 85 were retested after an interval of about two years.

The remaining 19 patients having dropped out because of following reasons : 7 physical deterioration, 5 test-technical, 2 psycho-mental, 2 unknown, 3 refused second test.

The 85 patients retested included 47 men and 38 women most of whom were outpatients. The mean age was 43 years, and the avarage duration of the disease was 12 years. The mean test interval was 24 months. The Expanded Disability Status Scale, at the first testing was 5,66 (sd. 1,86); and at the second testing it was 5,96 (sd. 2,02). It is important to note that during the observation period there was a significant increase in the E.D.S.S. ($p < 0,02$).

The battery of neuro-psychological tests consisted of :
- WAIS verbal and performental (Intelligence)
- ADM1 and ADM2 (Attention)
- Word fluency test
- Finger tapping
- 15 words of Rey (Memory)
- Checker-board
- Benton (F-form)

RESULTS

At the conclusion of the first testing period the group as a whole was evaluated. This confirmed the data of other cross-sectional studies carried out in other centres as well as our own.

We found a regression of cognitive functions compaired with the premorbid status after a disease duration of about 10 years. After the second testing period we detected no significant change in the groups' cognitive status which remained fairly constant over all modalities for an average period of 2 years.

In order to study the evolution in greater detail we created 3 subgroups. The first group (n = 24) had a disease duration of less than 90 months, the second group (n = 25) more than 180 months and the third group (n = 22) had an important impairment of cognitive function compaired to the premorbid level.

During a two year follow-up none of the subgroups developed a significant deterioration of cognitive function. The only group to show a tendency towards decreasing cognitive function was that with the shortest disease duration.

CONCLUSION

1. No alteration of cognitive function in patients with a 10 year history of M.S. was detected over a follow-up period of 2 years.

   This finding contrasts with most other neuro-degenerative diseases where cognitive deterioration is progressive.

2. In our study the evolution of cognitive functioning was un-related to the changes in physical handicap.

   During the 2 year survey the Disability Status Scale progressed significantly while the cognitive scoring remained stable.

3. In the subgroups, a tendency towards impairment of cognitive function was noted only in those patients with a disease duration of less than 7.5 years.

   The other subgroup (i.c. patients with disease duration of more than 15 years or patients with a serious cognitive deficit) showed no such change. This finding suggests that cognitive impairment is an early symptom of M.S..

4. These findings could have important implications regarding the information given to relatives and treatment strategy.

MAGNETIC NUCLEAR RESONANCE

© 1989 Elsevier Science Publishers B.V. (Biomedical Division)
Recent advances in multiple sclerosis therapy.
R.E. Gonsette, P. Delmotte, editors.

CHANGING ACTIVITY IN MS LESIONS: AN MRI STUDY.

AG KERMODE, PS TOFTS, AJ THOMPSON, P RUDGE, DG MACMANUS, BE KENDALL, IF MOSELEY, DPE KINGSLEY, WI McDONALD.

The Multiple Sclerosis NMR Research Group, Institute of Neurology, Queen Square, London WC1N 3BG, UK.

INTRODUCTION

The study of multiple sclerosis (MS) is complicated by both difficulties in clinical assessment of disease activity, and the occurrence of clinically silent lesions. Magnetic Resonance Imaging (MRI) is exquisitely sensitive in detecting the lesions of MS[1]. Gd-DTPA (Schering AG) enhanced T1 weighted MRI is a discriminating test for a defective blood-brain barrier[2], with lesions showing considerable variation in the pattern of enhancement[3].

Although probably of fundamental significance to the pathological development of the MS lesion, little is known of the changes in the blood-brain barrier in the active plaque over time. We therefore undertook to examine the natural history of blood-brain barrier disturbance in the MS lesion, and to confirm earlier reports that Gd-DTPA enhancement is a consistent early event in new lesions of relapsing/remitting MS[4]. This knowledge is essential for the use of MRI in monitoring treatment.

METHODS

Patients

We studied 11 patients with clinically definite MS[5], 2 male and 9 female, mean age 31 years. Seventeen dynamic Gd-DTPA studies have been performed. Three patients were scanned during a poly-symptomatic relapse, and had follow-up dynamic Gd-DTPA enhanced studies at 1 to 12 weeks. Two patients had un-enhanced MRI 10 and 28 days prior to Gd-DTPA study; six had earlier un-enhanced MRI's.

Imaging

Patients had an initial T2 weighted MRI (SE2000/60, 5mm slices) in a Picker 0.5T superconducting MR imager. The scanning plane was determined by 4 oblique pilots, facilitating reproducibility in follow-up studies. Un-enhanced T1 weighted MRI's (SE500/40, or later IR1020/40/500 and SE1020/40, all 5mm contiguous slices) were performed as a baseline. The patient remained in the scanner and a bolus injection of Gd-DTPA 0.1 to 0.2mmol/kg was given into previously inserted venous access. Immediately after Gd-DTPA injection serial MRI scans (SE500/40, or IR1020/40/500 in later studies) were performed producing eight axial images repeated at approximately 4 minute intervals. As the patient was not moved for Gd-

DTPA injection we avoided mis-registration errors when comparing the enhanced and un-enhanced images[6]. Attenuation was set manually.

Lesion intensity pre and post contrast was measured using a "region of interest" technique on a remote Sun 3 workstation running the Analyze image analysis software (Biodynamics Group, The Mayo Clinic, USA).

RESULTS

All patients had multiple periventricular and discrete lesions on the T2 weighted MRI. Eight patients had enhancing lesions. The maximum study duration was 384 minutes, with rest breaks, and mean study duration 167 minutes. There were 11 lesions known to be less than 5 weeks old; all enhanced. A further 9 of 13 lesions known to be less than 12 weeks old enhanced.

Ninety eight enhancing lesions were studied. Both the pattern and rate of enhancement varied with time. Some lesions enhanced rapidly and uniformly, often appearing less extensive than on the un-enhanced T2 weighted images. Most lesions over 5mm in diameter appeared as rings in the early post Gd-DTPA scans, but by 15 to 20 minutes most of these now appeared uniformly enhanced. The diameter of these "rings" was sometimes larger on the follow-up scan than on the first. By 5 hours after Gd-DTPA there was now faint enhancement spreading out from the initial enhancing areas into the larger region of high signal seen on the T2 weighted images.

Some of these large confluent lesions as seen on T2 weighted MRI were seen to decrease in size over three months on T2 weighted scans, after cessation of Gd-DTPA enhancement. The residual high signal lesions then resembled the areas outlined by Gd-DTPA enhancement in previous scans.

Maximum intensity of lesion enhancement occurred from 8 to 120 minutes after contrast injection. The mean time to peak enhancement was 29 minutes, and the great majority of lesions reached peak enhancement around this mean time. The time to peak enhancement in individual lesions was slower in follow-up scans several weeks later. Some lesions known to be recent from serial scans enhanced rapidly and uniformly.

DISCUSSION

The time of scanning MS patients after administration of Gd-DTPA can have a profound effect on image appearance. With 0.2mmol/kg to 0.1mmol/kg Gd-DTPA immediate post-contrast images characterised the pattern of blood-brain barrier disturbance within the lesions, with ring lesions being plentiful. After 10 to 20 minutes this detail is lost. Scanning over 60 minutes after Gd-DTPA may miss some smaller enhancing plaques.

The fact that other workers have seen rings less frequently may have been because first of all, partial volume effects may have made small ring enhancing lesions appear uniform, and secondly they may have selected their patients differently. Lastly, and probably more importantly, unless scanning begins immediately after injection of Gd-DTPA, the rings may be missed.

The enhancing area was often less extensive than the abnormality on T2 weighted images, and had decreased in size when the lesion no longer enhanced several months later. Isaac and others have also observed shrinking lesions[7]. This means that simply measuring the total volume of lesions as a monitor of treatment may be misleading in certain circumstances.

We detected 11 lesions known to be less than 5 weeks old. Combined with the results of Miller et al[4] we have now seen 23 lesions less than 5 weeks old, all of which enhanced. This provides further evidence that Gd-DTPA enhancement is a consistent feature of new lesions in relapsing/remitting MS.

We do not know over what period the maximum blood-brain barrier defect is reached in the lesion. It may be possible using dynamic Gd-DTPA enhanced MRI to quantitate the blood-brain barrier defect in individual lesions at any given point in time[8]. Dynamic Gd-DTPA enhanced MRI may be useful in investigating the pathophysiology of the MS lesion and of its therapeutic modifications.

What MRI parameters should be used to monitor treatment trials? It is generally agreed that the appearance of a new lesion on MRI is evidence of continued disease activity. Experimental studies provide compelling evidence that Gd-DTPA enhancement reflects active inflammation[9], and it may be useful not only in identifying renewed disease activity but in studying the mechanisms of action of putative treatments. We are unsure of the role of measuring total lesion volumes because of the existence of "shrinking" lesions. We are currently studying the role of each of these techniques in assessing therapy.

ACKNOWLEDGEMENTS

The scanner is supported by the Multiple Sclerosis Society of Great Britain and Northern Ireland, and also by the Medical Research Council of Great Britain. Gd-DTPA was provided by Schering AG. We are grateful to R Robb for providing Analyze image processing software.

REFERENCES
1.Ormerod IEC, Miller DH, McDonald WI, et al. The role of NMR imaging in the assessment of multiple sclerosis and isolated neurological lesions: a quantitative study. Brain 1987;110:1579-1616
2.Grossman RI, Gonzalez-Scarano F, Atlas SW, Galetta S, Silberberg DH. Multiple sclerosis: gadolinium enhancement in MR imaging. Radiology 1986;161:721-725
3.Kermode AG, Tofts PS, MacManus DG, et al. The early lesion of multiple sclerosis. Lancet 1988;2:1203-1204
4.Miller DH, Rudge P, Johnson G, et al. Serial gadolinium enhanced magnetic resonance imaging in multiple sclerosis. Brain 1988;111:927-939
5.Poser CM, Paty DW, Scheinberg L, et al. New diagnostic criteria for multiple sclerosis:

guidelines for research protocols. Ann Neurol 1983;13:227-231

6.Kermode AG, Tofts PS, McDonald WI, MacManus DG. Towards quantification of Gadolinium-DTPA leakage in multiple sclerosis. 7th Annual Meeting of Society of Magnetic Resonance in Medicine (San Francisco, August 1988), works in progress:21.

7.Isaac C, Li DKB, Genton M, et al. Multiple sclerosis: A serial study using MRI in relapsing patients. Neurology 1988;38:1511-1515

8.Tofts PS, Kermode AG. Measurement of blood-brain barrier permeability using Gd-DTPA scanning. 7th Annual Meeting Society Magnetic Resonance Imaging, February 1989, Los Angeles. Mag Res Imaging 1989;7(Suppl.1):150

9.Hawkins CP, Munro P, Kesselring J, et al. Gadolinium-diethylenetriamine-pentacetic acid and Gadolinium-protein markers used to study blood-brain barrier disturbance in vivo in experimental allergic encephalomyelitis. 7th Annual Meeting of Society of Magnetic Resonance in Medicine (San Francisco, August 1988) works in progress:103

© 1989 Elsevier Science Publishers B.V. (Biomedical Division)
Recent advances in multiple sclerosis therapy.
R.E. Gonsette, P. Delmotte, editors.

IMPORTANCE OF STANDARDIZATION IN MAGNETIC RESONANCE IMAGING EVALUATION OF MULTIPLE SCLEROSIS

JAN GHEUENS[1], FRANK L. VAN DE VYVER[2], LUC TRUYEN[1], PAUL M. PARIZEL[3], HENDRIK R. DEGRYSE[3], GREET V. PEERSMAN[2], ARTHUR M. DE SCHEPPER[3], JEAN-JACQUES MARTIN[1]

[1]Department of Neurology, [2]Research Group for Biomedical NMR, and [3]MR-unit, Department of Radiology, University of Antwerp, B 2610 Wilrijk (Belgium)

INTRODUCTION

Magnetic resonance imaging *(MR)* has become the method of choice to visualize lesions in multiple sclerosis *(MS)*. Apart from its application in the diagnosis of MS, MR is now used to evaluate the course of the disease and the effectiveness of therapeutic regimens. However, the correlation between clinical disability and MR-abnormalities is generally thought to be limited. Reported MR-results in MS are often difficult to compare, because of the variability of MR-systems and imaging techniques.

To assess the importance of standardization, we have compared two different MR-procedures for evaluation of MS. It was found that an extensive and standardized MR-protocol that included parasagittal with intermediate TR as well as axial images with long TR offered improved sensitivity, better evaluation of the intracranial infratentorial compartment and the cervical part of the spinal cord, and better correlation between clinical disability.and MR-results. Preliminary results of serial MR in a small group of MS patients are also reported.

MATERIAL AND METHODS

Patients

First, 98 patients *(62 female, 36 male)*with definite *(N 30)* or probable MS *(N 68)* according to Poser's criteria were studied with both MR-procedures in one session. The MR-results obtained in this group were analysed to compare the sensitivity of both MR-procedures.

Then, a group of 25 patients *(19 female, 6 male)*was studied separately. The mean age of these patients was 41 year *(SD 9 years)*. Age at diagnosis of MS in this group was 30 years *(SD 10 years)*. A total of 65 MR-examinations were performed in these patients, at least two per patient, with an average interval of 6 months. The neurological disability of the patients was scored according to Kurtzke's expanded disability status scale *(EDSS)*. The mean EDSS was 3.5 *(range 0 to 8.0)*.

MR-procedures

A superconducting MR-unit *(Magnetom, Siemens AG, Erlangen, FRG)* operating at 0.5 T with a 28 cm diameter head coil was used in all patients. Only spin-echo sequences were used. The image matrix was 256x256. Two imaging procedures were performed in one session. Procedure A included T1-weigthed parasagittal images and double-echo axial images with long TR. Procedure B consisted of double-echo parasagittal images with moderately long TR[1]. Further characteristics of the MR-procedures are given in **Table I**.

TABLE I: PARAMETERS OF MR-PROCEDURE

	PROCEDURE A		PROCEDURE B
	SEQUENCE 1	SEQUENCE 2	
TR *(msec)*	500	2500	1600
TE *(msec)*	30	35, 120	35, 90
Projection	parasagittal	axial	parasagittal
Slice thickness *(mm)*	5	7	5
Interslice gap *(mm)*	0	3.5	0
Number of slices	5	13	7
Number of acquisitions	2	1	2

MR-scoring system

To compare sensitivity of MR-procedures, the central nervous system was divided in 4 regions: supratentorial, brainstem, cerebellum and cervical spinal cord. A region was scored positive if at least 1 lesion was visualized. In addition, a score was given for the number of lesions *(0, 1, 2 or more than 2)*. Brain or spinal cord atrophy and patterns 0-2 periventricular hyperintensity were not taken into consideration[1]

To establish the correlation between MR-results and clinical disability, the total number and size of the MS lesions were taken into account as described[2]. A score of 1 was given to a lesion less than 0.5 cm diameter, 2 to a 0.5-1 cm lesion, 3 to a 1-1.5 cm lesion, 4 to a 1.5-2 cm lesion and 5 when the plaque size was greater than 2 cm. The final MR-score was the sum of the scores for individual lesions. Atrophy was not scored.

RESULTS

Quality of MR-images

Procedure B provides parasagittal MR-images in which the brain parenchyma and cerebrospinal fluid are isointense *(Fig. 1)*. This allowed clear demarcation of hyperintense periventricular foci from the cerebrospinal fluid, and good visualisation of brainstem, cerebellum and cervical spinal cord.

Sensitivity of the MR-procedures

In the supratentorial region, the sensitivity of both MR-procedures was comparable. However, the combination of procedure A+B was significantly more sensitive than procedure A to assess involvement of the brainstem, the cerebellum and cervical spinal cord (**Table II**).

Correlation of MR-score with EDSS

The regression line between MR-scores and EDSS for the 65 evaluations in the second group of patients *(N=25)* is shown in **Fig. 2**. The correlation coefficient was 0.68. *(p = 0.0001)*. This indicated that there was a significant correlation between the MR-scores and the EDSS score for MS patients as

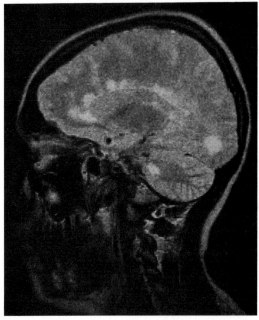

Fig. 1

Typical parasagittal MR-image obtained following procedure B. The normal brain parenchyma and cerebrospinal fluid are isointense, and periventricular lesions with prolonged T2 are clearly demonstrated as areas of high signal intensity.

TABLE II

NUMBER OF POSITIVE PATIENTS IN SEPARATE ANATOMICAL REGIONS

	PROCEDURE A	PROCEDURE A+B	P -VALUE
DEFINITE MS *(N=30)*			
Supratentorial	28	29	NS
Brainstem	13	21	< 0.005
Cerebellum	14	18	NS
Cervical spinal cord	0	18	< 0.001
PROBABLE MS *(N=68)*			
Supratentorial	52	56	NS
Brainstem	17	25	< 0.005
Cerebellum	14	25	< 0.001
Cervical spinal cord	3	25	< 0.001

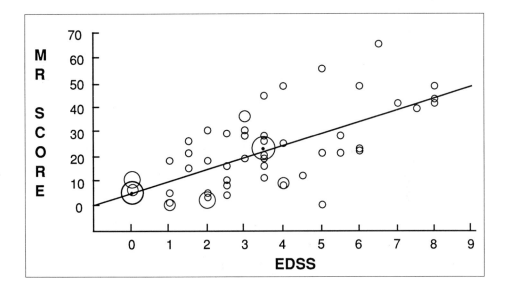

Fig. 2

Regression line of MR-scores versus EDSS-scores. Points with multiple coincidence are represented by bigger circles. The correlation coefficient was 0.68.

Preliminary results of serial MR in MS patients

Initial results indicated that in general, the MR-scores did not change in patients who were clinically stable. Clinical deterioration was accompanied by increased MR-scores in approximately half of the patients. However, patients who had improved clinically only rarely showed an improved MR-score.

DISCUSSION

The results indicated that the combination of procedures A and B provided improved sensitivity of MR-evaluation of MS patients[1]. In addition, the correlation of the MR-scores with the clinical disability scores thus obtained were better than what has been reported[3,4]. A tentative explication for these results is that procedure B allowed better identification of abnormal signals, because the normal brain parenchyma and the cerebrospinal fluid appeared isointense. Moreover, procedure B provided good visualisation of brainstem and cervical spinal cord in comparison with more generally used MR-procedures in which only axial images are obtained.

Our preliminary results on serial MR-studies have provided no evidence for subclinical MR-deterioration in patients who were clinically stable. At first sight, this appears in contrast with other reports[5,6]. However, others have studied patients preselected with clinically unstable disease, whereas we have not preselected the patients on clinical grounds. It is clear that clinically unstable patients may develop new lesions in anatomically silent regions that can be visualized on MR.

In general, our results indicated that sensitivity of MR in the evaluation of MS is greatly influenced by the choice of pulse sequences and imaging procedures that are used. Therefore, standardization of MR-procedures is mandatory if MR is to be used in diagnostic criteria for MS, assesment of evolution of the disease, and effect of treatment in multi-center trials.

REFERENCES

1. Van de Vyver FL, Truyen L, Gheuens J, Degryse HR, Peersman GV, Martin JJ (1989) Magn Res Imaging 7 (in press)

2. Huber SJ, Paulson GW, Chakeres D, Pakalnis A, Brogan M, Phillips BL, Myers MA, Rammohan KW (1988) J Neurol Sci 86: 1-12

3. Edwards MK, Farlow MR, Stevens JC (1986) Am J Neurorad 7: 595-598

4. Uhlenbrock D, Seidel D, Gehlen W, Beyer HK, Haan J, Dickmann E, Zeit T, Herbe E (1988) Am J Neurorad 9: 59-67

5. Isaac C, Li DKB, Genton M, Jardine C, Grochowski E, Palmer M, Kastrukoff LF, Oger J, Paty DW (1988) Neurology 38: 1511-1515

6. Kappos L et al, this volume.

NEUROPHYSIOLOGICAL TECHNIQUES

© 1989 Elsevier Science Publishers B.V. (Biomedical Division)
Recent advances in multiple sclerosis therapy.
R.E. Gonsette, P. Delmotte, editors.

MAGNETIC STIMULATION OF THE MOTOR CORTEX IN EARLY MULTIPLE SCLEROSIS

ALAIN MAERTENS de NOORDHOUT[*], MARIANNE CHARLIER[o], PAUL J. DELWAIDE[*]

[*] University Department of Neurology, Hôpital de la Citadelle, Bd du 12° de Ligne 1, 4000 Liege (Belgium)

[o] Centre Neurologique de Fraiture

INTRODUCTION

Percutaneous magnetic stimulation of the motor cortex allows non-invasive and painless measurement of the conduction time in central motor pathways of fully conscious man (1). Recent reports have indicated that central motor conduction time (CMCT) is often prolonged in patients with multiple sclerosis (2-6). Hess et al. (4) observed CMCT lengthening in 79% of patients with definite MS and in 54% of those with probable MS. In that population of 83 patients, overall incidence of CMCT prolongation (72%) was higher than visual evoked potential abnormalities (67%). A good correlation was found between delayed CMCT and clinical signs of pyramidal tract involvement. Interestingly, CMCT was abnormal in 7 cases with fully normal clinical examination. Motor cortex stimulation thus seems to be a sensitive method to detect demyelinating lesions in the central motor pathways, even those without clinical manifestations.

The aim of the present study is to investigate this further in a selected group of MS patients with a short disease duration and showing little clinical evidence of pyramidal traction lesions.

PATIENTS AND METHODS

Thirty-four patients (19 female, 15 male, mean age: 32 ± 4.9 years) were studied. Following the criteria of Poser et al. (1983), 23 cases were classified as definite and 11 as probable multiple sclerosis. The mean duration of disease was 23 ± 8 months as estimated by retrospective clinical history. All patients showed clinically normal muscle strength in upper limbs. Brisk tendon jerks were observed in 32 of 68 limbs tested (47%), finger flexor jerks were increased on 39/68 sides (57%) and 17 arms (25%) exhibited some degree of spasticity. Finally, no sign of central motor dysfunction was found in 26/68 upper limbs (38%).

Muscle action potentials (MAPs) evoked in the first dorsal interosseous muscle of the hand (f.d.i.) were recorded with surface Ag-AgCl electrodes placed on the muscle belly and the first phalanx of the index finger, 3 cm apart from each other. Both sides were tested. In order to obtain MAPs of shortest latency and greatest amplitude, the subjects were instructed to hold a steady background voluntary contraction of f.d.i. (20% max). Facilitation of the responses during voluntary contraction seems to be mostly due to increased excitability of spinal motoneurones (7), although some effect at a cortical level cannot be ruled out (8). Responses to 8 maximal stimulations of the motor cortex were amplified and filtered (3Hz-3000Hz) and recorded on floppy disks for off-line analysis. Magnetic stimulation of the motor cortex was achieved with a Novametrix 200 stimulator. The 9 cm diameter stimulation coil was located over the vertex. To activate the right f.d.i., the current flowed clockwise in the coil seen from above. Mean latency, duration and morphology of the responses evoked by cortical stimulation were measured. CMCT was calculated by substracting peripheral motor conduction time (PMCT) from the total latency from cortex to f.d.i.. PMCT was obtained by percutaneous electrical stimulation over the spinous process of C7 vertebra (9). Recordings from MS patients were compared with those of a group of 34 age-matched normal subjects. In all patients, standard evoked potential studies were also performed (pattern-shift VEPs, median SEPs and BAEPs). The following parameters were taken into consideration: P100 latency for PSVEPs, N13-N20 interval for median SEPs, I-V interwave delay and V/I amplitude ratio for BAEPs. Results were considered abnormal if they exceeded 3 S.D. from the mean values of our laboratory. MRI scans of brain and spinal cord were obtained in 12 patients (6 definite and 6 probable MS).

RESULTS

Mean CMCT from cortex to C7 was 6.6 ± 0.5 ms in normal subjects. Peak-to-peak amplitude of MAPs evoked in f.d.i. was 3.9 ± 0.6 mV. In MS patients, mean CMCT was 12.5 ± 5.8 ms and MAP amplitude amounted 2.6 ± 1.3 mV. Both values were significantly different from those of normals ($p < 0.0001$ and $P < 0.001$ respectively, unpaired t).CMCT was abnormal (> 8.1 ms) in 24/34 MS patients (71%). It was prolonged on both sides in 20 patients and unilaterally in 4. Two additional patients had normal CMCT, but responses were abnormally small (> 3 S.D.) and/or very polyphasic on one side. Thus one or several characteristics of MAPs evoked in f.d.i. by cortical stimulation were abnormal in 26/34 MS cases (76%). A typical example of responses recorded from f.d.i. of a MS patient is shown in figure 1. This subject has prolonged CMCT from cortex to C7 (14 ms) and MAPs to cortical stimulation show reduced amplitude and very polyphasic morphology.

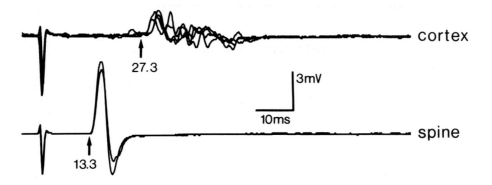

Fig. 1. MAPs recorded from f.d.i. of a patient with definite M.S., showing brisk finger flexor jerks on both sides. Upper traces are four superimposed responses to magnetic cortical stimulation. Lower traces are two superimposed responses to cervical electric stimulation. CMCT is 14 ms and responses to cortical stimuli are polyphasic and of reduced amplitude.

Figure 2 displays the relationship between CMCT and MAP amplitude on the 68 sides tested. Correlations with clinical findings were good. Responses were abnormal on 41/42 sides with some clinical signs of central motor dysfunction. Twelve patients in whom "pyramidal" symptoms were more prominent on one side

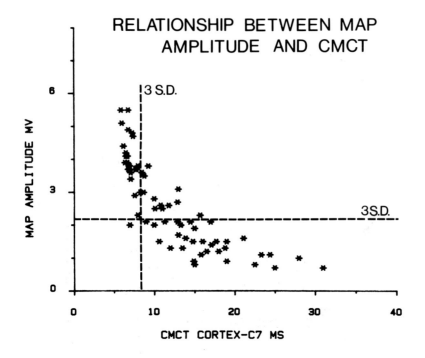

Fig. 2. Relationship between CMCT from cortex to C7 and peak-to-peak MAP
amplitude for the 68 sides tested. Most patients with CMCT longer than 12 ms
show responses of reduced amplitude, suggesting some degree of central motor
conduction block.

has longer CMCT on that side. Interestingly, cortical stimulation revealed
lesions of the central motor pathways in 5/26 clinically normal limbs (19%).

Results of multimodal evoked potential studies are shown on tables 1 and 2.
In the present series, incidence of motor evoked potential abnormalities was
higher (76%) than of any classic EP, including PSVEPs (65%). Considering cases
with abnormalities of a single EP modality, PSVEPs were isolatedly abnormal in
12% and motor EPs in 15%. Of the 12 patients who underwent MRI studies, 2 (one
definite and one probable MS) had abnormal responses to cortical stimulation
despite normal MRI scans. On the other hand, plaques could be disclosed on MRI
scans of 2 patients with normal responses to brain stimulation. In these
cases, plaques were located outside motor pathways.

Table 1 : **EVOKED POTENTIAL ABNORMALITIES IN 34 MS PATIENTS WITHOUT MUSCLE WEAKNESS**

MS CLASSIFICATION (POSER et al. 1983)			
	DEFINITE	PROBABLE	TOTAL
ABNORMAL PSVEPs ONLY	2/23 (9%)	2/11 (18%)	4/34 (12%)
ABNORMAL MEDIAN SEPs ONLY	0/23 (0%)	0/11 (0%)	0/34 (0%)
ABNORMAL BAEPs ONLY	0/23 (0%)	1/11 (9%)	1/34 (3%)
ABNORMAL MOTOR EPs ONLY	4/23 (17%)	1/11 (9%)	5/34 (15%)
FULLY NORMAL EP STUDIES	1/23 (4%)	2/11 (18%)	3/34 (9%)

Table 2 : **INCIDENCE OF MULTIMODAL EVOKED POTENTIAL ABNORMALITIES IN 34 MS PATIENTS WITHOUT MUSCLE WEAKNESS**

MS CLASSIFICATION (POSER et al. 1983)			
	DEFINITE	PROBABLE	TOTAL
PSVEPS	16/23 (70%)	6/11 (55%)	22/34 (65%)
MEDIAN SEPs	14/23 (61%)	5/11 (45%)	19/34 (56%)
BAEPs	10/23 (43%)	3/11 (27%)	14/34 (41%)
MOTOR EPs	19/23 (83%)	7/11 (64%)	26/34 (76%)

DISCUSSION

Before discussing the usefulness of magnetic cortical stimulation in the assessment of MS, some explanations must be given about the mechanisms of activation of central motor structures by this technique. There is strong evidence that when the stimulating coil is placed over the vertex, large diameter pyramidal neurones are activated transsynaptically via some cortical interneurones (10,11). This phenomenon explains why the latency of muscle responses evoked by magnetic cortical stimuli is 1.5-2 ms longer than with electric cortical shocks which seem to activate the axons of pyramidal cells directly (7). Moreover, collision experiments (8) and single motor unit studies (11) indicate that a single cortical shock can produce repetitive activation of pyramidal cells, leading to multiple descending volleys in the fast-conducting pyramidal axons. This also explains the different latencies of

MAPs produced during background voluntary contraction and at rest. At rest, the spinal motoneurones are relatively inexcitable and to be depolarized, they need the summation of two or more EPSPs corresponding to the arrival of successive descending volleys in central motor tracts. Voluntary contraction increases the excitability of spinal motoneurones, allowing them to fire in response to the earliest descending volley evoked by a cortical stimulus (6). These points have several implications for clinical studies. The same method of cortical stimulation as well as the same position and polarity of the stimulating coil must be used for all subjects tested to ensure reproducible conditions. Additionnally, responses of shortest latency and highest amplitude are always obtained when the subject holds a background contraction of the target muscle. Finally, with the method used here, CMCT is slightly overstimated, because it includes conduction within a short portion of peripheral motor structures. Indeed, it has been shown (9) that electric stimulation over the cervical column activates the motor roots some 2-3 cm distally to the spinal cord.

F.d.i. responses to magnetic stimulation of the motor cortex were abnormal in 76% of the MS patients of the present series, at least on one side. This proportion is very similar to that quoted by Hess et al. (4), in spite of the fact that the group selected here had a relatively short disease duration and did not show muscle weakness in the upper limbs. Correlations between abnormal motor evoked potentials and clinical signs of "pyramidal tract involvement" were good and the technique seems able to disclose clinically silent lesions in a relatively high (19%) proportion of cases. Prolongation of CMCT was the most frequently encountered abnormality, often associated with reduced amplitude and/or polyphasic aspect of MAPs. Additionnally, patients with longest CMCT usually showed responses of very low amplitude, suggesting that some degree of central conduction block was present. An alternative explanation would be that the descending volleys generated by a single cortical shock were too desynchronized to bring spinal motoneurones to their firing threshold. In 22 of 64 sides tested, CMCT was longer than 14 ms. This finding deserves some attention. Except in very severe forms of cervical spondylosis, we never observed such delays of central motor conduction in other conditions than MS.

In this series as well as that of Hess et al. (4) , motor evoked potentials were more sensitive than any classic EP modality, including PSVEPs. There were also more patients with isolated motor evoked potential abnormalitiés than with any other EP. Had we performed PSVEP, BAEP and SEP recordings only, the percentage of patients with normal EP studies would have been 24%, instead of 9% when adding cortical stimulation. Moreover, 2 patients with abnormal responses to brain stimulation had normal MRI scans. Provided the procedure is well standardized, magnetic stimulation of the motor cortex is easy to perform, fast and painless. No untoward effects have been reported so far. From the results of the present study and others, it seems that this new method should be used routinely in addition to other EP modalities for the paraclinical diagnosis of multiple sclerosis.

REFERENCES
1. Barker AT, Jalinous R, Freeston IL (1985) Lancet i:1106-1107

2. Cowan JMA, Dick JPR, Day BL, Rothwell JC, Thompson PD, Marsden CD (1984). Lancet ii: 304-307.

3. Hess CW, Mills KR, Murray NMF (1986) Lancet ii: 355-358

4. Hess CW, Mills KR, Murray NMF, Schriefer TN (1987) Ann Neurol 22,6: 744-760

5. Barker AT, Freeston IL, Jalinous R, Jaratt JA (1987) Neurosurgery 20: 100-109

6. Maertens de Noordhout A, Rothwell JC, Day BL, Thompson PD, Marsden CD (1989) Rev Neurol 145, 1: 1-15

7. Day BL, Rothwell JC, Thompson PD, Dick JPR, Cowan JMA, Berardelli A, Marsden CD (1987) Brain 110,5 : 1191-1210.

8. Hess CW, Mills KR,Murray NMF (1987) J Physiol (Lond.) 388: 397-420.

9. Mills KR, Murray NMF (1986) Electroenceph Clin Neurophysiol 63: 582-589.

10.Day BL, Thompson PD, Dick JPR, Nakashima K, Marsden CD (1987) Neurosci Lett 75:101:106

11.Day BL, Dressler D, Maertens de Noordhout A, Marsden CD, Nakashima K, Rothwell JC, Thompson PD (1989) J Physiol (Lond.) In press

© 1989 Elsevier Science Publishers B.V. (Biomedical Division)
Recent advances in multiple sclerosis therapy.
R.E. Gonsette, P. Delmotte, editors.

CENTRAL MOTOR CONDUCTION TIME : WHAT IS ACTUALLY MEASURED BY THIS PARAMETER ?

PAUL DELTENRE, PHILIPPE NOEL AND ANDRE THIRY.
Service de Revalidation Neurologique, Hôpital Brugmann, Place A. Van Gehuchten, 4, B-1020 Brussels (Belgium).

The recent availability of electrical (1) and magnetic (2) stimulators that allow percutaneous stimulation of the motor cortex and of the anterior spinal roots has triggered a major breaktrough in the electrophysiological assessment of the central motor pathways. The so-called Central Motor Conduction Time (CMCT) is computed by subtracting the latency of the muscular compound action potential evoked by anterior spinal root stimulation, from the absolute latency obtained after cortical stimulation (3, 4, 5).

A characteristic feature of brain stimulation is the facilitation effect that is induced by voluntary contraction. This facilitation has three main effects on the evoked EMG response : (A) a lowering of the treshold for excitation by brain stimulation, (B) an amplitude enhancement and (C) a shortening of the latency (6).

This paper reviews our present knowledge about the mechanisms underlying the latency reduction component since this latter effect obviously influences CMCT measurements.

It is well-known from animal data (7, 8) that when motor units are at rest, the voltage gap between the resting membrane potential and the firing threshold of the spinal motor neurone amounts to several millivolts. Because of their smaller amplitudes, single suprasegmental Excitatory Post Synaptic Potentials (EPSP's) have very little chance to close the gap and trigger the spinal motor neurone. There is evidence (9, 10) however, that single transcranial stimuli evoke multiple descending volleys (hence multiple EPSP's) after electrical as well as magnetic stimulation. Such multiple descending volleys allow sufficient temporal and spatial synaptic summation to trigger spike initiation. In resting conditions, the spinal motor neurone will fire on arrival of one of the last corticospinal volleys, the one that will bring the sum of the added postsynaptic potentials across the firing threshold. Bearing this in mind, it is anticipated that any circumstance that will depolarize the spinal cell sufficiently close to its firing threshold will allow one of the earlier corticospinal volleys to trigger the action potential with a shorter latency.

The effects of tendon vibration, a well-known source of almost pure powerful muscle spindle primary endings excitation, have recently been investigated (11). Although significant, the latency reduction was small and never matched what could be obtained by voluntary contraction.

Prestimulation of the mixed nerve at the wrist with a near treshold intensity (12) enhances the Compound Muscle Action Potential amplitude only when the interval separating the stimulus on the nerve from the one on the scalp is greater than 20 msec , a clearly suprasegmental latency, suggesting that the facilitation effect has taken place at the cortex, but here, no latency reduction is elicited.

It therefore seems that the facilitation due to voluntary contraction has something unique that allows marked latency reduction.
One obvious hypothesis about this unique feature of voluntary facilitation is related to the application of the size principle of Henneman (13).
This hypothesis has been substantiated by single unit recordings, showing that the first motor units recruited by voluntary contraction are the same that are recruited by weak magnetic stimuli, and that larger motor units are progressively recruited both by stronger voluntary contraction and by stronger magnetic stimulation (14). This means that in great contrast to what applies for direct peripheral nerve stimulation, cortical stimulation first recruits small peripheral motor units that have a slow conduction velocity. If for any reason, brain stimulation fails to recruit faster motor units it may well occur that the populations of motor units used to measure the peripheral and central latencies will be largely different !

Recently, Starr et al. (15) have shown that latency decreases of up to 6 msec were already present in the period preceding the onset of voluntary movement. Latencies were already shortened in the time slot between -80 and -20 msec before the onset of voluntary EMG, not to be further reduced later on when there was an additional amplitude enhancement during the + 20 to + 70 msec epoch. It therefore appears that the latency facilitation is largely independant of actual movement, hence of secondary afferent activity. Because the time course of their premovement facilitation approximates what is found in monkey pyramidal neurones of the primary and supplementary sensorimotor areas, these authors postulated the participation of intracortical facilitatory mechanisms to the premovement latency reduction. It is difficult to sort out the relative contributions of the cortical and spinal levels of facilitatory interactions in those data, but it must be kept in mind that the use of a ballistic type of voluntary movement may have favoured the effect of Henneman's size principle (16).

There is usually no difficulty in securing minimal latencies in normal cooperative subjects, and normative values for CMCT to small hand muscles exhibit small standard deviation values, as shown in the following table.

TABLE

CMCT for small hand muscles during voluntary facilitation :
(latency after magnetic brain stimulation) - (latency after electrical
stimulation of the motor roots).

Author		Mean in ms	(S.D.)
Hess et al. (5)		6.0	(0.76)
Maertens de Noordhout (17)		6.6	(0.70)
Personal data	right Abductor Dig. Min.	6.0	(1.11)
	left Abductor Dig. Min.	6.1	(1.07)

These small values raise the question of the reliability and specificity of prolonged CMCTs since it is expected after what precedes, that a defect in one of the mechanisms involved in the facilitation effect may prolong the CMCT by several multiples of its normative standard deviation value, in the absence of genuine conduction slowing.

The following conditions may cause CMCT prolongation : (A) demyelination of the corticospinal tract, (B) Selective loss or conduction block of the faster corticospinal neurons to the recorded motor units, (C) Failure of the cortical stimulus to recruit the faster motor units of the recorded muscle, (D) Abnormal level of tonic excitatory-inhibitory balance at the spinal motor neurones pool level, and (E) even slowing of conduction in the very proximal part of the anterior roots should be considered (18, 19). The finding of a prolonged CMCT is therefore not specific for any disease or pathological process. Two diseases pathologically so different as Amyotrophic Lateral Sclerosis and Multiple Sclerosis can produce superposable CMCT pictures with prolonged values in the 10-20 msec range along with reduced amplitudes and abnormally prolonged CMCTs have been found in diseases as varied as hereditary ataxia, stroke, hemispheric glioma and spondylotic cervical myelopathy (18).

If clinical neurophysiology of the central motor pathways is to provide information of differential diagnostic value, it remains to design the complementary tests that will investigate each isolatable individual mechanism contributing both at the spinal and cortical levels to the CMCT value.

64

REFERENCES

1. Merton PA, Morton HB, Hill DK, Marsden CD (1982) Lancet ii : 597-600.

2. Barker AT, Jalinous R, and Freeston IL (1985) Lancet i : 1106-1107.

3. Marsden CD, Merton PA, Morton HB (1982) J Physiol (Lond) 328:61.

4. Mills KR, Murray NMF (1985) Ann Neurol 18:601-605.

5. Hess CW, Mills KR, Murray NMF (1986) Lancet ii:355-358.

6. Rothwell JC, Thompson PD, Day BL, Dick JPR, Kachi T, Cowan JMA, Marsden CD (1987) Brain 110:1173-1190.

7. Amassian VE, Stewart M, Quirk GJ, Rosenthal JL (1987) Neurosurgery 20: 74-93.

8. Phillips CG (1987) in : Epicortical electrical mapping of motor areas in primates : discussion. Motor areas of the cerebral cortex. Ciba Foundation Symposium n° 132:5-20.

9. Amassian VE, Quirk GJ, Stewart M (1987) J Physiol (Lond) 394 : 119 p

10. Boyd SG, Rothwell JC, Cowan JMA, Webb PJ, Morley T, Asselman P, Marsden CD (1986) J Neurol Neurosurg Psy 49:251-257.

11. Claus D, Mills KR, Murray NMF (1988) EEG Clin Neurophysiol 69:431-436.

12. Deletis V, Dimitrijevic MR, Sherwood AM (1987) Neurosurgery 20:195-197.

13. Henneman E, Somjen G, Carpenter DO (1965) J Neurophysiol 28:560-580.

14. Hess CW, Mills KR, Murray NMF (1987) J Physiol (Lond) 388:397-419.

15. Starr A, Caramia M, Zarola M, Rossini PM (1988) EEG Clin Neurophysiol 70:26-32.

16. Desmedt JE (1983) In : Desmedt JE (ed) Motor Control Mechanisms in Health and Disease. Raven Press, New York, pp 227-251.

17. Maertens de Noordhout A, Rothwell JC, Day BL, Thompson PD, Delwaide PJ, Marsden CD (1989) Rev Neurol (Paris) 145:1-15.

18. Murray NMF (1988) In : AAEE/AEEGS Joint Symposium on Somatosensory Evoked Potentials and Magnetic Stimulation Proceedings pp 41-48.

19. Mills KR, Murray NMF (1985) EEG Clin Neurophysiol 18:601-605.

© 1989 Elsevier Science Publishers B.V. (Biomedical Division)
Recent advances in multiple sclerosis therapy.
R.E. Gonsette, P. Delmotte, editors.

THE ROLE OF MULTIMODALITY EVOKED POTENTIALS IN MONITORING OF MULTIPLE SCLEROSIS PROGRESSION.

A. GHEZZI, E. MAZZALOVO*, C. LOCATELLI, M. ZAFFARONI, S. MARFORIO, R. MONTANINI*, C.L. CAZZULLO

Centro Studi Sclerosi Multipla, Ospedale di Gallarate - Università di Milano
*Divisione Neurologica, Ospedale di Gallarate, Via Pastori,4 - 21013 Gallarate
(Italy)

INTRODUCTION

Cerebral evoked potentials (EPs) are sensitive tests in diagnosis of multiple sclerosis (MS) as they can disclose subclinical lesions of CNS. The possibility to measure neurological damage objectively has suggested the use of EPs in monitoring of the demyelinating process. However literature reports on this subject appear conflicting. Probably it depends on several factors, such as the duration of follow up, the extent of the different series, the particular type of test used, the criteria of evaluating EP modifications (literature data are widely discussed in a previous paper -1-). The last finding seems particularly important to us: in most studies the criteria are not specified (2-7), some Authors have purposed the test to test variability (8-10), or +2 SD the normal values (11), or ± 10% (12).

Our study was carried out in order to evaluate: 1) the test to test variability in normal subjects, 2) the modifications of EPs in relation to clinical modifications of the corresponding tested pathways, 3) the modifications of EPs in relation to disease evolution.

SUBJECTS AND METHODS

36 definite MS patients took part in the study; they were 19 females and 17 males, mean age 32.1 years (range 17-44), mean disease duration 7.9 years (range 2-20). Clinical status, scored with Kurtzke functional systems (FS), expanded disability status scale (EDSS) (13) and clinical history were assessed before each

Fig. 1: Diagrams showing the increase of limits of test to test variability in relation to the latency of evoked potentials (values in msec.).

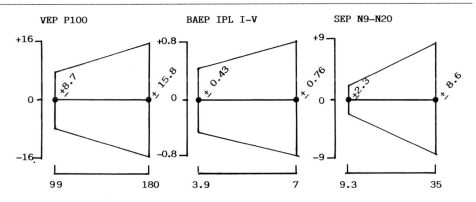

Table 1: Correlation between neurophysiological findings and clinical status of
the tested pathways in the first 18 months of follow-up.

| | | No. of patients with responses | | | |
| | | stable | | modified | |
		A	B	A	B
VEPs	P100	24	0	4	8
BAEP	IPL I-V	24	1	4	7
SEP	N9-N20	20	0	6	10

A   Correspondence with clinical status of the tested pathways
B No   "   "   "   "   "   "   "   "

session. EPs were recorded every 3 months, the follow-up lasted 18 months. The
methods were extensively described elsewere (9). Briefly: visual evoked potentials (VEPs) were recorded in response to a LED pattern reversal, brainstem auditory potentials (BAEPs) in response to monoaural alternating clicks 70 dB SL, so
matosensory evoked potentials (SEPs) in response to medial nerve stimulation. The
following measures were considered: VEP P100 latency, BAEP I-V interpeak latency
(IPL), SEP N9-N20 latency.

In a subgroup of 27 patients EPs were finally recorded after 3 years.

The limits of test to test variability were assessed in 10 normal volunteers,
whose responses were recorded 2-4 months after the first recording.

RESULTS

The limits of test to test variability at +3 SD the normal values were: 8.7
msec. for VEP P100, 0.43 msec. for BAEP I-V IPL, 2.3 msec. for SEP N9-N20. Considering that MS patient latencies are frequently delayed with respect to normal
values, the limits were adjusted proportionally for each patient, as shown in the
diagrams of Fig.1. Once defined the limits of test to test variability, we observed modifications of responses in MS patients after 18 months as shown in table 1.
Temporary modification were observed in two eyes testing with VEPs, in 2 arms testing with SEPs, in 1 side testing with BAEPs.
The latencies of EPs after 3 years were compared with the initial ones in relation to disease evolution. There were 15 patients whose final Kurtzke Scores were
higher than initial ones: they were classified as "progressive patients". In
other 12 patients the final scores did not change with respect to initial ones
(in one patient visual scale improved): they were classified as"stable patients".
Results are reported in table 2: latencies appeared statistically more delayed
at the end of the follow-up in the progressive group, in the stable group they
were slightly but not significantly more delayed.

DISCUSSION

A variability of responses in MS patients has been observed by several Authors
(2,3,5,9), but it seems important to define the normal limits of variability in
successive recordings. In our study they were assessed in normal subjects and
proportionally adjusted in relation to the values of each patient. So defined the
limits of test to test variability we observed that changes of response frequently
occurred with no correspondence with the clinical status of the tested pathway:
it can mean that EPs are sensitive test to appreciate the progression of lesions.
However it must be considered that demyelinated fibers are particularly sensitive
to chemical and/or physical changes (9), so fluctuations of latency can also

Table 2: final versus initial values of neurophysiological measures and clinical scores in stable and progressive patients (latencies in msec.).

		Stable MS	Progressive MS
VEP P100	I	123.7±30.2 *	133.4±21.8 **
VEP P100	F	131.3±33.1	156.5±35.3
BAEP IPL I-V	I	4.22±0.69 *	5.12±1.38 **
BAEP IPL I-V	F	4.31±0.84	5.78±1.29
SEP N9-N20	I	13.3±6.4 *	15.8±8.4 **
SEP N9-N20	F	14.6±8.9	22.4±9.9
Disability status	I	2.6±0.8 *	3.0±1.1 **
Disability status	F	2.4±0.7	5.5±2.4

I = Initial   * Paired t-test: $p > 0.10$
F = Final   ** Paired t-test: $p < 0.001$

reflect conduction failure of demyelinated fibers: in our series temporary changes occurred only in a few recordings, probably because of the restrictive limits of test to test variability.

In most studies the clinical-neurophysiological correlation has been investigate in relation to the appearance/disappearance of neurological symptoms or signs of the corresponding tested pathways but not in relation to the overall neurological status. In our study EP findings at the end of follow-up were analized in relation to disease evolution, assessed with Kurtzke scale: latencies increased only slightly but not significantly in stable patients, on the contrary they increased significantly in progressive patients.

To conclude, changes of EPs can occur with no relation with the status of the corresponding pathway but they appear to be closely correlated with the overall clinical evolution of multiple sclerosis.

REFERENCES

1) Ghezzi A, Caputo D, Zaffaroni M et al (1987) Multimodality evoked potentials in MS monitoring. Rivista Neurol 57:92-98
2) Aminoff MJ, Davis SL, Panithc HS (1984) Serial evoked potential studies in patients with definite multiple sclerosis. Arch Neurol 41:1197-1202
3) Davis SL, Aminoff MJ, Penitch HS (1985) Clinical correlations of serial somatosensory evoked potentials in multiple sclerosis. Neurology 35:359-365
4) Walsh JC, Garrick R, Cameron J et al. (1982) Evoked potential changes in clinically definite multiple sclerosis: a two year follow-up study. J Neurol Neurosurg Psych 45:494-500
5) Cohne SN, Syndulko K, Hansh E et al. (1982) Variability serial testing of visual evoked potentials in patients with multiple sclerosis. In: Courjon J, Mauguière F, Revol M (eds) Clinical applications of evoked potentials in Neurology. Raven Press N.Y., 559-566
6) Kjaer M (1982) The values of sequential evoked potential recordings in multiple sclerosis. In: CourjonJ, Mauguière F, Revol M (eds) Clinical applications of evoked potentials in Neurology. Raven Press N.Y., 567-569
7) Gambi D, Rossini PM, Marchionno L et al. (1982) Multimodal evoked potentials in multiple sclerosis: basal and follow-up data. In: Courjon J, Mauguière F,

Revol M (eds) Clinical applications of evoked potentials in Neurology. Raven Press N.Y., 551

8)Becker WJ, Richards IM (1984) Serial pattern shift visual evoked potentials in multipla sclerosis. Canadian J Neurol Sciences 11:53–59

9)Ghezzi A, Zaffaroni M, Caputo D et al. (1986) Evaluation of evoked potentials and lymphocyte subsets as possible markers of multiple sclerosis: one year follow-up of 30 patients. J Neurol Neurosurg Psychiat 49:913–919

10)De Weerd, Jokman EJ (1982) Changes in visual and somatosensory evoked potentials in patients with multiple sclerosis. In: Courjon J, Mauguière F, Revol M (eds) Clinical applications of evoked potentials in Neurology. Raven Press N.Y., 527–534

11)Likosky W, Elmore RS (1982) Exacerbation detection in multiple sclerosis by clinical and evoked potentials techniques: a preliminary report. In: Courjon J Mauguière F, Revol M (eds) Clinical applications of evoked potentials in Neurology. Raven Press N.Y., 535–540

12)Confavreux C, Mauguière F, Courjon J, Aimard G, Devic M (1982) Course of visual evoked potentials in multiple sclerosis: electroclinical correlations and patophysiological considerations in 25 patients. In: Courjon J, Mauguière F, Revol M (eds) Clinical application of evoked potentials in Neurology. Raven Press, N.Y., 541–550

13)Kurtzke JF (1965) Further notes on disability evaluation in multiple sclerosis with scale modification. Neurology (Minneap.) 15:654–661

BIOLOGICAL MARKERS

© 1989 Elsevier Science Publishers B.V. (Biomedical Division)
Recent advances in multiple sclerosis therapy.
R.E. Gonsette, P. Delmotte, editors.

BIOLOGICAL MARKERS OF DISEASE ACTIVITY IN MULTIPLE SCLEROSIS

C.J.M. SINDIC, M.P. CHALON, D. BOUCQUEY, C. LATERRE
Laboratory of Neurochemistry and Department of Neurology, 53-59, Avenue Mounier,
1200 Brussels, Belgium

The assessment of disease activity in MS is still mainly based on the clinical examination of the patient and the detection of either new symptoms and signs or the reappearance of previous symptoms and signs. Exacerbations may be hard to define, may be simulated by changes of body temperature or fatigue and must be distinguished from fluctuations of persisting symptoms. We also know that plaques may develop in areas within the central nervous system (CNS) without presenting any clinical signs or symptoms : longitudinal MRI studies have shown that new lesions can appear without clinical changes. It may be therefore illusory to expect an absolute correlation between the clinical assessment of disease activity and any biological marker.

Two types of biological markers of disease activity have to be considered : first, biological markers of the demyelinating process, that is, the quantitative determination of products of the myelin degradation, in CSF, in serum and in urine; second, biological markers of the inflammatory-immune process which is the suspected cause of myelin degradation. A CSF biological marker of disease activity is, however, less clinically useful to follow the disease course of individual patients as CSF examination requires an invasive procedure.

Considering first the putative biological markers of the demyelinating process, we know since the pioneering work of Cohen et al[1] that Myelin Basic Protein (MBP) immunoreactive material is present in CSF following myelin damage. But how does the MBP-like material get into the CSF? During the demyelinating process in active MS plaques, the myelin is taken up by macrophages and completely degraded intracellularly. However, one may speculate that proteinases and other lytic agents released by the macrophages cause the initial damage to the myelin sheath. As MPB is known to be extremely susceptible to such enzymes, proteolytic fragments, formed extracellularly, could escape phagocytosis and appear in the CSF. This may explain why not all antisera raised against intact MBP react with CSF MBP-like material. Recent works[2] have shown that the selection of antibody is crucial for sensitive detection of MBP-like material in CSF; the antiserum used should be able to recognize epitopes on MPB peptide 45-89. These studies indicate that the bulk of the MBP-immunoreactive material in CSF from MS patients consists of fragments that contain a dominant epitope located in amino acid residues 45-89. When comparing the MBP assay with an immunoassay specific for this peptide 45-89, Gupta et al[2] found a greater sensitivity with

the peptide assay (59% of positive samples as against 30% in the group of clinically definite MS) whereas the specificity was similar to the MBP assay (80.6 %
as against 82 %).

For reasons already discussed, it seems difficult to obtain a perfect correlation between CSF MBP-like material and any measure of clinical severity. Demyelination in clinically silent areas of the CNS still causes MBP elevation and the
exact time of lumbar puncture after an exacerbation could only be defined for
clinically relevant lesions. Nonetheless, in the study of Gupta et al[2], both
factors (timing of the lumbar puncture in relation to exacerbations and degree
of disability as expressed in the Kurtzke score) were significantly related to
high MBP levels only when MBP fragments were measured by the peptide assay
(p < 0.04).

In the same field, the results reported by C. Martin-Mondière et al[3] are significant. These authors were able to detect CSF MBP in some patients with an
active progressive form of the disease (3 out 15) and during exacerbations with
the presence of signs or symptoms not previously experienced by the patient.
Twenty-six of 29 cases were indeed positive during the period when symptoms were
most acute. In contrast, MBP was not detected in any patient with an inactive or
slowly progressive form of the disease, nor in any patient during exacerbations
with only recurrence of old signs or symptoms. In the latter case, MBP produced
by further chronic demyelination of old or established plaques could be completely degraded intracellularly by macrophages.

Since a lumbar puncture remains an invasive procedure not practical to use
routinely, the report by John Whitaker[4], that MBP-immunoreactive material is
present in urine of MS patients and controls, was a new and exciting finding.
The MBP-like material in urine is approximately 1,000 daltons and has chromato-
graphic and charge properties similar to those of peptide 80-89. The antiserum
used for the detection of this urinary material does not react either with intact
MBP or with MBP fragments in CSF. This implies that the MBP-like material is
altered, presumably degraded, in the kidney. The concentration of urinary MBP-
like material, in relation to the concentration of urinary creatinine, was
significantly higher in MS patients (22 ng MBP-like material per mg of creatinine)
than in patients with other neurological disorders or in controls. Variations
in the level of this urinary material during longitudinal studies of MS patients
may therefore provide a clinically feasible test for myelin damage.

Other putative biological markers of demyelination have been studied. A proteo-
lipid protein immunoreactive material in CSF and serum was detected by a radioimmunoassay[5] in spite of the relative insolubility of this protein, and the
reactivity was more marked in demyelinating diseases, encephalitis and strokes.
A procedure for quantifying the Myelin-Associated Glycoprotein (MAG) in CSF was

also developed[6]. Samples from normal volunteers and patients with demyelinating
diseases contained levels of MAG ranging from 2 to 13 ng/ml. It was not possible
to detect any additional release of MAG as a result of demyelination. Conflicting results have been reported about the CSF activity of some myelin-associated
enzymes[7-8]. The determination of such enzymatic activities would appear to be
unsuitable for the assessment of the activity of a demyelinating process. More
promising is the use of an enzyme linked immunosorbent assay for the determination of galactosylceramide in biological fluids and especially in sera[9]. Positive results were found only in sera from patients suffering from brain injury,
as in MS, strokes and brain tumours.

We have now to consider a second type of putative biological markers of disease
activity in MS, that is, markers of the inflammatory-immune process responsible
for myelin degradation. Pathological findings of lymphocyte-macrophage infiltration in the mutifocal sites of active myelin destruction are the key to the hypothesis that MS is an autoimmune disorder. The aim of many studies related to
the immune system and MS is to define specific immune aberrations that correlate
with clinical features of MS and disease activity.

A consistent finding in patients with chronic progressive MS is the inability
of the immune system to induce suppression, because of a reduced suppressor cell
activity. For example, in the work of Antel et al[10], the level of suppression
induced by the Concanavalin A activated suppressor cells on the mitogenic response of autologous peripheral blood lymphocytes is reduced in patients with
active disease ($3 \pm 8\%$) compared with stable patients ($30 \pm 8\%$), patients recove-
ring from a relapse ($62 \pm 5\%$) and controls ($40 \pm 5\%$). Since 1980, monoclonal
antibodies directed against membrane glycoproteins of T-cells were widely used
for the determination of respective percentages of helper/inducer (CD4) and cyto-
toxic/suppressor (CD8) T-cells. A decreased number of CD8[+] cells and hence an
increase in the CD4/CD8 ratio were reported in MS patients with acute exacerbation and/or with a progressive course of the disease by most investigators[11-12].
Longitudinal studies showed wide variations of the CD4/CD8 ratio in some MS
patients which coinceded in most, but not all, cases with a relapse or a progression of the disease. We obtained similar results in a study of 924 blood samples
from 213 MS patients[13].

It should be noted here that there is only a weak correlation, or even no
correlation at all in some studies, between the loss of functional suppression,
as tested for example by means of Concanavalin A activated T-cells, and the
decrease in the proportion of circulating CD8[+] cells. A major question in the
study of human autoimmune diseases is wether abnormalities in immunoregulation
and loss of suppression can be attributed to a particular T-cell subset. In
the CD4[+] subset of lymphocytes, there are at least two distinct subpopulations :

inducers of help for B cell antibody production and inducers of suppressor CD8[+] cells. This subset of suppressor inducer cells within the CD4[+] population may be detected by monoclonal antibodies such as the 2H4 antibody directed against the CD45 antigen. Recent studies showed indeed a selective decrease of this suppressor-inducer T-cell subset in progressive or active MS[14-15]. In addition, significant correlations were found between decreases in circulating CD4[+] 2H4[+] cells and loss of suppressor functions, as tested by the autologous mixed lymphocyte reaction and the amount of IgG synthesis by mononuclear cells plus pokeweed mitogen[16]. Longitudinal studies of the same subset were recently published by Rose et al[17]. These authors calculated a ratio of CD45[-] to CD45[+] cells and significant changes in this ratio were detected in 7 out 9 MS patients with active disease, but not in any of the control subjects. The increase in the CD45[-] to CD45[+] cells ratio within the CD4[+] population resulted from a simultaneous depletion in the number of CD45[+] cells and an increase in the number of CD45[-] T cells. However, it should be stressed that the CD45 antigen expression on CD4[+] cells may reflect only a state of cell activation rather than the demarcation of distinct subsets with fixed regulatory functions.

This leads us obviously to the question about the presence of circulating activated T-cells in MS. Activation of human T-cells by antigen or mitogen leads to the sequential appearance of specific cell surface structures that are normally either absent or present in very small quantities on resting T-cells. The best known marker of T-cell activation is the interleukin 2 (IL-2) receptor, a 60 kilodalton glycoprotein that is essential for T-cell proliferation.

In vivo circulating activated T-cells were indeed detected in MS by some workers sometimes with conflicting results[18-21]. Some[20-21] found a significantly higher percentage of IL-2 receptor positive T-cells, especially in acute relapse, whereas others[19] failed to find such a correlation but described an increase in peripheral blood lymphocytes bearing another T-cell specific activation antigen called Ta1.

More recently, a soluble form of the IL-2 receptor, first found in supernatants of activated T-cell cultures, was also detected at low levels in the serum of normal persons and at higher levels in conditions associated with lymphocyte activation such as infectious and autoimmune states. High levels of soluble IL-2 receptors were reported in sera from MS patients and longitudinal studies are now required to determine the usefulness of these levels in monitoring disease progression[22-23].

In addition to the presence of circulating soluble IL-2 receptors, high levels of IL-2 were also recently reported in MS sera[24-25]. In the study of Gallo et al[24], 6 sera and 9 CSF of 30 MS patients contained high levels of IL-2 and all the positive samples were from patients with a relapsing-remitting disease, not with a chronic progressive one. Trotter et al[25] found a direct correlation between serum levels of IL-2 and a poor prognosis after 18 months of observation. Other cytokines may be also involved in triggering exacerbations. For example, Beck et al[26] found an increase of the interferon-gamma and of tumour necrosis factor in a whole blood mitogen stimulation assay which preceeded clinical relapses by a maximum of two weeks.

A biological marker of the macrophage function within the CNS may be also relevant in the assessment of disease activity. For example, Neopterin is a factor known to be released from macrophages and monocytes after stimulation in vitro by gamma-interferon from activated T-cells. Using a sensitive radioimmunoassay, Fredrikson et al[27] were able to detect higher CSF levels in 10 out 12 MS patients during exacerbations in comparison with remissions. This significant elevation in CSF during exacerbations was not observed in the corresponding serum.

From this review, one may tentatively conclude that, on one hand, systemic immune dysregulations occur in MS, on the other, there is an ongoing immune process within the brain of MS patients. Especially during the first years of the disease, the systemic immune dysregulations are correlated with the clinical activity of the disease. The intrathecal ongoing immune process is reflected by CSF immune abnormalities, both at cellular and humoral levels, and would become more and more autonomous in escaping systemic immune regulations. Components of the intrathecal immune process are persistently activated and this may be associated with a progressive course of the disease. It is not possible to assess all the faces of the MS process by means of a single biological marker. These markers have to be correlated not only with clinical changes but also with the appearance of new lesions in MRI studies. In the meantime, we are still waiting for a biological marker related to the causal agent of the disease.

ACKNOWLEDGEMENTS

This work was supported by grants from the "Fonds de la Recherche Scientifique Médicale" (n°3-4529-79 and 9-4509-85) and from the "Groupe Belge d'Etude de la Sclérose en Plaques". D.B. had a fellowship from "Communauté Française de Belgique - Recherche médicale appliquée".

REFERENCES

1. Cohen SR, Herndon RM, McKhann GM (1976) N Engl J Med 295 : 1455-1457
2. Gupta MK, Whitaker JN, Johnson C, Goren H (1988) Ann Neurol 23 : 274-280
3. Martin-Mondière C, Jacque C, Delassalle A et al (1987) Arch Neurol 44 : 276-278
4. Whitaker JN (1987) Ann Neurol 22 : 648-655
5. Trotter JL, Wegescheide CL, Garvey WF (1983) Ann Neurol 14 : 554-558

76

6. Yanagisawa K, Quarles RH, Johnson D et al (1985) Ann Neurol 18 : 464–469

7. Raes I, Weissbarth S, Maker HS, Lehrer GM (1981) Neurology 31 : 1361–1363

8. Pitkänen ASL, Halonen TO, Kilpeläinen HO, Riekkinen PJ (1986) J Neurol Sci
74 : 45–53

9. Zalc B, Lubetzki G, Thuillier Y, Galli A (1988) Neurochem Int 13 : 37
(suppl 1)

10. Antel JP, Arnason BGW, Medof ME (1979) Ann Neurol 5 : 338–342

11. Bach MA, Phan-Dinh-Tuy F, Tournier E et al (1980) Lancet ii : 1221–1223

12. Reinherz EL, Weiner HL, Hauser SL et al (1980) N Engl J Med 303 : 125–129

13. Chalon MP, Sindic CJM, Boon L, Laterre EC (1987) Acta Neurol Belg 87 : 245–
260

14. Rose LM, Ginsberg AH, Rothstein TL et al (1985) Proc Natl Aca Sci USA 82 :
7389–7393

15. Morimoto C, Hafler DA, Weiner HL et al (1987) N Engl J Med 316 : 67–72

16. Chofflon M, Weiner HL, Morimoto C, Hafler DA (1988) Ann Neurol 24 : 185–191

17. Rose LM, Ginsberg AH, Rothstein TL et al (1988) Ann Neurol 24 : 192–199

18. Golaz J, Steck A, Moretta L (1983) Neurology 33 : 1371–1373

19. Hafler DA, Fox DA, Manning ME et al (1985) N Engl J Med 312 : 1405–1411

20. Bellamy AS, Calder VL, Feldmann M, Davison AN (1985) Clin Exp Immunol 61 :
248–256

21. Selmaj K, Plater-Zyberk C, Rockett KA et al (1986) Neurology 36 : 1392–1395

22. Greenberg SJ, Marcon L, Hurwitz BJ et al (1988) N Engl J Med 319 : 1019–1020

23. Adachi K, Kumamoto T, Araki S (1989) Lancet i : 559–560

24. Gallo P, Piccinno M, Pagni S, Tavolato B (1988) Ann Neurol 24 : 795–797

25. Trotter JL, Clifford DB, McInnis JE et al (1989) Ann Neurol 25 : 172–178

26. Beck J, Rondot P, Catinot L et al (1988) Acta Neurol Scand 78 : 318–323

27. Fredrikson S, Link H, Eneroth P (1987) Acta Neurol Scand 75 : 352–355

© 1989 Elsevier Science Publishers B.V. (Biomedical Division)
Recent advances in multiple sclerosis therapy.
R.E. Gonsette, P. Delmotte, editors.

CD4+ T LYMPHOCYTE SUBSETS IN MULTIPLE SCLEROSIS

FRANCIEN T.M. ROTTEVEEL, BART KUENEN, INGRID KOKKELINK, ANTHONY MEAGER[*] and
CORNELIS J. LUCAS
Central Laboratory of the Netherlands Red Cross Blood Transfusion Service and
Laboratory for Experimental and Clinical Immunology, University of Amsterdam,
Plesmanlaan 125, 1066 CX Amsterdam (The Netherlands). [*]National Institute for
Biological Standards and Control, Potters Bar (United Kingdom).

INTRODUCTION

Multiple sclerosis (MS) is characterized by demyelination of the central
nervous system (CNS). The demyelinated plaques are associated with perivascular
infiltrates consisting predominantly of T lymphocytes and monocytes (1,2). Traugott and Lebon (3) have previously demonstrated that Ia antigens are detectable
on astrocytes at the edge of active chronic MS lesions and in the adjacent
normal-appearing white matter. They also provided evidence for the presence of
interferon (IFN)-gamma in and around the lesions. CD4+ T cells and IL-2-produ-
cing cells were found at the same place. In most MS patients, there is a modest
cerebrospinal fluid (CSF) pleocytosis. The cells in the CSF are mainly T lymphocytes. Many of these T cells appear to have been activated in vivo (4-6).

In a previous study, we analyzed the heterogeneity of the CSF T cells. Examination of the genes that encode for the T-cell receptor for antigen, indicates
that among 30 T-cell clones from the CSF of two MS patients no sets of clones
with the same T-cell receptor rearrangements could be detected (7). These data
suggest that if there is an oligoclonal population of T cells, it represents a
relatively minor fraction of the total T cells in the CSF of MS patients.

Recently, we demonstrated the existence of two different subsets of human
CD4+ T-cell clones by phenotypical and functional characteristics (8). We used
the tools provided by that study to address the question whether one of these
subsets is predominantly present in the CSF of MS patients. Therefore, we
analyzed a large number of T-cell clones derived from CSF and peripheral blood
lymphocytes of three MS patients. We observed that most of the clones obtained
from the T cells in CSF are of the inflammatory, cytotoxic Th1 subtype. A possible role for the high number of the inflammatory CD4+ T cells in the CSF in
multiple sclerosis is discussed.

RESULTS AND CONCLUSION

Recently, we demonstrated the existence of two different CD4+ subsets by functional and phenotypical analysis of CD4+ T-cell clones derived from the peripheral blood of a healthy donor (8).

T lymphocytes obtained from the CSF and peripheral blood of three patients with clinically definite MS (Table 1) were cloned in a direct limiting dilution microculture system. Interestingly, relatively more CD4+ T-cell clones with anti-CD3-mediated cytotoxic activity can be derived from the CSF of MS patients as compared to peripheral blood of the same patient (Table 1). The percentage of CD4+ T-cell clones with cytotoxic activity obtained from peripheral blood of the three MS patients is similar to the percentage seen in the peripheral blood of healthy individuals (8). The T-cell clones with anti-CD3-mediated cytotoxic activity also produce vast amounts of IL-2, IFN-gamma and TNF-alpha,-beta. These data suggest that T cells in the CSF compartment represent a selectively increased population of inflammatory T cells. It is not clear whether CSF inflammatory T cells concern specific cells from CNS infiltrates or predomi- nantly inflammatory T cells from peripheral blood that have crossed the blood- brain barrier nonspecifically. It can be postulated that CD4+ cytotoxic T cells preferentially cross the blood-brain barrier via IFN-gamma or TNF, since TNF and IFN-gamma participate in the mobilization of mononuclear cells in the chronic inflammatory reaction by stimulation of the adhesiveness of endothelium for

TABLE 1

CLINICAL AND CSF FINDINGS

Patient	R13	V10	R12
Age, sex	48, m	36, m	27, f
State of disease	CP	CP	ER
Oligoclonal IgG	+	+	−
Cells/microlitre CSF	6	16	2
% cytotoxic CD4+ CSF			
T-cell clones	78	81	68
% cytotoxic CD4+ PBL			
T-cell clones	44	41	38

CP, chronic progressive; ER, exacerbating remitting.

circulating lymphocytes (9).

Normal CNS astrocytes are major histocompatibility complex (MHC) class II-negative and rarely express MHC class I antigen (10). In contrast, astrocytes with expression of MHC class I and class II antigens in the CNS of patients with MS have been observed (11). In chronic MS, IFN-gamma-producing cells, CD4+ T cells and MHC class II-positive astrocytes were consistently found at the lesion edge and also into the adjacent normal white matter (3). Interestingly, an increased production of IFN-gamma and TNF preceding clinical manifestations in multiple sclerosis was reported (12). Because cytokines such as IFN-gamma and TNF can induce MHC antigens in vitro on various neuroectodermal cells (10,13), it can be suggested that CD4+ T cells induce MHC antigen expression via production of IFN-gamma and TNF, and thus the possibility of local antigen presentation within the CNS is ascertained (14). Moreover, these CD4+ T cells can also be involved in the immunopathology because TNF can cause damage to the myelin sheath. In addition, macrophages can be attracted to and activated at the site of inflammation under the influence of T cell lymphokines, e.g. IFN-gamma (15). Therefore, we suggest that a subset of CD4+ T lymphocytes, via production of cytokines, could contribute to the immunopathology of multiple sclerosis.

ACKNOWLEDGEMENT

This study was financially supported by a grant from the Netherlands Foundation for the support of Multiple Sclerosis Research.

REFERENCES

1. Traugott U, Reinherz EL, Raine CS (1983) Science 219:308

2. Hauser SL, Bhan AK, Gilles F, Kemp M, Kerr C, Weiner HL (1986) Ann Neurol 19:578

3. Traugott U, Lebon P (1988) J Neurol Sci 84:257

4. Hafler DA, Fox DA, Manning ME, Schlossman SF, Reinherz EL, Weiner HL (1985) New Engl J Med 312:1405

5 Tournier-Lasserve E, Lyoncaen O, Roullet E, Bach MA (1987) Clin Exp Immunol 67:581

6. Bellamy AS, Calder VL, Feldmann M, Davison AN (1985) Clin Exp Immunol 61:248

7 Rotteveel FTM, Kokkelink I, Van Walbeek HK, Polman CH, Van Dongen JJM, Lucas CJ (1987) J Neuroimmunol 15:243

8. Rotteveel FTM, Kokkelink I, Van Lier RAW, Kuenen B, Meager A, Miedema F, Lucas CJ (1988) J Exp Med 168:1659

9. Cavender D, Saegusa Y, Ziff M (1987) J Immunol 139:1855

10. Wong GHW, Bartlett PF, Clark-Lewis I, Battye F, Schrader JW (1984) Nature 310:688

11. Traugott U (1987) J Neuroimmunol 16:283

12. Beck J, Rondot P, Catinot L, Falcoff E, Kirchner H, Wietzerbin J (1988) Acta Neurol Scand 78:318

13. Fierz W, Endler B, Reske K, Wekerle H, Fontana A (1985) J Immunol 134:3785

14. Traugott U, Scheinberg LC, Raine CS (1985) J Neuroimmunol 8:1

15. Mogensen SC, Virelizier JL (1987) Interferon 8:55

CLINICAL SIGNIFICANCE OF MONITORING MS THERAPY
BY A MYELIN-REACTIVE ACTIVE T-CELL TEST

EVAMARIA MAIDA
Neurological University Clinic of Vienna,
Lazarettgasse 14, A-1090 Vienna, Austria

INTRODUCTION

Following the demand for some technical examination, by which
the success of a treatment of MS might be estimated after a shorter
time than by clinical observations alone, a myelin-reactive active
T-cell test (MY-ATC) has been introduced at the Neurological University Clinic of Vienna in 1981 with the purpose of finding a
means for monitoring MS (1). The different ranges of application
of the test and the clinical consequences are described here.

MATERIAL AND METHODS

The MY-ATC is an easily performable blood examination, a modification of the unstimulated and myelin-antigen stimulated "early"
T-cell assays of Felsburg et al.(2), Hashim et al.(3) and Offner
et al.(4). For details see (1). Briefly, aliquots of blood mono-
nuclear cells are incubated without antigen (=unstimulated active
T-cells, ATC), with encephalitogenic peptide (=EP-stimulated active
T-cells, EP-ATC) and with galactocerebrosides (=GC-stimulated active
T-cells, GC-ATC). After a 5 min. incubation with sheep erythrocytes
the percentages of E-rosette forming cells are determined by micro-
scopy. Evaluation: %ATC; stimulation index SI-EP and SI-GC =
% EP-ATC (GC-ATC) : % ATC
Normal values: 22-34 % ATC, SI-EP(GC) < 1,25

Since 1981 6539 samples have been examined under different clinical aspects (1,5,6). For the numbers of patients, who belong to
the different groups of examinations see under "Results"and (5)

RESULTS AND CONCLUSIONS

1. When comparing MS intervals (457 patients) and times shortly
before and after relapses (134 and 208 patients) 3 observations
are of clinical importance, for details see (5):

1.1. Before a relapse %ATC is markedly going down (< 15%) and
SI-EP(GC) is going up (> 2,0 (> 1,8)). From a single examination

this can undoubtfully be recognized up to 5 days before a relapse.
The possibility to predict an increased tendency for a bout by
the MY-ATC is being used practically in situations, which are
connected with an increased risk for a relapse: since 1981
250 patients before vaccinations, operations, tooth extractions
and after delivery had been examined by the MY-ATC, 21 of whom
showed an increased tendency for a bout, which could be prevented
in all cases by postponement of the vaccination etc. or by pro-
phylactic administration of high-dose i.v. gammaglobulins in case
of delivery and acute operation, for details see (5).

1.2. During the first 5 days of an untreated relapse %ATC is
low ($<$ 15%) and SI-EP(GC) is normal or only slightly elevated
($<$ 1,6). Beyond that time %ATC remains low and SI-EP(GC) is going
up and down every few days in concordance with persistence of
clinical symptoms. We have seen that even after up to 3 months of
duration of bouts and patients improved, when treated at that time.
This observation points to the importance of early acute therapy
to stop the relapse and is being applied practically as another
part of a treatment concept of MS: since 1981 acute therapy is
started at the third or fourth day of a relapse after patients
had been requested to contact the clinic early in case of a relapse.
Furthermore, the MY-ATC helps to decide whether there is a treat-
able bout in unclear or long-lasting relapses and thus it also
helps to avoid unnecessary corticosteroid therapies.

1.3. MS intervals reveal a remarkable variability of findings
(%ATC 22 +/- 7, SI-EP 1,58 +/- 0,61, SI-GC 1,44 +/- 0,48). This
might be explained by clinically latent demyelinating activity
(latent bouts) and it is of clinical importance, when evaluating
the efficiency of a long-term therapy (see below).Furthermore,
interval findings of the MY-ATC are connected with the general
activity and thus with the prognosis of MS :

2. When doing follow-up examinations of the MY-ATC every 2 weeks
for 3 months (342 patients) a significant correlation was found
between relapse rate and the mean values of the individual patients
of %ATC (r= -0,77) and of SI-EP (r= +0,85) and SI-GC (r= +0,81).
4 groups of differently active MS could be divided (table 1).
Thus, follow-up examinations of the MY-ATC are useful for
prediction of prognosis and decision on the need for a long-term
therapy in the early stage of the disease and are applied as

another part of the treatment concept of MS.

Table 1. Results of follow-up examinations of the MY-ATC and
correlation with relapse rate

group relapse rate	m %ATC	m SI-EP	m SI-GC
1; n=52 1/> 5 years	27 +/- 5	1,16 +/- 0,19	1,12 +/- 0.18
2; n=98 1/ 2-5 years	22 +/- 4	1,35 +/- 0,23	1,31 +/- 0,22
3; n=125 1-2/year	20 +/- 3	1,70 +/- 0,21	1,59 +/- 0,23
4; n= 67 >=3/year	18 +/- 3	1,88 +/- 0,18	1,78 +/- 0,17

3. When evaluating 3 different types of acute therapies - corticosteroids i.v. pulse (1g, 5 days), p.o. (3 weeks, falling from
150 mg) and synth. ACTH (3 weeks i.v., 7 weeks i.m.) corticosteroids i.v. showed the best response: rapid normalization of
the MY-ATC in concordance with clinical remission, while ACTH
showed the weakest effect (normalization of MY-ATC and clinical
remission delayed or lacking). For details of the follow-up examinations see (5), a brief summary is given in table 2

Table 2. Comparison of MY-ATC findings during corticosteroid
i.v. pulse, p.o. and ACTH relapse therapy

therapy	%ATC	SI-EP	SI-GC
cort. i.v., n=76			
after 2 weeks	21 +/- 3	1,28 +/- 0,31	1,18 +/- 0,23
after 6 weeks	23 +/- 5	1,20 +/- 0,24	1,16 +/- 0,21
cort. p.o., n=47			
after 2 weeks	17 +/- 3	1,54 +/- 0,32	1,46 +/- 0,21
after 6 weeks	22 +/- 5	1,24 +/- 0,30	1,19 +/- 0,25
ACTH, n=24			
after 2 weeks	13 +/- 3	1,62 +/- 0,31	1,60 +/- 0,41
after 6 weeks	20 +/- 4	1,48 +/- 0,52	1,41 +/- 0,25

With regard to these observations corticosteroids, mostly i.v.
pulse, is being used since 1981 as another part of the treatment concept of MS.

4. When evaluating the efficiency of long-term therapies follow-
up examinations of the MY-ATC before and during the treatment
allowed to estimate   the success after a few months. It was the
purpose to achieve normal or nearly normal mean values in the MY-
ATC like in benign MS. Patients then showed no relapses during

the treatment. According to the different groups of MS activity
different types of long-term therapies have been tested. All
patients revealed no incapacities ((= grade 2 by Kurtzke DSS score).

4.1. group 3 (51 patients) showed MY-ATC values of 19 +/- 3 %ATC
and SI-EP(GC) 1,68 +/- 0,23 (1,61 +/- 0,22) before the onset of
therapy. 30 patients received 5g gammaglobulins i.v. every 3 weeks
for 2 years: 18 patients showed no further bouts, MY-ATC findings
were 25 +/- 4 %ATC and SI-EP(GC) 1,31 +/- 0,22 (1,26 +/- 0,15).
Azathioprin, 2 mg/kg for 2 years, was given to 21 patients of whom
13 showed no relapses. The MY-ATC values, although they were better
than before, showed a greater variation (24 +/- 6 %ATC, SI-EP(GC)
1,38 +/- 0,29 (1,29 +/- 0,25, possibly because MS was latently
going on in some of these patients. Non-responders of both groups
received a combination of the two substances (20 patients) of whom
16 showed a good response in the MY-ATC and clinically.

4.2. group 4 (63 patients) had either lymphocytapheresis (4 or
more pheresis under control of the MY-ATC every 10 weeks (6),
25 patients) or cyclosporin (initial high dose of 9 mg/kg for 6
weeks, 2 years treatment, 28 patients) or mitoxantrone (13 mg/m,
every 3 weeks, 10 patients since June 1988). MY-ATC results before
therapy were 18 +/- 4 %ATC, SI-EP(GC) 1,89 +/- 0,14 (1,74 +/- 0,16).
The best response was seen to cyclosporin (no bouts in 25 patients,
%ATC 26 +/- 5, SI-EP(GC) 1,30 +/- 0,13 (1,17 +/- 0,15)), followed
by lymphocytapheresis (no bouts in 18 patients, %ATC 23 +/- 4,
SI-EP(GC) 1,33 +/- 0,16 (1,29 +/- 0,11). 7 from the 10 mitoxantrone-
treated patients showed no bouts, but there was a great variation
in the MY-ATC (%ATC 24 +/- 5, SI-EP(GC) 1,37 +/- 0,26 (1,25 +/-
0,17)) pointing to the possibility of latent bouts during that type
of therapy. Altogether, the MY-ATC helped to treat patients more
effectively, individually and at an earlier time. The clinical
significance of monitoring MS by the MY-ATC became most evident,
when evaluating the influence of the treatment concept based on
early monitoring on MS progression in very active cases (group 4):
23 patients showed grade 1,8 +/- 0,8 by Kurtzke DSS score after
5,1 +/- 0,8 years, while 79 patients with the same MS activity,
who had not been treated in that way, showed grade 5,2 +/- 1,1
after the same time (5,3 +/- 0,7 years). In addition, the ealier
the monitoring and treatment concept was started, the better the
influence on MS progression (r=0,90): the best effects were seen,
when starting within the first year of MS.

REFERENCES

1. Maida EM (1981) Proc. 4th South-East Neuropsych. Conf., Halkidiki
2. Felsburg PJ (1976) J Immunol 116:1110
3. Hashim GA (1978) Neurochem Res 3:37
4. Offner H (1978) Acta neurol scand 57:380
5. Maida EM (1989) Proc Internat MS Conf, Rome 1988. Monduzzi Bologna
6. Maida EM (1986) Eur Neurol 25:225

© 1989 Elsevier Science Publishers B.V. (Biomedical Division)
Recent advances in multiple sclerosis therapy.
R.E. Gonsette, P. Delmotte, editors.

DETECTION OF ANTI-MYELIN BASIC PROTEIN NEUTRALIZING FACTOR IN THE CSF OF MS PATIENTS IN REMISSION

INGRID CATZ and K G WARREN

Multiple Sclerosis Patient Care and Research Clinic, University of Alberta, 9-101 Clin. Sci. Bldg., Edmonton, Alberta, Canada   T6G 2G3

INTRODUCTION

Previous research has shown that active phases of MS are assoc- iated with increased titers of intrathecaly produced anti-MBP in both free (F) and bound (B) forms (1,2). These autoantibodies are predominantly in F form in acute relapses and predominantly in B form when the disease is insidiously progressing (2,3). Longitudi- nal studies of clinically definite MS patients experiencing acute relapses demonstrate a gradual decline in F anti-MBP commensurate with a progressive rise of the B fraction, as these patients begin entering into the convalescent phase (4). This results in a rever- sal of F/B anti-MBP ratios from an initial value above unity to a value below unity (Fig. 1). Subsequently anti-MBP levels become undetectable, when remission is complete.

The distinct clinical profiles of relapsing-remitting and insidiously progressing MS permitted the development of 3 hypotheses:

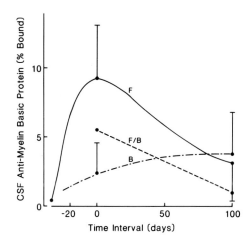

Fig. 1   Kinetics of F,B and F/B anti-MBP in acute relapses and subsequent convalescent phases.

Hypothesis 1: Active phases of MS are associated with increased CSF anti-MBP titers in both F and B forms.

Hypothesis 2: Remission phases of MS are associated with anti-MBP neutralization.

Hypothesis 3: Insidiously progressing non-remitting phases of MS are associated with inhibition of anti-MBP neutralization.

METHODS

Free and B anti-MBP levels were detected before and after CSF acid hydrolysis by a solid phase radioimmunoassay (1-3).

Anti-MBP neutralization (4) was detected in autologous and homologous experiments when CSF from patients in remission were reacted with CSF from patients with acute relapses (Fig. 2).

Inhibition of anti-MBP neutralization (4) was detected in the CSF of MS patients with chronic progressing MS (Fig. 3).

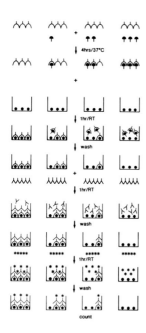

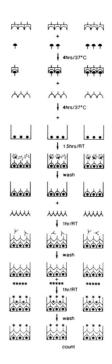

Fig. 2   Anti-MBP neutralization (ʎ = anti-MBP in acute relapses of MS ↑ = neutralizing factor in MS remission)

Fig. 3   Inhibition of anti-MBP neutralization (⩑ = inhibiting factor in progressing MS)

RESULTS

An anti-MBP neutralizing effect was observed in 36 of 37 autologous and homologous in vitro experiments when CSF with undetectable anti-MBP from a patient in remission was reacted with CSF with
high anti-MBP from a patient with an acute relapse of MS (Figs. 4
and 5). CSF from non-MS patients (negative control) substituted
for the remission sample had no neutralizing effect, while CSF from
other patients with acute relapses (positive control) had a cumulative effect (Figs. 4 and 5), confirming the validity of the assay.

Patients with chronically progressing MS are associated with persistence of elevated CSF anti-MBP titers (F/B ratios below unity)
over long periods of time (5). CSF from such patients produced
inhibition of anti-MBP neutralization (Fig. 6) in 29 of 31 individual experiments.

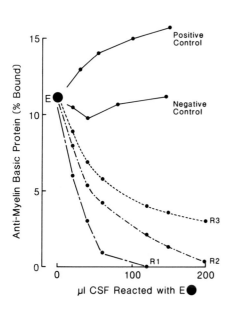

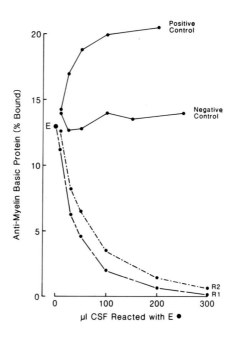

Fig. 4   Autologous anti-MBP   Fig. 5   Homologous anti-MBP
neutralization   neutralization

90

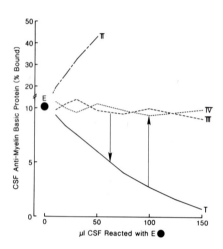

Fig. 6   Inhibition of anti-MBP neutralization

CONCLUSION

Acute relapses of MS are associated with pulsed intrathecal anti-MBP production resulting in a high (above unity) F/B anti-MBP ratio.

The remission phase of MS is characterized by undetectable CSF anti-MBP as well as a factor causing anti-MBP neutralization.

Chronically progressing MS is associated with steady state anti-MBP production. Anti-MBP is predominantly in B form resulting in a F/B ratio below unity. CSF from patients with progressing MS produces inhibition of anti-MBP neutralization.

REFERENCES

1. Catz I, Warren KG (1986) Can J Neurol Sci 13:21
2. Warren KG, Catz I (1986) Ann Neurol 20:20
3. Warren KG, Catz I (1987) Ann Neurol 21:183
4. Warren KG, Catz I (1988) J Neurol Sci 88:185
5. Warren KG, Catz I (1987) Clin Neuropharmacol 10:397

CONCLUDING REMARKS

© 1989 Elsevier Science Publishers B.V. (Biomedical Division)
Recent advances in multiple sclerosis therapy.
R.E. Gonsette, P. Delmotte, editors.

PARAMETERS OF DISEASE ACTIVITY

SPECULATIVE REMARKS ON DISEASE ACTIVITY

O.R. HOMMES
Nijmegen, The Netherlands

In today's presentations and discussions (5th ECTRIMS Congress, Brussels 1989) some important points appeared.

It has been clearly established now that there is a subclinical stage of the disease. Arguments are

- the presence of NMR lesions in clinically unaffected twins
- changes in the blood-brain barrier detected by NMR gadolineum enhancement at a clinically silent stage of the disease
- absence of correlation between NMR lesion volume and neurological status.

If there is a subclinical stage of the disease, this means that there is subclinical progression of the disease. And subclinical progression of the disease means subclinical disease activity.

Now it is important to relate this notion, disease activity, to our knowledge of the pathogenesis of multiple sclerosis in the central nervous system. The pathogenesis of multiple sclerosis is not monomorphic, but can be described in 5 different stages (fig. 1). Each of these stages can have, but must not have, relation to clinical phenomena. It can be surmised that the pathogenesis can stop for shorter or longer time, completely or incompletely, at each of the stages. It is assumed at the same time that each of these stages can supersede the forgoing one at any moment in the course of the disease. It also has to be assumed that several stages can exist at the same time.

Clinically, however, there may be a synchronicity of stages in certain phases of the disease. However it will be clear that what is called a clinical relaps, may be a heterogenic phenomenon. In these concluding remarks I would like to start the discussion on the association of several clinical and laboratory aspects of multiple sclerosis. The stages introduced here, could have their function in clinical diagnosis, in that they direct the attention not only to a point in the clinical course of the disease, but associate the immuno-biochemical, neurophysiological and imiging findings to it. The weight of the technical findings in assessing the stage of the disease may be, and has to be sometimes, greater than the clinical ones.

STAGE I. BLOOD-BRAIN BARRIER

This stage can clinically be silent, or present itself in signs and symptoms of low intensity and short duration of minutes, or hours. There is complete functional restauration. Clinically well known are fleeting visual and other sensory disturbances, pareses and ataxias.

In background of these disturbances probably is abnormal endothelial activity, leakage through the vessel wall of the postcappillary venules and consequently disturbance of the surrounding milieu by humoral factors such as albumen, other proteins, amino acids and minerals.

It is likely that this stage has an immunological cause.

In the CSF albumin and total protein are increased. There is no increased cell count, no intrathecal IgG synthesis and oligoclonal banding.

In the blood the anti-endothelial cell antibodies, the interferon-gamma and the TNF levels may be increased as well as IL_2 and IL_2R.

The NMR shows gadolineum enhanced lesions.

There is no conduction slowing in evoked responses.

STAGE II. INFILTRATION

This stage can proceed from stage I. Clinically it can consist of signs and symptoms that appear rather quickly (hours, days, may be up to one week), and disappear rather quickly without any clinical functional residue. This is a "relaps".

The difference between stage I and II is the time course and the intensity and severity of the clinical signs and symptoms.

It is assumed that the pathogenic process can stop at stage II and disappear completely. The pathogenic process is inflammatory, with perivascular infiltration of humoral and cellular aspects. It does not have to proceed into demyelination. The functional disturbance is caused by this infiltrate, by edema, secondary swelling of astrocytes, splitting of myelin lamellae, blocking of Ranvier-nodes, metabolic disturbance of oligodendrocytes. All these changes are assumed to be reversible; without demyelination. In the CSF there is intrathecal IgA and IgM, and later IgG synthesis, and oligoclonal banding. There is increased cell content of the lymphocytic type.

In the blood changes like in stage I may be found, or they may have disappeared already. The NMR shows lesions, that may or may not be enhanced by gadolineum, dependend on the functional closure of the blood-brain barrier, that can occur in this stage. Some conduction slowing may be found by evoked response study, but it is minimal. It may be completely absent.

This stage is part of an immunological reaction.

STAGE III. DEMYELINATION

This stage can proceed from stage II, earlier or later in the course of a "relapse". Clinically its most salient feature is the functional loss that increases over days or weeks, resulting from demyelination. The duration of the increase in clinical symptomatology is longer than that of relapses related to stage II.

The pathogenic process consists of all the cellular, humoral and enzymatic proteolytic activity known from demyelination. And this demyelination is, associated with bystander effects, the cause of functional loss.

This stage can proceed into remyelination, thus showing a slow but definite recuperation of function. It can also proceed into scarformation, thus showing hardly any functional improvement. In CSF the appearance of MBP from myelin breakdown, and neopterin from macrophage activity is the most important feature. Cells may be at a normal level. Intrathecal IgG is increased and there is oligoclonal banding.

In the blood no abnormalities are encountered. There is no gadolineum enhancement in NMR.

Evoked response studies show definite conduction slowing.

This is only partly an immunological stage.

STAGE IV. REMYELINATION

This stage appears as the slow recovery after a stage III relapse, and its main aspect is remyelination, that takes months to complete. The recovery of function is however not always complete.

Frequently there is an increase of symptomatology by fatigue and by rise of body temperature, consisting in the reappearance of the earlier symptoms and signs. They quickly disappear after resting or cooling. An example is the short-lived blinding of an eye, after recovery of an optic neuritis, by fatigue or increased temperature. This may be related to short, thin, incomplete internodes of remyelinating oligodendrocytes or Schwann cells (shadow plaques).

In the CSF there is intrathecal IgG synthesis, T cell, pleiocytosis and oligoclonal banding. In the blood no changes are found.

NMR shows no gadolineum enhancement of the lesions.

Evoked response studies show conduction slowing. This is not an immunological stage.

STAGE V. SCARFORMATION

This is the clinically residual stage after one or more inflammatory and demyelinating attacks, or after severe chronic inflammation and demyelination. There is a constant, stabilized functional deficit and disability, showing no signs of recovery. On the contrary: In the years a very slow functional decrease is observed.

This can be related to axonal loss in gliotic scars, so typical for burnt out plaques. The gliosis is an astrocyte type II sequence. The border of the gliotic field may serve as the place for new, extending, stage I, II and III immunological activities.

The CSF shows intrathecal IgG synthesis and oligoclonal banding, but at a low level. In the blood no changes are found. NMR shows no gadolineum enhancement of the lesions.

Evoked response studies show conduction slowing. This is not an immunological stage.

CLINICAL USE OF MS STAGES

The most important use of stageing MS will be found in its clinical pressure on doctors to realize that the pathogenic processes in MS patients are very different.

Another aspect of stageing MS is the prognostic factor, included in it, with regard to short terms outcome of a relaps.

Stageing MS could also be very important in the choice of experimental treatment. Corticosteroids are theoretically only of value in stages I, II and III, antimitotics only in stages II and III. For preventive measures antimitotics might also be used in stage I and in stages IV and V. The same hold for total lymphoid irradiation.

Interferons and COP-I may theoretically only be effective in stages II and III.

The stageing may also be important to direct attention in experimental medicin to the activation of remyelination in stage IV and prevention of axonal loss in stage V.

Very important the stageing may be in the design of clinical trials. Any clinical trial sofar executed certainly is a mixture of various stages, that in themselves will show very different characteristics with regard to the objectives of the trial. This especially holds for therapeutic trials.

The stageing may be usefull in the study of the course of the disease. There are ample indications now that the disease in its first years shows more inflammatory characteristics than later on. In later years scarformation may be more preponderant.

OBJECTIVE PARAMETERS OF DIFFERENT STAGES

From the various studies reported at this congress it is clear that objective parameters for disease activity are very important. But disease activity is not a unitary notion, as was discussed under pathogenesis. Only in stageing MS, the term disease activity will find its real meaning. In the blood-brain barrier stage (stage I), the activity of the disease process may be best characterized by the amount of leakage of the blood-brain barrier as demonstrated by total protein and total albumin and by gadolineum enhancement.

The infiltration stage (stage II), may be best characterized by pleiocytosis, increased number of T cells and increased CD_4/CD_8 rations of blood and CSF.

The demyelination stage (stage III) could find its main characteristics in increased CSF MBP and neopterin, as expression of macrophage activity and myelin breakdown.

The remyelination stage (stage IV) may find its expression in reduced conduction latency in ER studies.

The scarring stage (stage V) may be best delineated by the absence of most of the previous parameters. A parameter possitively indicating gliotic scarformation of course is strongly needed.

In table 1 a tentative list of parameters in various stages of MS is given

TABLE 1
Clinical, technical and laboratory aspects of several putative stages of Multiple Sclerosis pathogenesis.

```
TP              = Total Protein
MBP             = Myelin Basic Protein
IFN-gamma       = Interferon-gamma
TNF             = Tumor Necrosis Factor
IL2             = Interleukin 2
IL2R            = Interleukin 2 Receptor
anti endoth AB  = Anti-endothelial cell antibody
NMR gad         = gadolineum enhancement of NMR
ER              = Evoked Response.
```

STAGE		I BLOOD-BRAIN BARRIER	II INFILTRATION	III DEMYELINATION	IV REMYELINATION	V SCARFORMATION
Clinical	course	subclinical fleeting, short lived, hours	days, weeks	weeks, months	slow, months	stabile functional loss, increasing over years
	recovery	quick	slow	incomplete	slow	none
	residu	none	none	substantial	minor	slowly increasing
CSF	TP	+	±	-	-	-
	intrathecal IgG	-	±	+	+	+
	banding	-	+	+	+	+
	cells	-	+	±	-	-
	MBP	-	-	+	-	-
	neopterin	-	-	-	-	-
Blood/serum	IFN-gamma-TNF	+	±	-	-	-
	IL$_2$-IL$_2$R	+	+	-	-	-
	anti-endoth AB	+	±	+	-	-
	CD$_4$ subsets	+	+	-	-	-
	myelin reactive cells	+	+	-	-	-
	NMR gad	+	±	-	-	-
	ER slowing	-	-	+	+	+

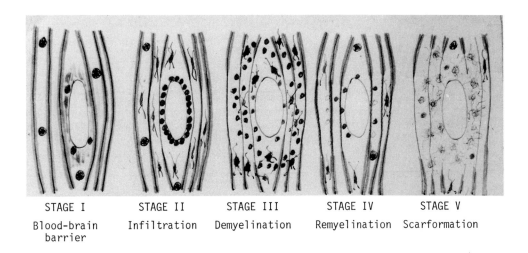

STAGE I	STAGE II	STAGE III	STAGE IV	STAGE V
Blood-brain barrier	Infiltration	Demyelination	Remyelination	Scarformation

Fig. 1. Various stages of disease activity in MS pathogenesis.

CONCLUSION

I am fully aware of the speculative aspect of these remarks, but at the same time feel that many of my thoughts may be shared by the audience. Disease activity in MS is different from one stage to another. The stages indicated here may not be defined to rigidly, by clearly enough to be recognized in clinical practice. The technical parameters allocated to them may be accessible to most neurologists.

TREATMENTS: RESULTS AND FUTURE PROSPECTS

CORTICOTHERAPY

© 1989 Elsevier Science Publishers B.V. (Biomedical Division)
Recent advances in multiple sclerosis therapy.
R.E. Gonsette, P. Delmotte, editors.

CORTICOSTEROIDS IN THE TREATMENT OF MULTIPLE SCLEROSIS

PROFESSOR D A S COMPSTON

University of Cambridge Clinical School, Neurology Department,
Addenbrooke's Hospital, Hills Road, Cambridge, CB2 2QQ.

Corticosteroids have been used successfully in the treatment of
Multiple Sclerosis for several decades but neither has the preferred
method of administration nor the indications for using corticosteroids been
firmly established. Most clinicians only use steroids during relapses but
new episodes are not always easily defined and many patients seek treatment
of persistent or slowly progressive disability with corticosteroids. Some
clinicians use corticotrophin whereas others prefer oral prednisolone or
dexamethasone but both these regimens are limited by adverse effects including weight gain and change in physical appearance. The evidence from
at least one double-blind placebo controlled trial and several open studies
is that high dose intravenous methylprednisolone is now the preferred means
of prescribing corticosteroids in patients with multiple sclerosis. Not
only are the beneficial effects comparable or better than those achieved
using corticotrophin but adverse effects are fewer and the spectrum of
patients who can expect to benefit is greater.

Milligan et al (1) treated 50 patients in a double-blind placebo controlled trial; 19/26 patients given methylprednisolone (0.5 grams intravenously by slow infusion over 20 minutes for 5 days) showed decreased
disability scores four weeks after starting therapy. 6/7 patients failing
to respond had chronic progressive disease. By comparison, 7/24 controls
had improved at four weeks whereas 16/24 were either unchanged or worse.
Overall these results showed a significant effect in favour of treatment
with methylprednisolone (t=-3.85; P 0.001). The main effect was in the
group treated with methylprednisolone during acute relapse, 8/13 of whom
had improved by up to 4.5 points on the Kurtzke expanded disability scale
within one week. In 7 further improvement occurred so that at four weeks
10/13 patients had improved by more than one point on the disability scale.
Patients given placebo treatment did not improve overall, although 2/9 improved spontaneously, as expected; new relapses occurred during the period
of observation but these were confined to those patients receiving placebo
treatment.

This study also demonstrated that patients with chronic progressive multiple sclerosis may improve following treatment with high dose intravenous methylprednisolone due to a selective effect on pyramidal function - the major cause of disability in this category of cases. 6/13 actively treated patients showed a reduction in disability score of more than one point on the Kurtzke scale at four weeks and in all instances this was due to improved pyramidal function. Sensory symptoms occasionally improved but other functional systems were unchanged. This effect was not observed in controls, two of whom suffered further disease activity during the period of observation.

Later follow up of these 50 cases confirmed that no significant adverse effects had developed during 1116 patient/months of follow up (2) and similar experience has since been reported in a larger retrospective view of 350 treatments, involving up to a 5 gram cumulative dose sometimes supplemented with oral prednisolone and occasionally involving six separate courses, given to 240 patients over a six year period (3). However, the initial clinical improvement seen both in patients with acute and chronic progressive multiple sclerosis is not maintained with time. Two years after treatment 4/24 actively treated patients had maintained their improvement whereas 8 were unchanged and 12 had deteriorated. Comparable figures in the placebo treated group were 6,8 and 10/24 (2). Since high dose intravenous methylprednisolone appears on the present evidence to be safe, some clinicians are prepared to give repeated doses and to supplement treatment with prolonged oral prednisolone. There is as yet no evidence that these regimens alter the course of the illness but further trials are expected.

After defining the clinical effects, attention has turned to the mechanism of action of high dose intravenous methylprednisolone in patients with multiple sclerosis (4). Analysis of cerebrospinal fluid sampled before and after treatment has shown that methylprednisolone lowers the content of inflammatory cells in spinal fluid to 33% less than expected on placebo treatment and there is also a reduction in intrathecal IgG synthesis, although neither result is statistically significant. Conversely there is evidence that intrathecal complement activation, previously demonstrated using indirect methods (5) is inhibited following intravenous steroid therapy. In vitro studies, using neonatal rat optic nerve oligodendrocytes, supplemented by cerebrospinal fluid analysis from patients with isolated and multiple episodes of demyelination, indicate that the immunopathogenesis of multiple sclerosis may ultimately involve complement dependent injury of oligodendrocytes and their myelin membranes. Scolding et al (6) have extended previous reports of complement activation by purified myelin (7) demonstrating that exposure of intact neonatal rat optic nerve oligodendrocytes to fresh rat serum results in antibody independent classical pathway activation of complement. Subsquently, Scolding and colleagues (8) have demonstrated that complement mediated oligodendrocyte injury is reversible, recovery occurring through the removal of membrane attack complex enriched vesicles. The vesicles appearing in the supernatant of cultured oligodendrocytes are identical to those subsequently recovered from cerebrospinal fluid in a high proportion of patients with multiple sclerosis but not individuals with mechanical nerve root irritation or intracranial mass lesions.

The intrathecal effects of methylprednisolone have also been examined indirectly using quantitative magnetic resonance imaging. 50 patients, treated electively at a time of clinical stability, in whom no overall reduction in score on the Kurtzke expanded disability status scale was demonstrated, were scanned before and after treatment. In 48/50 three or more cerebral white matter lesions were demonstrated and in 44/48 there were also lesions in the brain stem or cerebellum. There was no change in the appearance of these lesions after treatment in 36/48; new lesions developed in 9, in 7 old lesions appeared smaller, and in 2 both of these changes were observed. No area of white matter abnormality was seen to disappear. By contrast with the qualitative changes, quantitative studies showed a highly significant reduction in the T1 weighted signal from cortex and normal appearing white matter after treatment, and serial studies also demonstrated a significant sequential reduction in the T2 weighted signal. These findings indicate that there is a generalised reduction in water content throughout the central nervous system in patients with multiple sclerosis receiving high dose intravenous methylprednisolone consistent with an alteration in the inflammatory process (9).

Preliminary studies have been carried out on the function of lymphocytes or macrophages recovered from peripheral blood. Low molar concentrations of methylprednisolone were shown by Kirk and colleagues (10) to increase pokeweed mitogen stimulated IgG synthesis by unfractionated lymphocytes, in 20 patients with multiple sclerosis and 15 controls. In a further sample of 26 patients, IgG synthesis increased following treatment with methylprednisolone but the in vitro responsiveness of peripheral blood

106

mononuclear cells to methylprednisolone was uninfluenced. Phenotypic analysis of paired samples from 12 cases showed no alteration in CD4 or CD8 cells and their sub-populations. These results do not provide evidence that methylprednisolone adjusts the functional interaction of T and B cells in patients with multiple sclerosis. Subsequently Kirk et al (unpublished observations) have recovered cells adhering to coated polypropylene plates after mononuclear cell fractionation and incubated this macrophage enriched population, with different concentrations of methylprednisolone. Prosta-glandin E2, Leucotriene B4 and Thromboxane B2 were measured in the super-natants by radio immunoassay. In addition, samples were measured before and after a five day course of high dose intravenous methylprednisolone. Lower levels of each inflammatory cell mediator were detected in samples from patients with multiple sclerosis than controls but in both groups there was evidence for a dose dependent reduction in the release of macrophage mediators after incubation with methylprednisolone. The ability of cells to produce eicosanoids was also reduced in samples taken after a five day course of methylprednisolone by comparison with pre-treatment results. These studies provide evidence for a more marked effect on release of macrophage mediators by methylprednisolone both in vitro and in vivo than on functional interactions of T and B lymphocytes.

High dose intravenous methylprednisolone is the preferred method for administering corticosteroids in patients with multiple sclerosis both during relapse and the chronic progressive phase but a single pulsed treat-ment does not influence the long term course of the disease. More complex regimens involving elective retreatment or combined oral and intravenous steroids may prove more effective in this respect. Methylprednisolone appears to act by reducing oedema in the central nervous system perhaps through inhibition of local and infiltrating inflammatory cells.

REFERENCES

1. Milligan NM, Newcombe R, Compston DAS (1987) Journal of Neurology, Neurosurgery and Psychiatry 50: 511 - 516.

2. Compston DAS, Milligan NM (1988) Journal of Neurology, Neurosurgery and Psychiatry 51: 597 - 598.

3. Lyons PR, Newman PK, Saunders M (1988) Journal of Neurology, Neuro-surgery and Psychiatry 51: 285 - 287.

4. Compston DAS, Hughes PJ, Morgan BP, Gibbs J, Milligan NM (1987) Journal of Neurology, Neurosurgery and Psychiatry 50: 517 - 522.

5. Compston DAS, Morgan BP, Oleesky D, Fifield R, Campbell AK (1986) Neurology 36: 1503 - 1506.

6. Scolding NJ, Houston WAJ, Linington C, Morgan BP, Campbell AK, Compston DAS (1989) Nature (in press).

7. Vanguri P and Shin ML (1988) J. Biol. Chem. 263: 7228.

8. Scolding NJ, Morgan BP, Houston WAJ, Campbell AK, Linington C, Compston DAS. (1989) Journal of the Neurological Sciences 89: 289 - 300.

9. Kesselring J, Miller DH, MacManus DG, Milligan NM, Scolding N, Johnson G, Compston DAS, McDonald WI (1989) Journal of Neurology, Neurosurgery and Psychiatry 52: 14 - 17.

10. Kirk PF, Compston DAS (1989) Journal of Neuroimmunology (in press).

© 1989 Elsevier Science Publishers B.V. (Biomedical Division)
Recent advances in multiple sclerosis therapy.
R.E. Gonsette, P. Delmotte, editors.

EFFECTS OF HIGH-DOSE METHYLPREDNISOLONE THERAPY ON CEREBRAL MRI LESIONS OF MS PATIENTS

L. RUMBACH,* J.M. WARTER,* J.L. DIETEMANN,** E. BODIGUEL* and M. COLLARD*

* Clinique Neurologique, ** Service de Neuroradiologie, Hôpital Central, CHU, B.P. 426, 67091 - Strasbourg Cedex (France)

INTRODUCTION

It has been demonstrated that MS patients in acute exacerbation may improve more rapidly if they are treated with high doses of methylprednisolone [1]. Evoked potentials and immunological methods can be used to investigate patients with MS but no one abnormality correlates well with the time course of clinical symptoms. MRI is at present the most sensitive method for demonstrating MS cerebral lesions [2]. In a prospective study lasting one month, we have recorded serial MRI brain slices in methylprednisolone-treated patients and in patients in remission in order to compare lesions with clinical changes.

METHODS

Patients

Thirty clinically definite MS patients were divided into 2 groups similar as to distribution of age, sex and MS duration. The 17 Group 1 patients were in acute relapse and were treated with high doses of intravenous methylprednisolone, 20 mg/kg on day 1 and 15 mg/kg on day 3, followed by decreasing doses of oral prednisolone for the next 27 days. The 13 Group 2 patients had been in remission for the 3 preceding months. None of the 30 was being treated with immunosuppressive drugs. The clinical condition was assessed using the Kurtzke disability status scale (EDSS).

MRI

Two scans were obtained on each patient, at the beginning of the study month, before treatment started for Group 1, and at the end of the month. Images were obtained using a 0.5 T Magniscan 5000 scanner with a multi-spin echo sequence, TE 60 ms, RT 2 s. Several transversal slices were imaged, using 1 of the 2 protocols for the two MRI examinations of any one patient: either slices 4 mm thick separated by 8 mm, or 8-mm thick contiguous slices. Care was taken that the patient's head position was the same in repeat scans. All MRI results were judged after the study by a single naïve radiologist. Hypersignals only, their number, localization and size, were evaluated. Lesion number was sometimes difficult to determine if there were more than 5 near periventricular regions.

RESULTS

Clinically, all the treated patients in relapse reported diminished symptoms and this was borne out for some by their ratings on the EDSS. But in the untreated Group 2, neither symptoms nor signs had changed.

The first MRI was abnormal in all patients. There was little or no correlation between the number of lesions, their sites and the functional handicap. On the second scan 30 days later, lesions had changed in most cases (Table I). Seven of the 17 treated Group 1 patients had no change of lesions. In the other 10, new lesions appeared in new places, many lesions decreased in size, and some even disappeared in some patients. Four of the 13 untreated Group 2 patients showed no change of lesions. Some had fewer lesions, but in 6, new lesions appeared. In both groups, new lesions could appear and old ones disappear in the same patient.

DISCUSSION

This study confirms previous reports that high doses of methyl-prednisolone are beneficial clinically in acute MS exacerbations. It is thus ethically difficult to constitute two like groups in relapse, to be treated or not and then compared for MRI changes.

The serial MRI findings show that disease activity in MS is a dynamic process: lesion detected varied enormously with time. In both groups of patients, lesions disappeared and new ones appeared elsewhere.

The correlation between MRI and clinical signs was slight. Whereas in the treated group, symptoms improved, and often clinical signs too, in the untreated patients in remission there was no clinical change, yet the changing pattern of the MRI lesions was quite similar.

Finally, this study does not address the question of the nature of the histopathological processes inducing hyperbrilliant MRI lesions.

In conclusion, high doses of methylprednisolone appear to be beneficial to MS patients in acute relapse. But whereas serial MRI is indeed a good method of assessing dynamic disease activity, it is less reliable for judging the efficacy of therapeutic measures.

TABLE I

TOTAL CHANGE IN NUMBER OF PATIENTS PER GROUP OVER ONE MONTH
MRI lesions could appear and others disappear in the same patient

	Unchanged lesions	Lesions changed		
		Disappeared	Fewer	New
Group 1 treated n = 17	7	4	6	5
Group 2 untreated n = 13	4	3	3	6

REFERENCES

1. Milligan NM, Newcombe R, Compston DAS (1987) J Neurol Neurosurg Psychiatry 50:511-516

2. Young IR, Hall AS, Pallis CA, Legg NJ, Bydder JM, Steiner RE (1981) Lancet 2:1063-1066

INTERFERONS

© 1989 Elsevier Science Publishers B.V. (Biomedical Division)
Recent advances in multiple sclerosis therapy.
R.E. Gonsette, P. Delmotte, editors.

EFFECTS OF EXPERIMENTAL RECOMBINANT INTERFERONS
ON MULTIPLE SCLEROSIS

Kenneth P. Johnson, M.D. and Hillel S. Panitch, M.D.

Multiple Sclerosis (MS), first described by Charcot in 1877 (1), is a major crippling disease of young adults. Approximately 300,000 cases exist in the United States and over 60 percent are women. Clinically the disease is remarkably variable, appearing between the ages of 15 and 60 with a peak age of onset at approximately 30 years. Patients may experience any type of the central nervous system (CNS) symptom, however, weakness and sensory change of the extremities indicative of spinal cord disease or optic neuritis are the most common first complaints. Rapidly appearing exacerbations followed by gradual remission characterize the early years of the disease. Usually during the fifth decade, the disease pattern changes to one of chronic, increasing neurologic disability, often producing significant handicaps. As the disease progresses urinary dysfunction is almost universal secondary to spinal cord disease. Another frequent complaint is periodic severe fatigue which is more likely during periods of disease activity or when patients are exposed to increased ambient temperatures.

Pathologic change is restricted to the CNS and appears almost exclusively in the white matter. Discrete foci or plaques of varying size appear more or less randomly with some predilection for periventricular areas. Early on, these plaques have an inflammatory nature but over time they show demyelination, the central hallmark of the disease plus gliosis. Various lymphocytes always reside in the plaque and in perivascular cuffs and increased collections of immunoglobulins in the lesion are universally found as well.

The diagnosis of MS is made by observing the exacerbating remitting or progressive course and finding neurologic impairments on examination which must result from multiple, localized CNS lesions. The magnetic resonance imaging (MRI) scan almost always shows the lesions in cerebral white matter. Various evoked response tests aid in the detection of clinically silent lesions. Finally, spinal fluid immunoglobulin abnormalities can be detected in over 95% of cases if a search is made for an abnormal IgG index or the presence of oligoclonal IgG bands (2). Once other diseases are ruled out the diagnosis can be made with assurance relatively early in over 90% of cases. The differential diagnosis includes various neurologic infections such as neurosyphilis, Lyme disease and tropical spastic paraparesis produced by HTLV-1 virus infection. Brain tumors and cerebral vasculitis may at times confuse the picture and some cases of a more generalized autoimmune condition which includes CNS lesions, have been described.

Multiple sclerosis occurs primarily in the Caucasian population and occasionally affects several members in one family. Identical twins both show the disease more commonly than fraternal twins or other siblings (3). Certain HLA antigens are over represented in the MS population indicating that there is a genetic predisposition to the disease. Epidemiologic studies have shown that there is a geographic gradient with more cases in temperate areas; migration studies show that one's residence during the first fifteen years of life determine the prevalence of disease. True epidemics of MS have been described indicating that some environmental factor, probably acting during childhood, initiates the process in the genetically susceptible individual (4). The disease process itself is clearly immunologic in nature. The presence of immune active cells and immunoglobulin in plaques and spinal fluid plus the finding that T suppressor lymphocytes are deficient during exacerbations or during the chronic stages of disease all indicate the immunologic nature of the process. Exacerbations occur more frequently after banal infections suggesting that a perturbation of the immune system is likely to reactivate or create a new MS lesion (5). Recent evidence suggests that gamma interferon is a prime pathogenic factor in plaque initiation or activation as noted below. Indirect evidence has suggested that one or more viruses may contribute to the MS process but no convincing studies have settled this point.

Three human interferons (INF), alpha, beta and gamma, have been identified and all have antiviral activity as well as the ability to stimulate or modify various immunologic functions (6). Alpha and beta INF are quite similar and in fact use the same cell surface receptor. Gamma interferon is remarkably different in its immunologic functions and is known especially for its ability to stimulate the expression of DR histocompatibility antigen on the cell surface (7). By 1979 (8) it was known that MS patients often produce deficient amounts of various interferons and also show an abnormally low level of natural killer (NK) cells, a population known to be stimulated by interferons. These reasons plus the fact that MS has been indirectly linked to a past or persistent virus infection all suggested that interferons would be suitable candidates for therapeutic evaluation in MS.

We collaborated in the plans for the first controlled trial of INF therapy for MS and decided to explore systemic administration of alpha INF in an effort to reduce new attacks of disease (9). This route was chosen because there are systemically identifiable immunologic changes in MS and because interferons may cross the abnormal blood brain barrier at the site of an evolving plaque even though interferons cross the intact barrier poorly (10). Also there was a concern that repeated intrathecal injections of INF in a pharmacological vehicle may stimulate late progressive arachnoiditis. This first trial of alpha INF in MS, conducted in California, investigated natural interferon in a subcutaneous (sc) dose of 5 million units daily for six months. Twenty-four patients participated in a double blind, placebo controlled, crossover format. This small study did show a definite trend toward a reduction of attacks, however, persistent side effects precluded its consideration for long term use in exacerbating-remitting MS (9). At the University of Maryland we then initiated the second controlled trial of alpha INF using cloned interferon supplied by the Schering-Plough Corporation. Two million units of interferon were given sc three times a week for a one year to fifty MS patients while fifty others received placebo, again in a double blind format. Side effects were almost nonexistent and the number of attacks declined dramatically, however, the attack rate also declined in the placebo population precluding a claim of therapeutic efficacy (11). Of interest almost any form of therapy which has been evaluated for MS has shown a significant placebo effect (12).

In 1984 we were asked to initiate a study of recombinant gamma interferon again in exacerbating-remitting MS. Because of our concern of adverse immunologic stimulation, a small pilot trial was conducted involving 18 patients who received gamma INF intravenously in one of three doses, twice per week. During the one month study, seven patients experienced new attacks of MS indicating that gamma INF was a potent stimulator of new disease activity (13). While this experience was not useful therapeutically, it did indicate the central position that gamma INF probably plays in activation or initiation of disease activity in MS. As a result of this study, inhibition of gamma INF and its effects have become major therapeutic objectives in the search for new therapies for MS. Of interest all of the MS attacks experienced during the gamma INF trial were mild and all were clinically reversible within a three to four month period.

Currently we are engaged in a large clinical and scientific evaluation of recombinant Beta interferon in MS (14). A small pilot trial of beta INF supplied by Triton Biosciences, Alameda, California, has shown that remarkably large doses can be given sc with virtually no side effects. A pilot trial employing 30 patients indicated that 45 million units per dose, administered sc three times per week was well tolerated by young exacerbating-remitting MS patients. No increase in MS disease activity has been noted in this small study; in fact there is a clear trend towards reduction in new disease attacks. Following this two and a half year experience with beta INF, a large multicenter trial is now being conducted at ten participating centers, six in the U.S. and four in Canada. A total of 330 patients will be enrolled in a blinded, placebo controlled study in which one-third of the patients will receive 45 million units of beta INF sc every other day, another third will receive 9 million units and the rest will receive placebo. The trial is planned to last for two years and is enhanced by a number of clinical and laboratory evaluators including frequent MRI scans.

Studies in progress at the University of Maryland have shown that peripheral blood leukocytes from patients receiving beta INF have a decreased ability to synthesize gamma INF. This inhibitory effect on gamma INF and its functions seems to persist for prolonged periods of time. The preparation has also been shown to stimulate T suppressor cell activity, another potentially beneficial therapeutic function. Thus there is a clear immunologic and pharmacologic rationale for beta INF's potential effectiveness in MS.

The sequential studies described in this short report have encompassed over eight years of effort and have required the enrollment of over 250 courageous MS patients who have willingly accepted either therapeutic agents of unknown effects and toxicity or long term dosing with placebo. This series of studies has not as yet produced a clearly effective therapeutic agent for MS. However the studies and the accompanying scientific investigations have produced a great deal of fundamental information about the immunologic pathogenesis of exacerbating-remitting MS. In addition, the trials now underway rest on a firm foundation of scientific fact which provides great promise that interferons may find an acknowledged therapeutic role in the treatment of this highly variable, long term and, unfortunately, frequently disabling CNS disease of young adults.

References

1. Charcot JM: Lectures on the Diseases of the Nervous System: Delivered at La Salpetriere, Sigerson G(trans). London, New Sydenham Society, 1877-1889.

2. Johnson KP, Nelson BJ: Multiple Sclerosis: Diagnostic Usefulness of Cerebrospinal Fluid. Ann. Neurol. 2:425-431 (1977).

3. Compston, A: Genetic factors in the aetiology of multiple sclerosis. In: Multiple Sclerosis, McDonald WI, Silberberg DH (eds) . England: Butterworth & Co. (1986); 4:56-73.

4. Kurtzke JF, Gudmundsson KR, Bergmann S: Multiple sclerosis in Iceland. I. Evidence of a postwar epidemic. Neurology 32:143-150 (1982).

5. Sibley WA, Bamford CR, Clark K: Clinical viral infections and multiple sclerosis. Lancet 1:1313-1315 (1985).

6. Fleischmann WR Jr, Ramamurthy V, Stanton GJ, et al: Interferon: Mode of Action and Clinical Applications. In: Interferon Treatment of Neurologic Disorders, Smith RA (ed.): Marcel Dekker, Inc. New York (1988); 1:1-42.

7. Merrill JE, Targan SR: The Immunologic Basis for the Use of Interferons. In: Interferon Treatment of Neurologic Disorders, Smith RA (ed.): Marcel Dekker, Inc. New York (1988); 3:65-101.

8. Neighbour PA, Bloom BR: Absence of virus-induced lymphocyte suppression and interferon production in multiple sclerosis. Proc. Natl. Acad. Sci. USA 76:476-480 (1979).

9. Knobler RL, Panitch HS, Braheny SL, et al: Controlled clinical trial of systemic alpha interferon in multiple sclerosis. Neurology 34:1273-1279 (1984).

10.   Johnson KP: Systemic interferon therapy for multiple sclerosis: Design of a trial. Arch. Neurol. 40:681-682 (1983).

11.   Camenga DL, Johnson KP, Alter M, et al: Systemic recombinant alpha-2 interferon therapy in relapsing multiple sclerosis. Arch. Neurol. 43:1239-1246 (1986).

12.   Hirsch RL, Johnson KP: Placebo-induced enhancement of natural killer cell activity in a double-blind trial of recombinant alpha-2 interferon in multiple sclerosis patients. In: Neuroimmunomodulation. Proceedings of the First International Workshop of Neuroimmunomodulation, Spector NH (ed.). IWGN, Bethesda Maryland, 219-226 (1985).

13.   Panitch HS, Hirsch RL, Schindler J, et al: Treatment of multiple sclerosis with gamma interferon: Exacerbations associated with activation of the immune system. Neurology 37:1097-1102 (1987).

14.   Panitch HS, Johnson KP: Treatment of Multiple Sclerosis by Systemic Administration of Interferon. In: Interferon Treatment of Neurologic Disorders, Smith RA (ed.): Marcel Dekker, Inc. New York (1988); 9:209-240.

© 1989 Elsevier Science Publishers B.V. (Biomedical Division)
Recent advances in multiple sclerosis therapy.
R.E. Gonsette, P. Delmotte, editors.

A Pilot Trial of Recombinant Human Beta Interferon in the Treatment of Relapsing-Remitting Multiple Sclerosis

R.L. Knobler, J.I. Greenstein, K.P. Johnson, F.D. Lublin, H.S. Panitch, S.G. Marcus, S.V. Grant, T. DeRyk, J. Lombardi and E. Katz, Thomas Jefferson University, Philadelphia, PA, 19107; Temple University, Philadelphia, PA, 19140; University of Maryland, Baltimore, MD 21201 and Triton Biosciences, Inc., Alameda, CA 94501 (USA)

The pathogenesis of MS is generally believed to be due to an immunological response in a genetically predisposed individual, localized within the central nervous system white matter, and triggered by exposure to an environmental agent such as a virus. Type I (alpha, beta) interferons (IFN) merit investigation as a possible therapy in the treatment of multiple sclerosis (MS) based upon several properties. These include their antiviral properties which may reduce coincidental viral infections, their ability to restrict major histocompatibility complex (MHC) class II expression, and their capacity to induce suppressor cell function in assay systems.

Increased expression of class II molecules on endothelial cells and astrocytes in immune-mediated experimental models of MS, such as experimental allergic encephalomyelitis (EAE), as well as in MS tissue samples has been reported (Traugott et al 1985). Coincidental viral infections have been associated with an increase in exacerbations in relapsing-remtting MS (Sibley et al 1985). Immune responses to coincidental viral infection have been postulated to yield the release of immune modulators, such as gamma IFN, which may stimulate increased expression of MHC class II molecules on responsive cells.

A clinical trial with the administration of human recombinant gamma IFN in relapsing-remitting MS patients led to increased exacerbations. In these patients a notable feature was the recurrence of prior symptoms with their exacerbations (Panitch et al 1987).

These and similar studies of autoimmune disorders implicate aberrant expression of MHC class II molecules in the pathogenesis of these disorders (Steinman et al 1986). Therefore, it is desireable to look for therapies that will both reduce coincidental viral infections with their consequences on the activation of immune responsiveness and MHC class II expression, as well as having a direct impact on the reduction of MHC class II expression.

Alpha and beta interferons have each been shown to antagonize the action of gamma IFN in the induction of MHC class II expression (Ling et al 1985). Joseph et al. (1988), studied the effects of exposure to human recombinant beta IFN on the expression of MHC class II molecules induced by gamma IFN on human glioblastoma cells grown in primary culture. Beta IFN was able, in a dose dependent fashion, to antagonize and effectively block the expression of MHC class II molecules induced by gamma IFN. The most effective blocking occurred when the glioblastoma cells were pretreated with beta IFN and then exposed to both beta and gamma IFN. These results indicated the importance of both the timing of exposure and dosage of beta IFN in obtaining antagonism to the effects of gamma IFN. Of additional importance, however, was the observation that when low concentrations of beta IFN were used in conjunction with gamma IFN synergism rather than antagonism was observed.

These findings help to provide a perspective for the evaluation and interpretation of clinical responses to the treatment of patients with these agents. It is important to note that the maximum interferon dosage used clinically is limited by the occurrence of modest but recognizable side effects at higher doses which can have an impact on attempts to produce effective double-blinding (see below). The possibility of undesireable synergistic effects at lower dosages provides another concern. It was for the purpose of addressing this dilemma that the pilot study of human recombinant beta interferon in the treatment of relapsing-remitting MS was undertaken as a measure in the planning of a larger scale clinical trial.

In an earlier randomized, double-blind, placebo-controlled, crossover trial of systemic natural alpha IFN in 24 patients with exacerbating-remitting MS, patients with a strictly exacerbating-remitting course showed a reduction in the frequency and severity of exacerbations (Knobler et al 1984). In contrast, those with exacerbations superimposed upon a chronic progressive course did not benefit from this treatment, primarily because side effects that included fever, malaise and fatique made them feel much worse. It was later shown that the Cantell preparation of natural human alpha interferon used could lead to side effects in some individuals through the production of immune complexes (ICs). These ICs were due to the generation of antibodies reacting with residual Sendai virus proteins used in the preparation of the IFN and retained in the final formulation (Rice et al 1985). The encouraging, albeit inconclusive, results of this and other preliminary studies of beta IFN (Jacobs et al 1981) but not gamma IFN therapy in MS, coupled with the availability of more highly purified preparations, warranted further clinical trials of IFN in MS.

A single available human recombinant beta IFN (Betaseron) was chosen for study over the multiplicity of available forms of human recombinant alpha IFN. Thirty patients with clinically definite relapsing-remitting MS for less than 15 years, and at least 2 relapses in the preceding 2 years, were entered into this randomized, double-blinded, 3 center, phase I pilot study, to test the safety and dosage tolerance of Betaseron. Groups of 6 patients, in five groups, received either 90 million international units (mIU), 45 mIU, 22.5 mIU, 4.5 mIU or placebo administered subcutaneously 3 times weekly for two 12 week cycles. Beginning with cycle 3 all patients randomized to active drug were switched to 45 mIU.

Analysis after upto a two-year treatment period revealed that no exacerbations were triggered by Betaseron. Side effects that occurred included injection site erythrema and soreness at the onset of treatment, which was related to dose, but declined within 2 weeks, as did other minor transient side effects such as headache, fever, chills, lightheadedness, paresthesias and diarrhea. Laboratory abnormalities included transient mild leukopenia, proteinuria and elevation of hepatic enzymes. Dose reduction from 90 to 45 mIU to avoid side effects of persisting malaise and fatigue, and thus ensure blinding, were required initially for some patients who had already been experiencing fatigue prior to entering into the study. This strategy was then applied to all patients after the second 12 week cycle, since treatment was generally better tolerated at the lower doses. Exacerbation rates through the second 12 week cycle are indicated in Table 1.

Table 1. Exacerbation Rates through 12 weeks of Treatment

Dose	Fraction with Exacerbations	Number of Exacerbations	Rate Per Year**
Placebo	4/6	5	1.8
4.5	3/7*	3	1.1
22.5	3/6	5	2.1
45	2/10*	2	0.6
90	0/6	0	0.0

*   Five patients had dose reductions and have therefore been counted in the denominator of the group into which they were transferred.

**   Annualized rate for the first 24 weeks of treatment (2 cycles).

124

These results indicate that subcutaneously administered Betaseron is safe and well tolerated in relapsing-remitting MS patients, and provides guidelines for development of a dosage regimen. Full details of this Pilot Trial will be reported after the completion of a three year analysis. However, based on the present findings of safety and dose responses to BETASERON, a 10 center, phase II/III trial of 9 mIU, 45 mIU or placebo, subcutaneously, every other day, is currently underway to test efficacy of this form of beta IFN in the treatment of relapsing-remitting multiple sclerosis. The outcome of this latter study will help to clarify the usefulness of subcutaneous beta IFN in the treatment of relapsing-remitting multiple sclerosis.

References

Jacobs, L, J O'Malley, A Freeman and R Ekes. 1981. Intrathecal interferon reduces exacerbations of multiple sclerosis. Science 214: 1026-1028.

Joseph, J, RL Knobler, C, D'Imperio and FD Lublin. 1988. Down-regulation of interferon-gamma-induced class II expression on human glioma cells by recombinant interferon beta: Effects of dosage treatment schedule. J. Neuroimmunol. 20: 39-44.

Knobler, RL, HS Panitch, SL Braheny, et al. 1984. Controlled clinical trial of systemic alpha interferon in multiple sclerosis. Neurology 34: 1273-1279.

Ling, PD, MK Warren and SN Vogel. 1985. Antagonistic effect of interferon beta on the interferon gamma induced expression of Ia antigen in murine macrophages. J. Immunol. 135: 1857-1863.

Panitch, HS, RL Hirsch, AS Haley and KP Johnson. 1987. Exacerbations of multiple sclerosis in patients treated with gamma interferon. Lancet 1: 893-895.

Rice, GPA, EL Woelfel, PJ Talbot, et al. 1985. Immunological complications in multiple sclerosis patients receiving interferon. Ann. Neurol. 18: 439-442.

Sibley, WA, CR Bamford and K Clark. 1985. Clinical viral infections and multiple sclerosis. Lancet 1: 1313-1315.

Steinman, L, MK Waldor, SS Zamvil, et al. 1986. Therapy of autoimmune disease with antibody to immune response gene products or to T-cell surface markers. Ann. N.Y. Acad. Sci. 475: 274-284.

Traugott, U, LC Scheinberg and CS Raine. 1985. On the presence of Ia-positive endothelial cells and astrocytes in multiple sclerosis lesions and its relevance to antigen presentation. J. Neuroimmunol. 8: 1-14.

© 1989 Elsevier Science Publishers B.V. (Biomedical Division)
Recent advances in multiple sclerosis therapy.
R.E. Gonsette, P. Delmotte, editors.

INTERFERON-α AND TRANSFER FACTOR IN THE TREATMENT OF MULTIPLE SCLEROSIS: A DOUBLE-BLIND, PLACEBO-CONTROLLED TRIAL*

AUSTIMS RESEARCH GROUP
c/- Professor J.G. McLeod, Department of Medicine, University of Sydney, N.S.W. 2006, Australia

INTRODUCTION

In order to define further the roles of leucocyte IFN-α and TF in the treatment of MS, the AUSTIMS trial (Australian trial of TF and IFN-α in MS) was devised as a collaborative (multicentric), prospective, randomised, double-blind, placebo-controlled, non-crossover study of TF and IFN-α involving initial enrolment of 182 MS patients and treatment for a 3-year period.

PATIENTS AND METHODS

Patients

182 patients (112 female, 70 male) with symptoms and signs of clinically definite MS (1) and without serious intercurrent illnesses were accepted into the trial. Eighty-five percent of patients had MS for less than 10 years and all patients had clinical evidence of disease activity in the three pre-trial years. Patient disability was assessed with the Kurtzke disability status score (DSS)(2); at the initial assessment, 82% of patients had DSS scores of less than 4 which represented mild to moderate disability. After fulfilling these selection criteria, patients were randomized into three groups; 60 patients received IFN-α , 61 TF and 61 placebo. Patients, attending staff and neurologists were blinded to the treatment given. The protocol for the trial was approved by Medical Ethics Review Committees in all participating centres and written informed consent was obtained from all patients.

Each trial patient underwent a full neurological assessment performed by a neurologist before entry, after two months, and six months, and every three months of treatment thereafter for the duration of the trial. All neurological assessment forms were later reviewed by one neurologist (J.G.McL). At each examination the

* This paper was originally published by Elsevier Science Publishers b.v. in MULTIPLE SCLEROSIS RESEARCH. Proceedings of the International Multiple Sclerosis Conference held in Rome, 15-17 September 1988.

patients' disability was assessed on the Kurtzke DSS. Abnormalities in each of the functional systems (FSS) (pyramidal, cerebellar, brainstem, sensory, bowel-bladder, visual, mental, and other) (2) were also graded to indicate neurological impairment. Patient disability was further assessed on the Ambulatory Status Scoring System (ASSS) which, as an adaptation of the DSS, emphasised the impact of the patient's neurological dysfunction on performing the tasks of daily living. The number of relapses since the previous examination and adverse drug reactions were recorded.

Preparation and administration of interferon-α , transfer factor, and placebo

IFN-α (human leucocyte IFN) was produced by the Commonwealth Serum Laboratories (CSL) according to the method of Cantell and Hirvonen (3) from the buffy coats of healthy blood donors and purified by monoclonal antibody affinity chromatography (Celltech Ltd, UK). Transfer factor was produced as described previously (4). The concentration of TF was adjusted so that each 1ml contained 2.0×10^8 cell-equivalents and one unit of TF was arbitrarily defined as 4×10^8 cell-equivalents. Placebo consisted of a sterile buffered salt solution containing 0.5% human albumin which was also present in the IFN-α preparation.

IFN-α , TF and placebo were stored in 1 ml vials at -20°C until used. Each patient received either 3×10^6 units of IFN-α , 0.5 units of TF or 1 ml of placebo subcutaneously twice weekly for two months, then once weekly for 10 months, then fortnightly for 24 months.

Statistical Analysis

The base-line characteristics of the study population in the three treatment arms were compared with analysis of variance for continuous variables and Chi-square tests for discrete variables.

Differences in accumulation of disability between treatment groups were statistically evaluated in a number of ways. First, the significance of the differences in Kurtzke DSS and ASSS between treatment groups was assessed with unconditional multiple logistic regression (5) using odds ratios as the parameters. The simple dichotomy of worse versus no-worse was chosen as the primary outcome variable for the study.

Secondly, each patient's disability after three years of treatment was compared with his own initial disability and recorded as 'better' (by 1 or more points on the Kurtzke DSS), 'unchanged' or 'worse' (by 1 or more points on the Kurtzke DSS). The difference in distribution between treatment arms of patients within the categories, better or unchanged, and worse, was compared by Chi-square analysis with two degrees of freedom.

Thirdly, the mean of the change in DSS score for the patients in each group was compared by analysis of variance. The data for the three groups were also analysed using the Kruskal-Wallis statistic.

The mean number of types of adverse drug reactions per patient in each treatment group and the difference in the mean number of exacerbations of MS experienced by patients in each group was assessed for significance with 95% confidence intervals. An exacerbation was defined as a worsening of symptoms or signs or occurrence of new neurological symptoms or signs that persisted for at least 24 hours (6).

Analysis of results was performed on an intention to treat basis; all patients who commenced therapy, regardless of whether they completed the trial, were included in the statistical analysis of neurological status. The analyses were based on changes in status between the commencement of therapy and the final assessment, which, for most patients, was 36 months after commencing therapy. For all statistical analyses the level of significance was taken as $p < 0.05$.

RESULTS

182 MS patients were randomised into one of the three treatment arms: the IFN-α-treated , TF-treated or placebo group. The subjects in each of the treatment arms were similar with respect to age, sex, clinical course, clinical disease type, mean duration of disease, initial Kurtzke DSS score and the presence of HLA DR2.

153 (84%) of the 182 patients completed the trial (42/60, 53/61 and 58/61 patients in the IFN-α , TF and placebo groups respectively). Of the 29 patients who withdrew, 18 (62%) were receiving IFN-α , eight (28%) were receiving TF and three (10%) were receiving placebo. This represented a significant difference between treatment groups. Patient withdrawal from the IFN-α group occurred because of unacceptable adverse effects reported as fever, rigors, fatigue and/or transient worsening of neurological symptoms (13), perceived progressive neurological deterioration (2), myocardial infarction (1), commencement of chemotherapy for carcinoma of the lung (1), or a belief that the therapy was of no

128

benefit (1). Withdrawal from TF therapy occurred because of
pregnancy (2), perceived neurological deterioration (1), sudden
death (1), thrombocytopenia (1) or personal reasons (3). Withdrawal
from the placebo group occurred because of perceived neurological
deterioration (2), and loss to follow up (1).

When unconditional multiple logistic regression was performed on
the Kurtzke DSS and ASSS scores neither the crude odds ratio for
IFN-α (odds ratio with 95% confidence intervals = 0.79 (0.38-
1.62)) nor that for TF (1.70 (0.83-3.48)) reached a significant
difference from the placebo group.

When patients were assessed as better, worse or unchanged on the
DSS (Table 1), improvement was seen in 15%, 16%, and 26% of
patients in the IFN-α , TF and placebo groups respectively. The
difference was not significant (Chi-square=4.293, 2DF, p<0.25).
Similarly better, worse or unchanged analysis of the ASSS revealed
no significant difference between treatment groups (Chi-square=
1.559, 2DF, p<0.5)

TABLE 1
NUMBER OF PATIENTS WHOSE CLINICAL DISABILITY WAS BETTER, WORSE OR
UNCHANGED DURING THE TRIAL §

	INTERFERON-α	TRANSFER FACTOR	PLACEBO
BETTER *	9	10	16
UNCHANGED	26	15	17
WORSE *	24	36	28

* Change by ⩾1 on Kurtzke DSS   § Data unavailable on one patient

The mean change in DSS over the trial period of 0.59, 1.10 and
0.52 for IFN-α , TF and placebo groups respectively was not
significantly different (F=2.540, p>0.05). Similarly no
significant difference in change in ASSS between treatment groups
was demonstrated (F=2.384, p>0.05). The change in the DSS and the
ASSS, when analysed with the Kruskal-Wallis statistic, also

revealed no significant difference between treatment groups. The mean number of relapses during the three years of therapy for each group was 1.53, 2.11 and 1.97 for IFN-α , TF and placebo groups respectively. Using 95% confidence intervals derived for the ratio of observed to expected events (the number of expected events being the total number of relapses divided by the total number of trial participants) there was no significant difference in the mean number of relapses in each treatment arm.

The mean types of adverse drug reactions per patient were 5.42, 0.85 and 1.05 for the IFN-α , TF and placebo treated groups respectively. Patients in the IFN-α -treated group experienced significantly more types of adverse drug reactions than expected (the number of expected events being the total number of adverse drug reactions divided by the total number of trial participants).

DISCUSSION

Neither IFN-α nor TF significantly altered the rate of progression of MS compared to that of controls as measured by the Kurtzke DSS, the ASSS or the relapse rate. This conclusion was unaffected by the method of statistical analysis used.

The present study was prospective, double-blind, placebo-controlled, and involved 182 patients observed over a 3 year period. In addition, the composition of patients within each of the treatment arms was similar for demographic and prognostic variables. Therefore the negative result was unlikely to be a function of inadequate trial design.

Patients treated with IFN-α had significantly more different types of adverse drug reactions than those treated with TF or placebo. These reactions contributed to the significantly greater number of withdrawals in the IFN-α -treated group.

As a result of this study, it appears that neither IFN-α nor TF from cohabiting donors given subcutaneously modifies significantly the course of MS. This result may reflect the need for a more intensive dosage schedule or an alternative route of administration of therapy. With both treatments, efficacy presumably could be enhanced if their action could be directed specifically against the environmental agent that contributes to the disease.

ACKNOWLEDGEMENTS

The AUSTIMS Research Group includes the following people:

130

Professors J.G.McLeod and A.Basten, Drs J.A.Frith, S.R.Hammond, J.C.Walsh, and D.B.Williams, and Ms C.Van der Brink (Sydney); Drs I.R.Mackay, B.R.Chambers, G.Harris and G.Symington (Melbourne); Dr J.F.Hallpike and Professor J.Bradley (Adelaide); Drs P.T.Yeo and R.M.Lowenthal (Hobart); Dr K.M.R.Grainger and Professor R.L.Dawkins (Perth); Dr G.Danta (Canberra) and Dr A.C.Reid (Brisbane).

We gratefully acknowledge the assistance of Sr Pamela Crossie, Sr Claudia Charlton, Mrs Alison Morgan and Ms Kerri Gallagher (Sydney); Mrs Brenda Bradley, Ms S. Bayly and Sr Kathryn Bromson (Adelaide); Sr Bronwyn Jones, Ms Elizabeth Collins, Ms Angelena Iscaro, Dr B.D. Tait and Mrs Beryl McLachlan (Melbourne); Sr Anna Fasoli, Sr Kate duPlessis and Ms Sue Alexander (Canberra); Sr Doreen Walker, Sr Robyn Loughhead, Mrs Sally Sullivan, Mr Russell Lawrence and Mrs Fiona Wojtas (Hobart); Sr Di Coxon, Dr Guy Grimsley, Mr A. Jones, Prof. B. Armstrong and Dr D. English (Perth).

AUSTIMS was funded by the Commonwealth Government through the Commonwealth Serum Laboratories, Australia (CSL) and a grant from the National Multiple Sclerosis Society of Australia.

Our thanks are due to Drs J. Colebatch, P. Colville, J. Sutherland and R. Stark and Prof. R. H. Lovell of the Independent Review Committee for their advice.

The authors would also like to acknowledge the commitment and continued support of the patients and their families who helped to make this study possible.

REFERENCES

1. Rose A, Ellison G, Myers L, Tourtellotte W (1976) Neurology 26:20-22
2. Kurtzke J (1965) Neurology 15:654-661
3. Cantell K, Hirvonen S (1977) Texas Reports on Biology and Medicine 35:138-144
4. Basten A, McLeod J, Pollard J, et al. (1980) Lancet 1(Nov):931-934
5. Cox D (1970) The analysis of binary data. Methuen, London
6. Schumacher G, Beebe G, Kibler R, et al. (1965) Ann NY Acad Sci 122:552-568

CYCLOSPORINE A

© 1989 Elsevier Science Publishers B.V. (Biomedical Division)
Recent advances in multiple sclerosis therapy.
R.E. Gonsette, P. Delmotte, editors.

THE USE OF CYCLOSPORIN IN MULTIPLE SCLEROSIS.

Peter Rudge

National Hospital, Queen Square, London, United Kingdom.

Introduction.

   Cyclosporin (CsA) is a naturally occurring undecapeptide produced by the fungus

Tolyplocadium inflatum (*Trichoderma polysporum*) which has profound immune modulating

effects acting primarilly upon T-cell mediated immune events [1, 2] at a pre-translational

level [3]. It has become the immunosuppressant of choice in organ transplantation [4].

However many early experiments showed that it efficiently suppressed experimental allergic

encephalomyelitis (EAE) if given prophylactically and reduced the severity of the disease if

given after immunisation ie. therapeutically [5]. Further, it protected animals from EAE

induced by passive transfer of competent lymphocytes [6]. As a result of this animal work two

trials of the use of CsA in multiple sclerosis (MS) were set up in Europe both of which are

completed and have been published [7, 8]. A third trial in the United States of America (USA)

has finished but the results are not yet published in a definitive form. The following is a brief

review of these data.

MS trial results.

<u>German study [7]</u>

In this double blind controlled trial a total of 167 patients with a variety of types of clinically

definite MS were treated for 2-2.5 years with either CsA 5mg/kg/day or azathioprine 2.5

mg/kg/day. There was no placebo group.   No significant difference in outcome was seen on any

measure of progression or relapse rate.

<u>British/Dutch study [8].</u>

This study was a double blind placebo controlled trial conducted at two centres (London and

Amsterdam) it which it was intended to give an initial dose of CsA of 10 mg/kg/day for 2 months

followed by 22 months of CsA 8 mg/kg/day. Forty-three patients completed the trial in London

compared with 37 patients in Amsterdam. There were marked differences in the type of patient entered at the two centres; those in London were younger, had had more relapses and were more disabled than those in Amsterdam. Further, the dose of CsA actually received in London approximated to the protocol while that in Amsterdam was on average less than 5 mg/kg/day. The results indicated a beneficial effect of CsA in London where there were significantly fewer relapses of lesser severity in the treated group and the rate of progression of disability was less in that group. In addition there was evidence of a reduction of immunoglobulin synthesis in the cerebrospinal fluid (CSF) [8, 9]. In contrast no benefit of CsA was seen in the Dutch patients.

USA study.

This is the largest trial comprising an entry of 547 patients with progressive MS. It is a double blind placebo controlled trial of 6 mg/kg/day CsA, adjusted to keep the blood levels at 300-500 ng/ml for 2 years. No definitive results are published but it is understood that there has been a dropout rate of 33% in the placebo and 44% in the CsA groups. Little difference in outcome is apparent; indeed the only significant result has been the time it has taken for the patients to lose the ability to walk even though the rate of decline through the Kurtzke scale has not differed between the two groups.

Interpretation of the three trials.

All three trials have deficiencies. The German study is fatally flawed by the absence of a placebo group so that it is impossible to know if the two drugs were equally useful, harmful or neutral. The British/Dutch study suffers from the two centres having different types of MS patients given different doses of CsA rendering combined analysis impossible with consequent reduction in the power of the trial. The USA study is flawed by the enormous dropout rate greatly reducing its power. Further it is unwise to use the criterion of time to attain a given state if the patients are not seen on a regular basis even though they are all ultimately reviewed.

The author thinks these data are best interpreted as showing that CsA retards the progression of the disease if given in sufficient dosage. Since little of the drug enters the central nervous system (CNS) the progress of the disease is not halted. There is evidence that activated lymphocytes are greatly reduced in the peripheral blood but persist in the CSF [10]. As we know activated lymphocytes readily cross the blood brain barrier [11] it is possible that CsA can reduce acqusition of competent cells from the periphery whilst doing nothing to such cells already resident within the CNS thereby slowing, but not halting, the disease. Such a mechanism would account for the results obtained.

Conclusion.

These trials have been disappointing in that the effect of CsA upon MS is small even at high dosage. If a drug is to be considered as therapy it must have a high therapeutic index ie. a low toxicity. This is not the case with CsA. All authors report a large number of side effects most prominent of which are marked, and perhaps not totally reversible, nephrotoxicity [12], a variety of neurological disturbances including fits and tremor, and hypertrichosis of sufficient severity to preclude the use of CsA for such small gain.

A second even more worrying point concerns the possiblity that CsA makes MS worse. While the initial work with EAE showed a beneficial effect of CsA upon the disease it is now apparent that chronic relapsing experimental allergic encephalomyelitis (CREAE), possibly a better model for MS, is made worse and this is particularly the case if the dose is low [13,14,15,16]. The mechanism of this deleterious effect is unknown but it is possible that low dose CsA given to MS patients could be harmful - indeed in the German study 4 patients on CsA were withdrawn because of rapid deterioration.

It thus appears that CsA is not a useful drug in MS since to give it in sufficient dose causes unacceptable side effects and lower doses run the risk of exacerbating the disease for which it was given. The latter may not apply to other cyclosporins [14] but the problem of toxicity remains.

References.

1. Borel JF, Feurer C, Gubler HU, Staehelin H. Biological effects of cyclosporin A: a new antilymphocytic agent. Agents Action (1976) 6:468-475.

2. Borel JF. Immunosuppression: building on Sandimmune (cyclosporine). Transplant Proc (1988) 20(suppl 1) :149-153.

3. Thomson AW, Webster LA. The influence of cyclosporin A on cell-mediated immunity. Clin exp Immunol (1988) 71:369-376.

4. Calne RY. Cyclosporin in cadaveric renal transplantation: 5 year follow up of multicentre trial. Lancet (1987) 2:506-507.

5. Bolton C, Borel JF, Cuzner ML, Davison AN, Turner AM. Immunosuppression by cyclosporin A of experimental allergic encephalomyelitis.J Neurol Sci (1982) 56:147-153.

6. Bolton C, Allsopp G, Cuzner ML. The effect of cyclosporin A on the adoptive transfer of experimental allergic encephalomyelitis in the Lewis rat. Clin exp Immunol (1982) 47:127-132.

7. Kappos L, Patzold U, Dommasch D et al. Cyclosporine versus azathioprine in the long-term treatment of multiple sclerosis results of the German multicentre study. Ann Neurol (1988) 23:56-63.

8. Rudge P, Koetsier JC, Mertin J et al. Randomised double blind controlled trial of cyclosporin in multiple sclerosis. J Neurol Neurosurg Psychiat (1989) 52:559-565.

9. McLean BN, Rudge P, Thompson EJ. Cyclosporin A curtails the progression of free light chain synthesis in the cerebrospinal fluid of patients with multiple sclerosis. J Neurol Neurosurg Psychiat (1989) 52:529-531.

10. Calder VL, Bellamy AS, Owen S et al. Effects of cyclosporin A on expression of IL2 and IL2 receptors in normal and multiple sclerosis patients. Clin exp Immunol (1987) 70:570-577.

11. Wekerle H. Intercellular interactions in myelin-specific autoimmunity. J Neuroimmunol (1988) 20:211-216.

12. Mispelblom-Beyer JO, Donker AJM, Koetsier JC. Renal function three months after discontinuation of cyclosporine in patients with multiple sclerosis. Kidney Int (1988) 34:560.

13. Suckling AJ, Baron PW, Reiber H. Chronic relapsing experimental allergic encephalomyelitis: cyclosporin A treatment of relapsing and remitting disease. J Clin Lab Immunol (1986) 21:173-176.

14. Feurer C, Chow LH, Borel JF. Preventive and therapeutic effects of cyclosporin and valine^2-dihydro-cyclosporin in chronic relapsing experimental allergic encephalomyelitis in the Lewis rat. Immunol (1988) 63:219-223.

15. Polman CH, Matthaei I, de Groot CJA, Kaetsier JC, Sminia T, Dijkstra CD. Low-dose cyclosporin A induces relapsing remitting experimental allergic encephalomyelits in the Lewis rat. J Immunol (1988) 17:209-216.

16. Mertin J, Mertin LA. Experimental allergic encephalomyelitis and immunosuppression. Proceedings of joint meeting of the German Neurological Society and Neurological Societies of the Benelux Countries. (1987). eds: Poeck HK, Hacke W, Schneider R. Springer, Heidelberg. 38-48.

AZATHIOPRINE

© 1989 Elsevier Science Publishers B.V. (Biomedical Division)
Recent advances in multiple sclerosis therapy.
R.E. Gonsette, P. Delmotte, editors.

MULTIPLE SCLEROSIS AND IMMUNITY - THE NEED FOR A NEW CONCEPT

JUERGEN MERTIN

Department of Neurology and MS Centre, St. Gallische Hoehen-
klinik, CH-8881 Walenstadtberg (Switzerland)

INTRODUCTION

The first meeting on immunological treatment in multiple sclerosis
(MS) that I attended in Belgium was held in 1977 not far from here,
in Melsbroek. Some of the therapeutic trials presented and discussed
at that meeting showed results favouring immunosuppressive treatment (1). They were, unfortunately, all based on uncontrolled
trials. Nevertheless, they were encouraging and thereby gave great
hope for the future: we urged all investigators who planned new
trials to adhere to a design of strict scientific control, i.e.
randomisation and double blind procedure. It was hoped, thereby,
that immunosuppression would be established as a generally recommen-
dable treatment for MS.

TRIALS OF AZATHIOPRINE

In the meantime, a number of such controlled trials have been
completed, I myself taking part in two of them employing azathioprine (AZA) as immunosuppressant. In the first of these trials 43
patients with a relapsing-remitting clinical course were included
(2). Short-term treatment with a combination of antilymphocyte
globulin, prednisolone and AZA was followed by 14 months treatment
with AZA alone, bringing the duration of the overall treatment
period to 15 months.

The results revealed a marginally beneficial effect on relapse
rate and clinical progression. There were significant effects on
in vitro lymphocyte function (3) and on visual evoked potentials
(VEP) in favour of the group receiving suppressive treatment (2).
Serious side effects were noted, especially during the initial
phase of the treatment.

The second trial I want to refer to was the British and Dutch AZA
trial (4). This, so far largest, double-blind controlled study
included 354 patients with relapsing-remitting and progressive
course of the disease.

After three to four years of treatment with 2.5 mg/kg of AZA or
placebo substance daily, there was a distinct, but non-significant

therapeutic effect in favour of the AZA-treated group. There were
also fewer relapses and steroid-treated relapses in the AZA group
than in the placebo group. Clinical subgroups in which AZA is
particularly beneficial, could not be identified. A series of side
effects were observed. These side effects, together with the
only marginal therapeutic success, led to the conclusion, that
immuno- suppression with AZA cannot be recommended for general
use in the treatment of patients with MS (4).

DISCUSSION

The same conclusion, I think, has to be drawn when one looks at
the results of other trials of immunological treatments or procedures reported here or at other recent meetings, particularly in
terms of therapeutic and unwanted effects as well as inconvenience
of drugs taking. The only exception seems to be treatment with
copolimer I (COP I), which during a 2 year treatment phase gave a
dramatically reduced relapse rate and, more important, halted
increasing impairment in patients with very active relapsing-
remitting clinical course of the disease (5). In the meantime,
however, Bornstein and coworkers have submitted the results of their
second trial, this time on patients with clinically fast progressing
disease (6,7). Within a treatment period of 2 years further progression was halted in 56% of the COP I treated patients. This would
have been a remarkable success had not the same held true for 49%
of the saline-treated patients in the control group - there was, as
would be expected, no statistically significant difference between
the 2 groups.

There are two possible ways to deal with this astounding observations. The one is that we simply ignore them and carry on trying
out any new immunologically active substance brought on to the
market. However, the other way to look at these results would be
to take them as a cornerstone in our thinking about the cause of MS
and a respective causal therapy. For many immunologists MS is a
disease of the immune system, in which autoaggression is more or
less accidentally directed against the central nervous system (CNS).
In a recent publication Hafler and Weiner have argued in this way
(8). An important basis for this argument is the widely held
 conviction that the immune system is an entirely self-regulating
entity. In the same issue Calder and her colleagues (9) have
 presented a different hypothesis, namely that MS is a localised

immune disease of the CNS, in which CNS-local T lymphocytes
sensitised against brain antigens are triggered into expansion and
thereby into pathological inflammatory and demyelinating activity -
"by as yet unidentified factors" including possibly "intercurrent
infection or stress". If we take their argument further and
postulate that the immune response is not in essence controlled
by self-regulatory feed back mechanisms of the immune system
itself, but submitted to a superior control excerted by the CNS,
then we could explain a placebo effect of 49% via the activity of
hypothetical suppressive factors, which are generated by the CNS
under the influence of stimuli that could include psychological
events. Calder et al have stressed in their article that "there
is a need to focus research on the immunological events within
the CNS rather than the peripheral blood". In the context of such
CNS-focussed research it may be possible to identify factors which
are the true immunoregulators, and with their manipulation we
may learn to influence MS more effectively than to date. I very
much hope, that such new concepts will stimulate increasing
interest and thereby possibly also increasing experimental support,
in order that they may not remain in the realm of speculation.

ACKNOWLEDGEMENTS

The author is supported by the Swiss Multiple Sclerosis Society.
He wants to thank Ms. L. Gmuer for her help in preparing the
manuscript.

REFERENCES

1. Delmotte P, Hommes OR, Gonsette R, eds. (1977) Immuno-
    suppressive treatment in multiple sclerosis. European Press,
    Ghent

2. Mertin J, Rudge P, Kremer M, Healey MJR, Knight SC, Compston
    A, Batchelor JR, Thompson EJ, Halliday AM, Denman M, Medawar
    PB (1982) Lancet ii: 351-354

3. Knight SC, Harding B, Burman S, Mertin J (1981) Clinical and
    Experimental Immunology 46: 61-69

4. British and Dutch Multiple Sclerosis Azathioprine Trial Group
    (1988) Lancet ii: 179-183

5. Bornstein M, Miller A, Slagle S, Weitzman M, Crystal H,
    Drexler E, Keilson M, Merriam A, Wassertheil-Smoller S, Spada
    V, Weiss W, Arnon R, Jacobsohn I, Teitelbaum D, Sela M (1987)
    The New England J. of Medicine 317: 408-414

144

6. Bornstein M, Miller A, Slagle S, Weitzman M, Crystal H, Drexler E, Keilson M, Merriam A, Spada V, Rolak L, Appel S, Brown S, Harati Y, Weiss W, Arnon R, Jacobsohn I, Teitelbaum D, Sela M (1988) Proceedings Internat. MS Conference, Rome 15.-17. Sept. 1988 (in press)

7. Miller A, Bornstein M, Slagle S, Crystal H, Drexler E, Keilson M, Spada V, Weiss W, and Weitzman M, Bronx, NY; Appel S, Brown S and Rolak L, Houston, TX; Arnon R, Jacobsohn I, Teitelbaum D and Sela M, Rehovot, Israel (1989) Neurology (Abstract) 39 (Suppl.) : 356-357

8. Hafler DA, Weiner HL (1989) Immunology Today 10:104-107

9. Calder V, Owen S, Watson C, Feldman M, Davison A (1989) Immunology Today 10:99-103

CYCLOPHOSPHAMIDE

© 1989 Elsevier Science Publishers B.V. (Biomedical Division)
Recent advances in multiple sclerosis therapy.
R.E. Gonsette, P. Delmotte, editors.

ORAL CYCLOPHOSPHAMIDE TREATMENT IN MULTIPLE SCLEROSIS

C. LATERRE, C.J.M. SINDIC, H. HEULE
St-Luc Hospital, Neurology Department, Avenue Hippocrate 10, Brussels, Belgium

Long-term, low-dose, oral cyclophosphamide therapy was chosen for several reasons : first of all because long-term remissions can be induced and maintained in a high number of patients in which autoimmune phenomena are established or suspected - among them rheumatoid arthritis and Wegener's granulomatosis, secondly because the oral way is comfortable in yet ambulatory patients, thirdly because by this regimen alopecia and nausea are avoided.

PATIENT POPULATION

Between 1971 and 1982, a trial of continuous oral treatment of 36 month's duration by cyclophosphamide was proposed to 80 (36 males, 44 females) clinically definite MS patients (Mc Alpine's criteria + CSF oligoclonal IgG) divided in two groups on the basis of the course of the disease :
Slowly or chronic Progressive (SP): 46; and Relapsing Progressive (RP): 34.

The patients of the first group presented with a progressive, relentless course of the disease for several years - progressive from the onset or progressive after a period of relapsing-remitting or relapsing-progressive evolution. The patients of the second group were selected because of high relapse rate uncontrolled by corticosteroids and of severity of residual symptoms heralding the progressive phase. The mean age at onset of disease was 28   8 years in the RP group and 37 ± 11 in the SP group; the mean age at entry in the trial was respectively 33 ± 8 and 46 ± 9. The follow-up was 3 and 7 years for the patients taken as a whole, 10 years and more for 48 patients treated between 1971 and 1978.

METHODS

Severity of symptoms was graded according to the extended Kurtzke disability status scale (DSS). All patients had a DSS of 3 or more at the beginning ot the trial. The daily doses of cyclophosphamide (calculated mean: 73 mg-SD : 18) were progressively adjusted in each case to obtain a blood leucocyte count between 4000 and $5000/mm^3$ controlled monthly.

RESULTS

Clinical evaluation was performed at the end of the 3 years treatment and 7 and 10 years after the beginning of the trial (Table I).

148

TABLE I

CHANGE IN DISABILITY SCALE

Category	N° cases	Total dose of cyclophosphamide (g)	Improvement or stabilization		
			End of trial	7 years	≥ 10 years
COMPLETE TRIAL					
I. RP	30	95 $\pm$ 27	26/30 (86%)	23/29(+1†) (76%)	7/11(+3†) (50%)
II. SP	23	80 $\pm$ 23	11/23 (48%)	3/23 (13%)	1/6 (+7†) (8%)
TRIAL STOPPED BETWEEN 18–36 MONTHS					
III. SP	3	58 $\pm$ 10	0/ 3	0/ 3	0/2 (+1†)
TRIAL STOPPED BEFORE 18 MONTHS					
IV. RP	4	9 $\pm$ 4	2/ 4	1/ 4	1/2
V. SP	20	29 $\pm$ 17	6/19 (+1†) (30%)	4/19 (21%)	3/10(+6†) (19%)

† = death.

Several patients stopped the trial before the end of its course. We have divided therefore our patient population in 3 categories : complete trial – trial stopped between 18 and 36 months and trial stopped before 18 months (Table I). Thirty patients in the RP group completed the trial – only 4 stopped during the first year. In contrast, among the 46 patients of the SP group, 23 completed the trial, 3 dropped out between 18 and 36 months and 20 during the first 18 months. The reasons for discontinuing treatment were: discouragement due to the apparent ineffectiveness of the treatment : 12, hemorrhagic cystitis : 5, patient preference for another type of treatment: 3, recurrent herpes simplex : 2, gastrointestinal intolerance: 2, influenza : 1, thrombocytopenia : 1, unexplained rise of acid phosphatase : 1.

The total dose of cyclophosphamide is indicated for each category and the results are summarized in term of improvement or stabilization. Categories I,II and V (Table) are interesting to analyze furthermore. If we compare the % of improvement or stabilization between categories I and II, the difference is obvious. In category I only a small % of the patients worsened during the trial and 7 years later; the effectiveness of treatment is still observed although at a lesser degree, 10 years later.

In the first category, a dramatic effect is observed on the relapsing rate (Table II) :

TABLE II

RELAPSING RATE IN RELAPSING PROGRESSIVE COURSE (Category I)

N°cases	Number of relapses			
	During 3 years before trial	During 3 years of trial	Between 3 and 7 years after trial	Between 7 and $\geq$10 years after trial
30	79	0	8	2
			6 remitting	1 remitting
			2 followed by progressive course	1 followed by progressive course

EVOLUTION TO SLOWLY PROGRESSIVE COURSE IN CATEGORY I

N° cases	During trial	Between 3 and 7 years after trial	Between 7 and $\geq$ 10 years after trial
30	4	3	1

Indeed, total number of severe relapses calculated on the whole of this group which was 79 during the 3 years preceding the trial fall to 0 during the trial. Hereafter we observed 8 relapses between 3-7 years, 6 remitting and 2 followed a by progressive course and 2 between 7 and 10 years, 1 remitting and 1 followed also by a progressive course. However, some patients in this category experienced progressive course in spite of this intensive treatment, 4 during trial, 3 between 3 and 7 years after trial, 1 between 7 and 10 years. We cannot compare the category of relapsing progressive MS which fulfilled the trial with the same population which dropped out before 18 months and considered as matched controls because the number of cases in the two series are too different. But we are justified to compare category II and V because the intention to treat was exactly similar (Table I). The % of stabilized cases is perhaps slightly different at the end of trial in favor of category II but the ratio is inverted after 7 and 10 years.

We have now to analyse the cause of deaths in patients which fullfilled the trial and in patients which dropped out for reasons previously detailled (Table III).

It is quite possible that immunosuppressive therapy played a role in the cases of tuberculosis, septicemia and kidney carcinoma. It is unquestionable that this role was decisive in cases of myeloid leukemia. Turning our attention to this patients we must note that three of them refused to stop the treatment which was prolonged of respectively 40 months – 15 months – 18 months. Consequently we limite now strictly the duration of the treatment to 24 months.

150

TABLE III
CAUSES OF DEATH

| | COMPLETE TRIAL | | INCOMPLETE TRIAL | |
	N° cases	Years after beginning trial	N° cases	Years after beginning trial
Score 10 Kurtzke	4 - V.H.	10	6 - I.E.	5
	- H.A.	11	- S.P.	13
	- V.C.	12	- D.Y.	7
	- W.V.	9	- C.A.	8
			- M.Y.	10
			- V.J.	13
Tuberculosis	1 - B.M.	8		
Septicemia	1 - D.J.	4		
Carcinoma of kidney	1 - K.R.	9		
Myeloid leukemia	4 - B.Y.	11		
	- T.S.	11		
	- F.J.	7		
	- D.J.	6		
Suicide			1 - V.N.	12
TOTAL	11/53 (20%)		7/27 (26%)	

CONCLUSIONS

The continuous oral immunosuppressive therapy by cyclophosphamide produced clinically important beneficial effets (100% excerbationfree patients during the trial and 73% post-treatment) in the group of "Relapsing Progressive" course of the disease. In this group, stabilization of the disability was obtained in 86% of the cases during the three years's treatment. This stabilization was still observed in 76% 7 years later and in 50% 10 years later. In contrast, in the group of "Slowly Progressive" course, stabilization of the disability was obtained in 48% of patients during the trial, in only 13% 7 years later and in 8% 10 years later. This poor result added to the toxicity of the drug allows to contest the value of immunosuppressive therapy in slowly progressive MS.

Patients will have to be treated at early stage of the disease. Fixed disabilities make the effectiveness of immunosuppressive therapy difficult to detect.

OTHER IMMUNOSUPPRESSIVE TREATMENTS

© 1989 Elsevier Science Publishers B.V. (Biomedical Division)
Recent advances in multiple sclerosis therapy.
R.E. Gonsette, P. Delmotte, editors.

THE TREATMENT OF MULTIPLE SCLEROSIS WITH HYPERBARIC OXYGEN: A LONG-TERM STUDY

ERIC P. KINDWALL, MICHAEL P. McQUILLEN, BHUPENDRA O. KHATRI, HARVEY W. GRUCHOW, MARILYN L. MacARTHUR

Department of Hyperbaric Medicine, St. Luke's Medical Center, and Department of Neurology, The Medical College of Wisconsin, Milwaukee WI 53226 (USA)

Reports that patients with multiple sclerosis (MS) may benefit from treatment with oxygen have appeared in the literature for more than 30 years. Hyperbaric oxygen (HBO) as a methodology for enhancing delivery of oxygen to tissue was first employed in MS 10 years ago. Patients with MS began to flock to HBO centers for treatment after the results of a controlled clinical trial were published by Fischer and co-workers in 1983 (1). In Fischer's trial, outcome in 17 patients who received 100 per cent oxygen was compared with that in 20 patients given 10 per cent oxygen, all at a pressure of 2 atmospheres absolute for 90 minutes once daily for a total of 20 treatments; the patients who received the 100 per cent oxygen reported improvement in mobility, equilibrium, fatigue, tremor, and bladder control, but no changes were recorded in their neurological examinations. While the improvement was mild and short-lived, and the sample size quite small, it was imperative that a study be devised to gather meaningful data from the treatment given to the large number of MS patients who sought HBO after publication of Fischer's study.

In practical point of fact, several studies were begun. Many of them were controlled in a randomized, blinded fashion as with the Fischer trial; in none of these were Fischer's results duplicated (e.g., 2). This study was based on the postulate of Schumacher (3) that a valid way to test the efficacy of any therapy in MS was to enter patients with a definite diagnosis of MS and follow them for 2 years after the imposed treatment; if an overwhelming majority fail to get worse over this observation period, the efficacy of the treatment would be manifest. Kurtzke's Expanded Disability Status Scale (EDSS) (4) was used to assess severity. Patients could enter the study only on referral by their

neurologists. All neurologic evaluations had to be carried out by Board-
eligible or Board-certified neurologists. Data from all patients with MS treated
with HBO at a participating institution had to be entered into a Registry,
maintained by the Department of Neurology at The Medical College of Wisconsin.
Between February, 1983, and January, 1987, 312 patients were entered by 170
neurologists in 22 institutions. The majority of patients (71 per cent) had
chronic, progressive MS; a small number (10 per cent) had relapsing-remitting
problems, with the remainder (19 per cent) chronic and stable. Protocol called
for an initial 20 treatments in either a monoplace or a multiplace chamber on a
daily basis, followed by monthly booster treatments for 2 years. Drop-out rate
was high: only 62 per cent finished the initial 20 treatments; 18 per cent
finished 1 year of booster therapy, and only 7.3 per cent finished 2 years of
monthly boosters. There was a mean deterioration in EDSS of 0.93, or almost a
full step from the beginning of treatment until the last evaluation. There was
no difference in outcome between those who had the shortest and longest periods
of time between onset of symptoms and HBO treatment. Treatment pressures made no
difference in outcome. Changes in EDSS bore no relation to the use of booster
treatment. Patients who were reasonably well off at the onset of treatment
(initial EDSS of 1 or 2) deteriorated by an average of 1.7 steps. Those patients
whose initial EDSS was greater than 2 deteriorated an average of 0.82 steps
(p=0.028). Temporary improvement in bladder function occurred in 19.5 per cent,
but was maintained in only 5.5 per cent at 2 years. Long-term worsening was
reported by 7.5 per cent. Worsening occurred in all categories of disease
treated, most significantly (p 0.01) in those patients with chronic progressive
disease. There was no significant change in the working status of patients
following HBO treatment.

Although patients in this study were treated with protocols reported to
produce benefit, we were unable to substantiate any useful long-term effect of
HBO in MS.

1. Fischer BH, Marx M, Reich T (1983) Hyperbaric oxygen treatment of multiple sclerosis. A randomized placebo-controlled double-blind study. NEJM 308: 181-6.

2. Wiles CM, Clarke CRA, Irwin HP, Edgar EF, Swan AV (1986) Hyperbaric oxygen in multiple sclerosis: a double-blind trial. Brit med J 292: 367-71.

3. Schumacher GA (1974) Critique of experimental trials of therapy in multiple sclerosis. Neurology 24: 1010-4.

4. Kurtzke JF (1983) Rating neurologic impairment in multiple sclerosis: an expanded disability scale (EDSS). Neurology 33: 1444-52.

© 1989 Elsevier Science Publishers B.V. (Biomedical Division)
Recent advances in multiple sclerosis therapy.
R.E. Gonsette, P. Delmotte, editors.

157

PLASMA EXCHANGE IN CHRONIC PROGRESSIVE MULTIPLE SCLEROSIS: A LONG-TERM STUDY

BHUPENDRA O. KHATRI, MICHAEL P. McQUILLEN, GREGORY J. HARRINGTON, DONNA SCHMOLL

Department of Neurology, The Medical College of Wisconsin, Milwaukee WI 53226
(USA)

Plasma exchange (PE) has been used in multiple sclerosis (MS) since 1980 in conjunction with a variety of immunosuppressive drugs regimens (ISDT). This approach to therapy in MS is based on several assumptions -- first, that MS is an autoimmune disorder; next, that PE is an effective means of removing antibodies and other proteins from the circulation; and finally, that ISDT will prevent a rebound reformation of that which is removed. Two controlled clinical trials have demonstrated benefit from PE + ISDT in MS -- the first (1), in the chronic progressive form of the disease (CPMS); and, most recently (2), in patients in the midst of an acute attack of MS. Major criticisms of this therapeutic regimen include concerns that:

1. its efficacy over the long term has not been established;

2. the need for retreatment is not clear;

3. long-term toxicity is not known; and

4. the issue of how to select the patient who stands the best chance of responding is not settled.

This analysis -- involving the use of PE + ISDT in 200 CPMS patients over the past 7 years at The Medical College of Wisconsin -- addresses these concerns.

All patients received PE once a week for 12 weeks. If improvement in disability status (as measured on Kurtzke's Expanded Disability Status Scale -- EDSS) (3) was recorded, PE was generally continued at gradually increasing intervals until no further improvment was noted. During each PE, a plasma volume equivalent to 5 per cent of the patient's body weight was exchanged with 5 per cent albumin solution and normal saline using a continuous flow PE machine. All patients received oral cyclophosphamide (1.5 mg per kg body weight per day, rounded off to the nearest 50 mg tablet); oral prednisone (1 mg per kg body weight per alternate day, in gradually declining doses after the 15th week); intramuscular pooled human serum immune globulin (40 ml in 4 divided injections, 2 each at 24 and 48 hours after each PE); and whatever other therapy (e.g. muscle relaxants; bladder stimulants or suppressants; antidepressants; physical therapy) they were being given before PE.

The patients in this series were quite disabled at entry: 90 per cent were at EDSS 6.0 or greater. Improvement -- as defined by a gain of 1 or more steps in the EDSS -- was significant at the conclusion of therapy and during follow-up, as can be seen from the following Table:

N	Follow-up (yr)	Mean Improvement in EDSS
200	0	0.956 (a)
178	1	0.843 (a)
165	2	0.667 (a)
139	3	0.604 (a)
67	4	0.642 (b)
36	5	0.292
12	6	0.650

a. comparing EDSS with pre-PE EDSS, p 0.001
b. same comparison, p 0.01

A minority of patients (n=43) received more than one course of PE + ISDT during follow-up. These were patients who had improved and stabilized initially, but then began to worsen at a variable time after their initial course. A short course -- usually 5 weekly PEs, followed in a few (n=4) by maintenance PE (once every 6 to 10 weks) -- restored or stablized improvement in the majority (n=35). Cytotoxic drugs were omitted; concommitant prednisone therapy was at half the original ISDT dose. The patients who received 3 or more courses of PE were significantly (p 0.001) younger and had more aggressive disease than those who were given only 1 course of PE.

Complications were minor (e.g., difficult vascular access; transient hypotension; excessive tiredness during the day after PE; reversible menstrual irregularities and foot swelling; and minimal hair loss), for the most part. Hemorrhagic cystitis that responded to adjustment of the dose of cyclophosphamide, occurred in 3 patients. One woman, age 58 years at entry, developed carcinoma of the breast 3 years after she stopped taking cyclophosphamide (100 mg per day for 5 months).

Significant predictors of improvement include age at the time of treatment; duration of disease; and degree of decline in EDSS before initiation of PE + ISDT. These clinical variables can be used to predict outcome in a given patient, according to the following Table:

Chance of 1 or more step EDSS improvement following PE + ISDT

	More aggressive course			Less aggressive course		
	Duration of MS			Duration of MS		
Patient Age	3 yr	3-7 yr	7 yr	3 yr	3-7 yr	7 yr
33	95%	86%	68%	76%	36%	26%
33-40	66%	77%	63%	56%	76%	20%
40	77%	95%	77%	55%	54%	39%

"more aggressive course" = worse by 1 EDSS step in previous yr; "less aggressive course" = worse by 1 EDSS step in previous year

From this analysis we conclude that:

1. PE + ISDT is an effective and long-lasting form of therapy for patients with severe CPMS;

2. the need for retreatment after an initial successful course of PE + ISDT appears limited to young patients with very aggressive disease;

3. complications are minor, reversible, or rare; and

4. significant predictors of improvement with PE + ISDT in CPMS include age at time of treatment, duration of disease, and degree of decline in EDSS before initial treatment.

160

1. Khatri BO, McQuillen MP, Harrington GJ, Schmoll D, Hoffman RG (1985)
    Chronic progressive multiple sclerosis: double-blind controlled study of
    plasmapheresis in patients taking immunosuppressive drugs. Neurology 35:
    312-19.

2. Weiner HL, Dau P, Khatri B, Petajan J, Birnbaum G, McQuillen M, Fosburg M,
    Fieldstein M, Orav J (1989) Double blind study of true versus sham plasma
    exchange in patients being treated with immunosuppression for acute attacks
    of multiple sclerosis. Neurology 39, in press.

3. Kurtzke JF (1983) Rating neurologic impairment in multiple sclerosis: an
    expanded disability scale (EDSS). Neurology 33: 1444-52.

© 1989 Elsevier Science Publishers B.V. (Biomedical Division)
Recent advances in multiple sclerosis therapy.
R.E. Gonsette, P. Delmotte, editors.

MITOXANTRONE : A NEW IMMUNOSUPPRESSIVE AGENT IN MULTIPLE SCLEROSIS

R.E. GONSETTE, L. DEMONTY

National Center for MS, Vanheylenstraat, B 1910 Melsbroek, Belgium

INTRODUCTION

There are more and more accumulating evidences that intensive immuno-suppression with cyclophosphamide (CY), or with Total Lymphoid Irradiation (TLI) can be of some benefit in patients with Multiple Sclerosis (MS). However because of immediate side-effects and long-term risks, there is a need for better tolerated immunosuppressive agents.

MATERIAL AND METHODS

Mitoxantrone (MX), a new anticancer drug, crosses the blood brain barrier to some extent (1) and, among immune effects that might be potentially useful in MS, it exerts a marked influence on the humoral immune system through a direct reduction in B Cell number (2). Where the cellular immune component is concerned, MX abrogates Helper activity and enhances Suppressor function (3).

MX is definitely more effective than CY in suppressing EAE in rats (4), mice (5) and Guinea pigs (6). Both clinical and pathological changes are reduced.

A very low acute and chronic toxicity is the main interest of MX (7). Myelo-suppression is the major dose-limiting toxicity in cancer therapy. White blood cells are the most sensitive hematopoietic tissue, but thrombocytopenia is usually mild. Nausea and vomiting are less pronounced than with CY. Hair thinning is observed in 20 % of the cases. Complete alopecia is exceptional.

Cardiotoxicity of MX, an anthraquinone, is very mild. Patients who received adjuvant chemotherapy with MX did not show any increased rate of second tumors compared with a control group (8). MX has little effect on reproductive function and amenorrhea has been reported in only one case in the literature (9). In our experience however, two patients had amenorrhea likely due to MX administration.

A marked and prolonged lymphopenia of about 1000 per ml seems to be required to halt the progression of the disease after TLI (10) or CY immunosuppression (11). Due to its strong immunosuppressive activity, it is to be expected that MX can provoke the same strong immunosuppression as CY or TLI, with less side-effects and lower long term risks.

Since November 1987, MX has been used in 18 MS patients to evaluate the clinical tolerance and safety as well as the effects on lymphocytes subsets.

No special criteria for inclusion were requested. All patients were in an active phase. Two patients with a wearing off effect during CY treatment were switched to MX as well as a third one who became intolerant to CY.

Patients received intravenous infusions of 14 mg/m² MX over 30 min, repeated every 3 weeks. Dose adjustment was performed according to WBC and platelet count at the start of each cycle. Treatment continued until lymphopenia was equal to or lower than 1.0 x 10/µl, and/or until until CD4 cells and B cells absolute values were lower than the 1st percentile of a normal population. Blood cells count and lymphocytes typing are performed every one or two weeks.

As a mean, a lymphopenia of 1000 is obtained with 3 to 4 infusions. Subsequent booster injections are given according to the evolution of lymphocytes count. The lowest values of blood cells are observed after 8-10 days. One patient had a severe leucopenia (< 2000) after the first infusion. No patient experienced toxicity with platelets. In the long-term MX appears to exert a selective effect on lymphocytes since WBC return to normal level whereas lymphocytes remain below the 5th percentiles in most patients.

A selective and quite immediate effect on B and HLA-DR+ cells was evident after the second or even the first cycle. At the end of the treatment, the mean reduction of B and HLA-DR+ cells was definitely more pronounced (by 90 %) than for other subsets (by 50 %). CD4 and CD8 cells are equally affected, but a mild and relative sparing of CD8 cells was usually noted at the end of treatment.

DISCUSSION

Eightteen patients have been treated so far with a follow-up for over 6 months in 8 and about 1 year in 4 and a lymphopenia of 1000 or below was obtained in all patients.

An immunosuppression with CY or TLI is likely unselective and, if we assume that the percentages of various subsets remain unchanged, it is to be expected that whith a lymphopenia of 1000, each subset is decreased below the first percentile of a normal population. (Table)

TABLE

LYMPHOCYTES SUBSETS PERCENTILES

	Percentages in healthy people	Healthy people 1st percentile	Non specific immunosuppression lymphocytes = 1000	Mitoxantrone immuno- suppression
Lymphocytes	-	1003	1000	971
T Lympho	70.0	859	700	764
CD4	41.6	431	416	432
CD8	27.0	261	270	290
B cells	10.0	85	100	35
HLA-DR+	14.4	81	144	103

As a matter of fact, MX provokes the same intense immunosuppression than CY or TLI, but with much less side-effects. Nausea and vomiting are definitely less pronounced than with CY and no alopecia has been observed so far. No adverse effect on MS evolution was observed in patients treated with MX, and all of them are stabilized so far.

CONCLUSION

With a follow-up for 1 year and over in 18 MS patients treated with MX it has been demonstrated that this strong immunosuppressive agent is as effective as CY or TLI in producing a severe and sustained lymphopenia as well as in decreasing various lymphocytes subsets and even more in reducing B and HLA-DR+ cell count. The good immediate and long-term tolerance of MX has been confirmed.

In conclusion, it appears that MX markedly reduces the burden of immuno-suppression in MS and that further clinical studies are warranted to investigate its potential beneficial effects on the progression of the disease.

ACKNOWLEDGEMENTS

Investigation supported by funding from the Belgian Research Group.

REFERENCES

1. Lu K, Savaraj N, Loo TL (1984) Pharmacological disposition of 1,4-dihydroxy-5-8-bis[[2[(2-hydroxyethal)amino] ethyl]amino]-9,10-anthracenedione dihydrochloride in the dog. Cancer Chemother Pharmacol 13:63-66

2. Fidler JM, DeJoy SQ, Gibbons JJ Jr (1986) Selective immunomodulation by the antineoplastic agent Mitoxantrone. I. Suppression of B lymphocyte function. J Immunol 137:727-732

3. Fidler JM, DeJoy SQ, Smith FR III, Gibbons JJ Jr (1986) Selective immunomodulation by the antineoplastic agent Mitoxantrone. II. Nonspecific adherent suppressor cells derived from Mitoxantrone-treated mice. J Immunol 136:2747-2754

4. Ridge SC, Sloboda AE, McReynolds RA, Levine S, Oronsky AL, Kerwar SS (1985) Suppression of experimental allergic encephalomyelitis by Mitoxantrone. Clin Immunol Immunopath 35:35-42

5. Lublin FD, Lavasa M, Viti C, Knobler RL (1987) Suppression of acute and relapsing experimental allergic encephalomyelitis with Mitoxantrone. Clin Immunol and Immunopath 45:122-128

6. Bisteau M, Devos G, Brucher JM, Gonsette RE (1989) Prevention of subacute experimental allergic encephalomyelitis in Guinea-pigs with desferrioxamine, isoprinosine and mitoxantrone. In Press

7. McDonald M, Posner LE, Dukart G, Scott SC (1985) A review of the acute and chronic toxicity of Mitoxantrone. Future trends in chemotherapy 6:443-450

8. Hortobagyi GN, Buzdar AU, Marcus CE, Smith TL (1986) Immediate and long-term toxicity of adjuvant chemotherapy regimens containing doxorubicin in trials at M.D. Anderson Hospital and Tumor Institute. NCI Monogr 1:105-109

9. Shenkenberg TD, Von Hoff DD (1986) Possible Mitoxantrone-induced amenorrhea. Cancer Treat Rep 70:659-661

10. Cook SD, Devereux C, Troiano R, Zito G, Hafstein M, Lavenhar M, Hernandez E, DolingG PC (1987) Total lymphoid irradiation in multiple sclerosis : blood lymphocytes and clinical course. Ann Neurol 22:634-638

11. Gonsette RG, Defalque A, Demonty L, Bohy E (1988) Serial determinations of lymphocytes subsets in multiple sclerosis : correlation with disease evolution and treatment in 364 patients. In: Confavreux C, Aimard G, Devic M (eds) Trends in European Multiple Sclerosis Research. International Congress Series 772, Excerpta Medica, Amsterdam, pp 195-201

SYMPTOMATIC TREATMENTS

© 1989 Elsevier Science Publishers B.V. (Biomedical Division)
Recent advances in multiple sclerosis therapy.
R.E. Gonsette, P. Delmotte, editors.

THE ROLE OF AEROBIC EXERCISE IN MULTIPLE SCLEROSIS

RANDALL T. SCHAPIRO AND JACK H. PETAJAN
The Fairview Multiple Sclerosis Center, Minneapolis, Minnesota,
The University of Utah, Salt Lake City, Utah, and The Jimmie
Heuga Center, Vail, Colorado (USA)

INTRODUCTION

Rigorous studies into the role of rehabilitation in multiple
sclerosis (MS) are few in number. This allows for the great
diversity of opinion as to the role of exercise in MS. Adding to
the confusion is the problem that what one person calls
"exercise" may well be quite different from another. There are
fundamentally four broad categories of exercise: 1) stretching,
2) balance/coordination, 3) strengthening, and 4) aerobic. Some
would also include relaxation, meditation etc.

Despite a lack of literature, many practioners who care for
people with MS agree that a rigorous stretching program may help
decrease muscle tone and increase comfort. It also aids in the
prevention of contractures and increases mobility.

The majority of rehabilitation specialists would also likely
agree that balance and coordination exercises do little to
actually change the poor balance sometimes seen in MS. They may
allow, however, for the learning of some compensatory techniques
which may allow for easier living despite the coordination
problem.

Because the problem with strength in MS lies not within the
muscle but within the nerve conduction system centrally, it is
virtually impossible to strengthen a muscle made weak by MS
demyelination. Most would, however, agree that some form of
active resistive exercise can prevent the disuse atrophy that so
often accompanies the weakness of MS. One must be extremely
careful to avoid fatigue which can, in fact, increase the
weakness.

In the arena of aerobic exercise there has clearly been a
change of philosophy in recent years. This change has come about
despite virtually no studies or objective experiments into the
role of aerobic exercise in MS. In the not so distant past the
use of aerobic exercise in MS was decried. Problems cited

included rapid induction of fatigue, increasing sensory symptoms
(L'hermitte's sign, Uhthoff's phenomena), increasing weakness,
and even fear of progression of the disease process. These
concerns were emphasized despite clear evidence that in static
neurologic diseases including spinal cord trauma, cerebral palsy,
and stroke aerobic exercises were not only safe, but allowed for
improvements in disability.

It is well accepted that aerobic exercise can aid in increasing
strength to the bones, improving weight control, increasing
energy, decreasing depression, and allowing for increased self
esteem and a feeling of "fitness". Endorphins have been
speculated for some of the subjective improvements seen but the
fact is that the mechanisms for improvement remain unclear.

MATERIAL AND METHODS

We performed one of the only controlled studies involving
aerobic exercise in MS reported in the literature. Fifty
patients were matched for age, sex, and disability status into
two groups of 25 each. Each was studied at baseline with a
resting electrocardiogram (ECG) followed by a cardiac exercise
(stress) test utilizing the Schwinn Air-Dyne ergometer. Ratings
of perceived exertion (RPE) were taught to each subject and
utilized to correspond to a target heart rate training zone of
approximately 65-80% of maximum achieved heart rate.
Psychological status was monitored by both observation and the
Sickness Impact Profile (SIP).

After the 50 participants were tested, they were each told into
which group (exercise versus control) they had been randomly
placed. The exercise group received an individualized written
exercise prescription based on his/her data. Each was told to
exercise approximately 15-30 min four to five times per week for
16 weeks. After that time all participants were retested.

RESULTS

The improvement in cardiovascular fitness was modest, with a
majority of subjects in all categories of disability improving by
the smallest measurable increment (25W). The exercisers did

improve over the non exercisers in work load achieved and graded
exercise time. They experienced a relatively modest training
effect of approximately 10%. Normal sedentary individuals
training for a period of 16 weeks should experience a 20-30%
increase in work load achieved.

TABLE 1

GRADED EXERCISE TIME

Group

Experimental	10.13 (4.64)	
Controls	9.85 (4.46)	

Post Exercise

Experimental	10.24 (4.51)	
Control	9,74 (4.26)	

TABLE 2

WORK LOAD ACHIEVED

Severity

Pre/post exercise

Pre-

Experimental	114.6 watts
Controls	116.7

Post-

Experimental	127.1
Controls	117.1

There were several unexpected problems associated with the
methodology utililized which are important for others doing
exercise studies in MS to keep in mind. Compliance means
everything in fitness studies. Thus great pressure was put on
the exercisers to be compliant. The objectivity of exercise
testing in some way obviates the errors that may arise from the
fact that more attention is paid to the exercising group. One
might expect that because of a desire to do well (cognitive
dissonance) a bias might exist toward the exercise performances.
During the testing, however, the exact opposite occurred. The MS
exercisers were especially tense and the tension made their MS

symptoms transiently worse thereby decreasing their objective
scores. The MS "non exercisers" appeared to feel no pressure to
perform and that coupled with the knowledge of how the test was
to be done had few performance problems.

Psychological testing failed to distinguish between the groups
but again the stress factor appeared to be playing a negative
role, pulling down the exercisers from what may have been
improvement.

While it is rare to hear a physician decry aerobic exercise in
MS today. Our study demonstrated that people with MS can
exercise aerobically and potentially benefit from the aerobic
exercises as other groups have. There is, however, much more
objective work to be done.

GENERAL REFERENCES
1. Young A (1983) Exercise in the prevention of disease and
disability. In: Gray M, Fowler GH eds. Preventative Medicine in
General Practice. New York: Oxford University Press 160-78.
2. Schapiro RT, Petajan JH, Kosich D, Molk B, Feeney, J (1988) J
Neuro Rehab 2:43-49.

© 1989 Elsevier Science Publishers B.V. (Biomedical Division)
Recent advances in multiple sclerosis therapy.
R.E. Gonsette, P. Delmotte, editors.

THE USE OF NEUROMUSCULAR STIMULATION IN THE TREATMENT OF MULTIPLE SCLEROSIS

JENNIFER WORTHINGTON AND LORRAINE DE SOUZA

ARMS Research Unit, Central Middlesex Hospital, Acton Lane, London, NW10 7NS.

INTRODUCTION

Investigations into the therapeutic use of low frequency neuromuscular stimulation (NMS) in multiple sclerosis (MS) patients have been limited. In order to determine the effects of NMS, first, a pilot study, and then, single case experimental design studies were carried out. We wished to use NMS in conjunction with a therapeutic exercise programme, and were interested in those benefits which could be sustained when stimulation was withdrawn. It is only when the benefits of treatment are translated into everyday living that therapeutic intervention has an impact on reducing disability for patients.

The pilot study, previously reported(1) was conducted on 10 patients. The results showed that when NMS was applied to the quadriceps and hamstring muscle groups and/or to the ankle dorsiflexors, and then withdrawn for a period, significant improvements were maintained in the range of movement measures but not functional ability. These mixed results may be due to the diversity of symptoms and disabilities found in the patients we selected for the pilot study.

On closer examination of the pilot group general indications for selecting patients for treatment became apparent. Patients who seemed to gain the most benefit from NMS were those who had stable MS symptoms, were able to walk, and either had a moderate degree of spasticity or weakness. On this basis two patients were selected for single case experimental design studies to determine the effects of NMS on a specific functional ability – walking.

METHODS

The stimulation parameters, equipment, and assessment techniques have been previously described(1).

For these studies a single case A-B-A-B-A design with withdrawal of treatment was used(2). During Phase A patients carried out physiotherapeutic exercise programmes, both at the clinic and at home. During Phase B treatment consisted of NMS in addition to home exercise programmes. Both of these patients had been attending our Unit for regular assessment and treatment for three years prior to the start of the study.

172

RESULTS

The first patient is a 56 year old female with a 21 year history of MS. She has moderate extensor spasticity of both legs and can walk 200 metres using one stick. Figure 1 shows changes in range of lower limb movement. Despite regular physiotherapy she has shown a 25%-40% loss in range of lower limb movements over the 3 years prior to the start of NMS. During the first application of stimulation she improved her lower limb movement by 14%, thus reversing the trend towards deterioration. When stimulation was withdrawn she shows a loss of lower limb movement, although not to baseline levels. This is again reversed on the second application of stimulation.

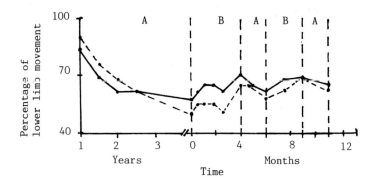

Fig. 1. Changes in voluntary range of lower limb movement (percentage) for patient 1. A = exercise only, B = period of NMS (this applies to other graphs shown). ── = right lower limb, ─── = left lower limb.

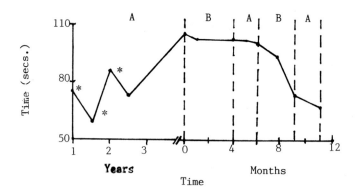

Fig. 2. Walking times over a distance of 50 metres for patient 1. * = no walking aids used.

Figure 2 shows the same patient's walking times over a distance of 50
metres. Over the 3 years prior to the start of stimulation she has shown
an increase in the amount of time taken to walk the same distance, increasing
from 73 to 104 seconds. In addition, she also began using a walking stick.
When stimulation is started, initially there are no changes in her walking
time, but improvement is evident during the second period of NMS. By the
end of the study she has decreased her walking time to 67 seconds.

The second patient is a 50 year old female with a 36 year history of MS.
She presents with weakness in all limbs and is able to walk 20 metres with
bilateral upper limb support. In Figure 3 a 40% loss in range of movement in
her right leg over the three year baseline is apparent. In addition, she has
shown very little voluntary movement in assessment positions in her left leg.
During the subsequent application and withdrawal of NMS her pattern of response
is similar to that shown by the first patient. She shows an improvement of
21% in movement of the right leg and 11% in the left leg when stimulation was
first given, followed by either loss or gain of lower limb movement corresponding to the treatment with NMS.

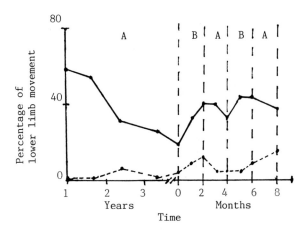

Fig. 3. Changes in voluntary range of lower limb movement (percentage) for
patient 2. ▬ = right lower limb, --- = left lower limb.

Figure 4 shows the changes in walking ability for the second patient. As
this patient did not walk the same distance or use the same walking aids over
this time a method of scoring functional mobility(3) was used. And again the
pattern is very similar to the first patient, with a 3 year history of deterioration followed by improvement during the second period of NMS. Here she
increased her walking distance from 20 metres, shown by "B" on the graph, to

174

50 metres, indicated by "C". Concurrently she also increased her speed of walking by 100 seconds.

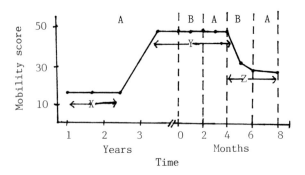

Fig. 4. Mobility score for patient 2. X = walks 50m using 1 stick, Y = walks 20m using bilateral upper limb support, Z = walks 50m using bilateral upper limb support.

CONCLUSION

The improvements in range of lower limb movements shown by these two patients appeared to be related to the application of NMS. These improvements seem to occur early in the treatment phase, while changes in walking ability are not evident for several months. The changes in walking ability do not seem to be a placebo effect as they did not occur initially. Although improvements were small, they did reverse the trend towards deterioration that both patients had shown on assessment during the 3 years prior to the start of the study. Further investigation is required to determine if the benefits from NMS can be maintained long-term.

REFERENCES

1. Worthington JA, DeSouza LH Low frequency neuromuscular stimulation in patients with multiple sclerosis. In: The CIBA Satellite Symposium on neuromuscular use and disuse: Basic concepts and clinical implications. Demos Pubs., New York. (in press).

2. Barlow DH and Hersenm (1984) Single case experimental designs. Pergamon Press, New York.

3. Worthington JA and DeSouza LH (1988) A method of scoring functional mobility in multiple sclerosis patients. Presented at the Society for Research and Rehabilitation, Bath, July, 1988.

© 1989 Elsevier Science Publishers B.V. (Biomedical Division)
Recent advances in multiple sclerosis therapy.
R.E. Gonsette, P. Delmotte, editors.

MAGNETOTHERAPY IN MULTIPLE SCLEROSIS

ANDRAS GUSEO

Department of Neurology, Central Hospital of County Fejer
Szekesfehervar (Hungary)

INTRODUCTION

Since M. Benedict[1] in the last hundre years it has been proved
many times that pulsing electromagnetic field /PEMF/ therapy is
useful in many neurological and other diseases. The Messmer experience and the fact that biophysicist couldn't explain how such
low energy low frequency pulsing electromagnetic field can cause
some change in membrane electron structure and in membrane potentials /irritability/, could be the reason that the treatment have
been neglected and forgotten. In the last twenty years interest
turned again toward action of magnetic field because of intensive
space research and better neurophysiological facilities. New generation of equipments using electric and magnetic field have been
developed for diagnostic and therapeutic purposes. We learned how
TENS alleviate pain syndrome, repetitive spinal cord stimulation
the spasticity and pain etc. "It may now be considered as a scientific fact, that electromagnetic fields, far below the levels producing heat, have major biological actions".[2]

A new equipment have been developed in Hungary in 1983. Pain
syndromes due to spondylarthrosis and muscle spasm were treated
very efficiently. Some of our MS patients, who took part in the
treatment, mentioned, that their spasticity decreased, urinary
incontinence and their everyday activity improved significantly.
That was the moment we started a systemic investigation in MS
patients, wether the pusling electromagnetic field has any measurable action on symptoms of MS.

MATERIAL AND METHODS

The electromagnetic device constructed by Gyuling and Bordacs
/GBM/ have been used for the treatment trials. The equipment
differs from any other PEMF equipment in the shape of its wave
form, which may be responsible for its superior effect in many
diseases including MS. Patients were treated in lieing position
once dayly for 15-45 minutes and for 1-3 body regions. A modified
Kurtzke DSS was used to measure actual disability. The results
found before

found before and after 15 treatments were compared. Normal and maximaly extended stepps needed to walk 10 meters and time to walk normaly and fast as possible 10 meters have been measured every day. Thermography, electromyography and intestinosonography have been used to demonstrate effects of PEMF.

RESULTS

More than 230 MS patients have been treated since 1984 by PEMF in our Department. The following physiological effects have been demonstrated after PEMF treatment:

1. Frequency dependent enhancement of infrared radiation of the human body. In MS the paretic cold extremities warmed up.
2. Increase in muscular irritability. Positive effect on the decrement /fatiguability/ of neuraly evoked high frequency short duration electromyogram.
3. Frequency dependent enhancement of small intestine motility.[4]
4. Temporary frequency dependent change in EEG.
5. Increase in cerebral perfusion in animal experiments.

Double blind clinical trials showed a positive action of PEMF on various symptoms of MS.[3] The following symptoms have been influenced by PEMF therapy:

1. Decrease of spasticity using low frequency and increase using high frequency, and decrease of contractures in some cases.
2. Improvement in bladder incontinence for several months.
3. Decrease of pain caused by spasticity as well as cure of trigeminal neuralgias, improvement in migraine and cervico-genic headache.
4. Improvement in power and endurance in upper motor neuron lesions.
5. Improvement in lazy bowel symptom.

70-80% of all treated MS patients improved after the treatment, the rest was non reacting. Sometimes their improvements was not measurable by gross neruological investigation, but their walking was better, safer, more stable, they could climb the stairs again, they could stay longer out of bed, they could make execises more easily. The effect lasted for several weeks or months. The effect of the treatment was more pronounced in less severly affected patients /Kurzke DSS 3-6/, however in patients who were bedridden for years a positive change have been seen too. No harmful side effects have been noted.

DISCUSSION

Without knowing the exact mode of action of the PEMF treatment
its usefulness have been demonstrated in many symptoms of MS.
It enables a better rehabilitation.

Comparing the effects of PEMF to those of the functional electric
stimulation /FES/ or to direct spinal cord stimulation by implanted
electrodes, the results are very similar, almost identical.

Putting all the above mentioned results into the rehabilitation
program, this new kind of physiotherapy gives the opportunity of
a quicker rehabilitation of MS patients. It widens the spectrum of
usable physiotherapy methods, can be combined easily with other
methods. If necessary, in chronic diseases the treatment can be
prolonged for months or years without complications. Taking into
consideration that the treatment is safe, no harful side effects
have been observed in the last 5 years using correct parameters,
the tratment can be used at home, sparing all traveling and
waiting inconveniences in a physiotherapy outpatient department.

SUMMARY

Low frequency, low energy pulsing electromagnetic field has
been proved to be effective in decreasing spasticity, urinary
incontinence, small intestine motility and influencing muscle
power and endurance /fatiguability/ in multiple sclerosis. The
method is safe, no harmful side effects have been observed in the
last five years. It can be used successfully in every rehabilitation center as well as in patients home. About 20% of all treated
patients were non reacting.

REFERENCES
1.   Benedict M (1885) Zur Magneto-Therapie. Wiener Medizinische
     Blatter 8: 1119
2.   Becker RO (1987) Guest Editorial. Nesletter J. Bioelectricity
     2:1
3.   Guseo A (1987) Pulsing electromagnetic field therapy in Mul-
     tiple Sclerosis by the Gyuling-Bordacs device: Double blind
     cross over and open studies. J. Bioelectricity 6: 23-35
4.   Guseo A (1989) The effect of pulsing electromagnetic field
     on small intestine motility. J. of Bioelectricity (in press)

CONCLUDING REMARKS

© 1989 Elsevier Science Publishers B.V. (Biomedical Division)
Recent advances in multiple sclerosis therapy.
R.E. Gonsette, P. Delmotte, editors.

TREATMENTS - RESULTS AND FUTURE PROSPECT

JUERGEN MERTIN

Department of Neurology and MS Centre, St. Gallische Hoehen-
klinik, CH-8881 Walenstadtberg (Switzerland)

It is a difficult task to give a resumé of all the treatments we
have heard about today. I intend to meet this task by first saying
something about symptomatic treatments, and thereafter I shall refer
to experimental causal therapies.

When we and our patients at times deplore the slow progress in
multiple sclerosis (MS) research and the failures in the development
of therapy we automatically refer, in the latter case, to causal
therapies, and ignore thereby the fact that in the field of
symptomatic treatment great advances have been made during the past
decades. These advances are best highlighted by the remarkable
increase in the mean life expectancy of MS patients, which with
about 30 years after diagnosis can be considered to be almost
normal. This success is due to developments - be they concencerned
with the general management of the patients or with advances in
pharmacology - which allow us to counteract efficiently the complications of the disease.

In terms of management we have learned that disease - produced
physical, psychological and social inactivities have to be counteracted, that the MS patient needs to be as active as possible.
Pharmacological development has brought effective treatment of
infections and inflammations, and drugs to reduce spasticity. I
belief that we still have not fully utilized the possibilities
given by these new developments, and further research on methods of
symptomatic treatment may help not only to lengthen the life span
but also to further improve the quality of life of the MS patients.

Nowadays, most of the meetings on MS are dedicated primarily to
basic research on aetiology, pathogenesis and experimental
therapies. The amount of reported progress from one meeting to the
other seems to me often negligable. We have, therefore, decided for
once to break with tradition and to dedicate the next ECTRIMS-
meeting primarily to the field of MS rehabilitation (besides cell
biology and virology). This meeting is planned for autumn next year
in Switzerland. We hope that the interest in this venue will be at
least as great as that in previous ECTRIMS meetings.

Now to the field of experimental causal therapies: none of the therapies we have heard about today appears to me to be so convincing that we could go home and treat most of our patients with it. It is my strong belief – as I have tried to convey in my earlier presentation – that basic research on MS needs to be targeted on the CNS itself. In terms of immunology that does mean a need for neuroimmunology rather than immunoneurology. With such a change it may be possible to develop more specific and thereby more effective treatments.

This afternoon you have heard a presentation reporting about effective suppression of EAE with sulfasalazine. Although EAE in a disease caused primarily by alteration of the systemic immune response, the suppressive effect of this substance could still be due to an influence on immunoregulatory activities of the CNS. We know nowadays that derivatives of arachidonic acid have transmitter function in the brain, and sulfasalazine is known to interfere with production of such derivatives. Another promising substance is mitoxantrone discussed today by Dr. Gonsette. With these examples I want to stress that we have to be openminded – we cannot stop performing trials of new drugs till the arrival of a new and better concept explaining the causes of MS. With such therapeutic pragmatism we could still "strike lucky" as has happened quite often in medical science. But one has to be clear, in my opinion, of the very important role of the systemic immune response in EAE (witness for example the success of T cell lines inducing this disease) and aware that, therefore, drugs which successfully supress the experimental disease may have little or no therapeutic value in MS. So, parallel to continuing efforts in experimental treatments with "conventional" immunemodulatory drugs, search is needed for substances able to modulate the CNS local immune response and also for new models which allow us to recognise the effectiveness of such substances.

Such approaches are a thing of the future: what about the patients we are confronted with now? How do we treat, for example, the young patient presenting with relapsing-remitting disease? In this case I personally think that besides exploiting the possibilities of symptomatic treatment, azathioprine is still the drug of choice, because of its limited side effects, both short and long term, in the light of present knowledge.

EXPERIMENTAL APPROACH OF MS THERAPY

© 1989 Elsevier Science Publishers B.V. (Biomedical Division)
Recent advances in multiple sclerosis therapy.
R.E. Gonsette, P. Delmotte, editors.

ADOPTIVE TRANSFER EXPERIMENTAL AUTOIMMUNE ENCEPHALOMYELITIS: ROLE OF MACROPHAGES AND REACTIVE OXYGEN SPECIES

KURT HEININGER[1] , BÄRBEL SCHÄFER[1] , HANS-PETER HARTUNG[1] , WALTER FIERZ[2] , KLAUS V. TOYKA[1] , HANS LASSMANN[3]

[1] Dept. of Neurology, University of Düsseldorf, West Germany;
[2] Dept. of Internal Medicine, Section of Clinical Immunology, University of Zürich, Switzerland; [3] Neurological Institute, University of Vienna, Austria

INTRODUCTION

The pivotal role of T helper lymphocytes in the pathogenesis of experimental autoimmune encephalomyelitis (EAE) has been established (1). Adoptive transfer of myelin basic protein (MBP)-specific T cells can induce EAE in naive recipient animals but the pathogenetic mechanisms remain unclear. In vitro findings suggested that T cells by themselves could bring about the functional deficit either by killing of astrocytes (2) or by directly interfering with nerve conduction (3).

We investigated effector mechanisms of adoptive transfer EAE (AT-EAE) in vivo by blockade of macrophages. Global blockade was achieved by silica, a macrophage toxin. Macrophages exert many of their effector functions by the release of reactive oxygen species. Selective blockade of macrophages was therefore induced by the administration of catalase, a scavenger of oxygen radicals (4).

Here we present evidence that macrophages are important effector cells in AT-EAE and that reactive oxygen species released by macrophages may be the predominant mediators of myelin damage.

MATERIALS AND METHODS

AT-EAE was induced by intravenous injection of 3×10^6 MBP-specific T line cells in naive Lewis rats. Groups of 6 animals received intraperitoneal (i.p.) injections of 200 mg of silica either on days 0, 2, and 4 or on day 4 after T cell transfer (a.t.). In another set of experiments i.p. injections of 15000 units of catalase were given daily starting on day 1 a.t. Control groups received i.p. injections of physiological saline. The course of the disease was followed by clinical and electro-physiological monitoring as described (5). On day 7 a.t. the animals were perfused and spinal cord specimen taken for quantitative morphological evaluation (6).

RESULTS

Effects of silica

Sham-treated AT-EAE rats developed a fulminant disease by day 4 a.t. and were moribund by day 7. Electrophysiological measure-ments revealed a marked delay of latencies of F and H waves and of lumbar and cervical somatosensory evoked potentials (SEP) (fig.1). Quantitative morphological analysis showed a marked meningeal and perivascular infiltration of mononuclear cells.

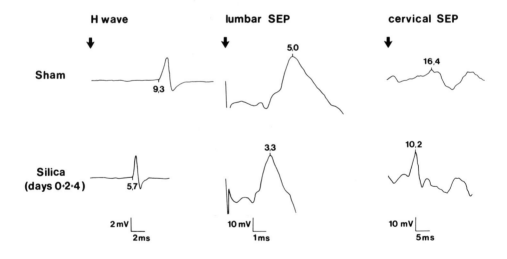

Fig. 1. Effect of silica on electrophysiological findings in AT-EAE. Redrawn original recordings of H waves, lumbar and cervical SEP from representative animals either sham-treated or treated with silica on days 0, 2, and 4 a.t. Note change of gain and time scales. Numbers indicate latencies in milliseconds.

In contrast, only two of the 6 animals treated with silica on days 0, 2, and 4 a.t. exhibited a limp tail while the other 4 rats remained normal. Electrophysiological findings were quite normal (fig. 1). Quantitative evaluation of inflammatory cells at the lumbar spinal cord level revealed that perivascular infiltration of mononuclear cells was greatly reduced in these animals (fig. 2).

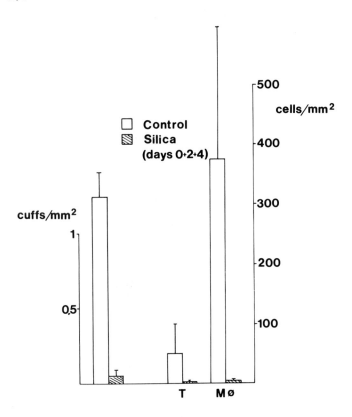

Fig. 2. Reduction of perivascular cuffs and infiltrating mononuclear cells in AT-EAE rats by treatment with silica (days 0, 2, and 4 a.t.). Note that macrophages are the predominant infiltrating cell type in AT-EAE. T = T cells, M0 = macrophages (see also ref. 6 for further details).

Even a single injection of silica on day 4 a.t. provided almost total protection from clinical, electrophysiological and morphological signs of CNS inflammatory disease (data not shown).

Effects of catalase

Catalase was also very effective in attenuating the clinical
and electrophysiological abnormalities of AT-EAE. On day 7 a.t.
3 of the animals had a mild paresis of the hind limbs, 3 only a
limp tail, while controls were tetraplegic. Latencies of F and
H waves, lumbar and cervical SEPs in catalase treated rats were
delayed by a mean of 15 to 20 % while sham-treated control
animals showed a slowing of 40 to 50 % (fig. 3).

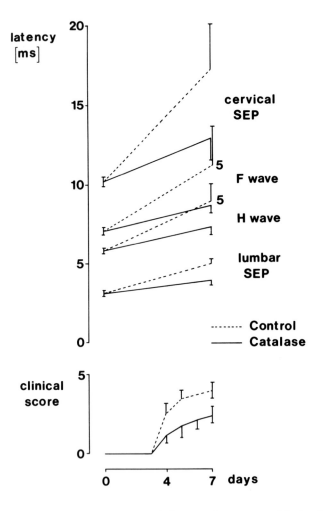

Fig. 3. Effects of treatment with catalase on clinical and
electrophysiological findings in rats with AT-EAE (see also ref.
5 for further details).

Surprisingly, upon histochemical analysis catalase treated rats showed the same amount of perivascular cuffs and infiltrating mononuclear cells as sham-treated animals.

DISCUSSION

The macrophage toxin silica greatly suppresses adoptive transfer EAE. These findings suggest that macrophages are the predominant effector cells in AT-EAE. Effector functions of the transferred T helper cells as suggested by in vitro findings seem to play a minor role in vivo. Silica treatment markedly reduced immigration of macrophages and T cells into the CNS parenchyma. Because silica does not influence T cell function directly this finding indicates that macrophages may also be important for the recruitment of endogenous T cells to the CNS, presumably by the mediation of interleukin-1 and/or tumor necrosis factor.

While catalase had a marked effect on the clinical and electro-physiological signs of AT-EAE it could not reduce infiltration of mononuclear cells to the CNS tissue. Some recent findings could provide an explanation for this differential effect. We have shown that the functional deficit in AT-EAE is based on paranodal demyelination which could be detected by electrophysio-logical techniques but escaped standard morphological analysis (5). We suggest that this paranodal demyelination is caused by reactive oxygen species and can consequently be attenuated by catalase. On the other hand reactive oxygen species seem not to take part in the cascade of events leading to the formation of the inflammatory infiltrates and therefore this cannot be prevented by catalase. Infiltration per se may not be sufficient to cause considerable functional deficit.

Our results shed light on the role of reactive oxygen products in the pathogenesis of inflammatory demyelinating CNS disease. Blocking of these oxygen species by a variety of so-called scavengers during active phases may prove effective in the treat-ment of these diseases including the human disorder multiple sclerosis.

ACKNOWLEDGEMENTS

Supported by Gemeinnützige Hertie Stiftung, Deutsche Forschungsgemeinschaft SFB 200,B5, Swiss National Foundation (3.998-086), and the Austrian Science Research Fund (P 5354).

REFERENCES

1. Ben-Nun A, Wekerle H, Cohen IR (1981) The rapid isolation of clonable, antigen-specific T lymphocyte lines capable of mediating autoimmune encephalomyelitis. Eur J Immunol 11:195-199

2. Sun D, Wekerle H (1986) Ia-restricted encephalitogenic T lymphocytes mediating EAE lyse autoantigen-presenting astro-cytes. Nature 320:70-72

3. Yarom Y, Naparstek Y, Lev-Ram V, Holoshitz J, Ben-Nun A, Cohen IR (1983) Immunospecific inhibition of nerve conduc-tion by T lymphocytes reactive to basic protein of myelin. Nature 303:246-247

4. Hartung H-P, Schäfer B, Heininger K, Toyka KV (1988) Suppression of experimental autoimmune neuritis by the oxygen radical scavengers superoxide dismutase and catalase. Ann Neurol 23:453-460

5. Heininger K, Fierz W, Schäfer B, Hartung H-P, Wehling P, Toyka KV (1989) Electrophysiological investigations in adoptively transferred experimental autoimmune encephalo-myelitis. Brain 112:in press

6. Lassmann H, Brunner C, Bradl M, Linington C (1988) Experi-mental allergic encephalomyelitis: the balance between encephalitogenic T lymphocytes and demyelinating antibodies determines size and structure of demyelinated lesions. Acta Neuropathol (Berl) 75:566-576

© 1989 Elsevier Science Publishers B.V. (Biomedical Division)
Recent advances in multiple sclerosis therapy.
R.E. Gonsette, P. Delmotte, editors.

SUPPRESSION OF EXPERIMENTAL ALLERGIC ENCEPHALOMYELITIS (EAE) IN LEWIS RAT BY NEUROTROPIN® TREATMENT

Mitsuru Naiki and Seishi Suehiro.
Department of Immunology and Allergy, Institute of Bio-Active Science, Nippon Zoki Pharmaceutical Co., Ltd., Hyogo, Japan

INTRODUCTION

Neurotropin® is a non-protein extract from the cutaneous tissue of rabbit inoculated with vaccinia virus and contains biologically active substances formed by neuroimmuno-inflammatory reactions. In several animal models with either suppressed or elevated immune responses, Neurotropin exerts immunomodulatory effects (1-2).

Experimental allergic encephalomyelitis (EAE) in Lewis rats is a model for human autoimmune disease, multiple sclerosis (MS), and is characterized by mononuclear cell infiltration and demyelination within the central nerves system (CNS). The adoptive transfer experiments suggest the role of T lymphocytes which are sensitized to MBP in the induction of EAE (3-4). On the other hand, Lewis rats recovered from EAE become resistant to active induction of disease (5) and the resistance can be adoptively transferred into naive rats with the lymph node cells from recovered rats (6), suggesting that the suppressor cells may regulate the induction of EAE (7). Because of immunoregulatory properties of Neurotropin, the ability of Neurotropin to suppress the development of EAE in Lewis rats immunized with MBP in CFA was examined.

MATERIALS AND METHODS

Treatment with Neurotropin

Neurotropin was obtained from Nippon Zoki Pharmaceutical Co., Osaka, Japan. It was administered i.p. daily at dose of 10, 20, or 40mg/kg body weight (b.w.) for 11 days postinoculation.

EAE induction and clinical assessment of rats

Synthetic peptide corresponding to the encephalitogenic determinant of guinea pig myelin basic protein (GP-MBP, residues # 68-84) in PBS (0.1mg/ml) was emulsified in an equal volume of complete Freund's adjuvant (CFA) containing 2.5mg/ml of Mycobacterium tuberculosis H37Ra (Difco Laboratories, MI, USA). Lewis rats (♀, 160-170g) were sensitized by inoculating 0.1ml of emulsion in the right hind footpad. Control rats received 0.1 ml of emulsion without GP-MBP. Rats were observed daily for clinical signs of disease. A clinical index (CI) was used to grade animals on a scale of 0-4 as follows: grade 0, no tail weakness; grade 1, distal tail weakness; grade 2, loss of tail tone; grade 3, hind leg weakness; grade 4, no hind leg movement accompanied by incontinence.

Delayed-type hypersensitivity (DTH)

One µg of GP-MBP or 20µg of OVA in 10µl of PBS was injected intradermally in right ear of Lewis rats 15days after immunization with 5µg of MBP or 100µg of OVA in CFA, respectively. The opposite ear was injected with an equal volume of PBS and served as a control. The thickness of each ear was measured 24hr postchallenge and DTH was expressed as the difference in thickness between the antigen-injected and PBS-injected ears.

In vitro proliferative response of lymph node T cells

Draining popliteal lymph nodes were aseptically removed from rats 15 days after immunization and nylon T cells were prepared. Nylon T cells ($2x10^5$) were cultured with MBP (1µg/ml) or Con A (2.5µg/ml) in the presence of irradiated (2,500R) thymocytes as antigen presenting cells ($2x10^6$) for 5 days or 3 days, respectively. The cultures were pulsed with 0.5µCi [^{3}H]-Thymidine for last 6hr of incubation.

Adoptive transfer of Suppressor cell

Single cell suspensions were prepared from draining popliteal lymph nodes 30 days after immunization with MBP in CFA. Lymph node cells were adoptively transferred i.v. into the lateral tail vein of syngeneic recipients. The recipient rats were immunized with MBP in CFA 24hr after cell transfer.

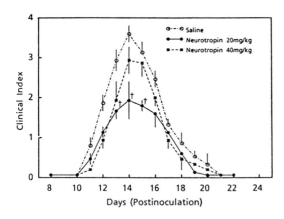

Fig. 1. Clinical scores of Lewis rats treated with Neurotropin.

RESULTS

To clarify the effect of Neurotropin on the induction of EAE, Lewis rats were treated daily with Neurotropin for 11 days after immunization. As shown in Figure 1, Neurotropin treatment at 20mg/kg b.w. significantly suppressed the induction of EAE as compared with control rats. However, Neurotropin treatment at 40mg/kg b.w. had no effect on the EAE induction in this system. Although data are not shown, Neurotropin treatment at 10mg/kg b.w. suppressed the EAE at the same degree as that of 20mg/kg b.w.. Furthermore, histological evaluation also indicated that

Neurotropin suppressed perivascular infiltration of mononuclear cells (data not shown).

To examine whether the suppressive effect of Neurotropin results from the modulation of the immune responses, the DTH response against MBP was measured. Neurotropin treatment at both 10 and 20mg/kg b.w. significantly suppressed the DTH response as compared with control rats when administered daily for 11 days after immunization with MBP in CFA (Table 1). This result suggests that Neurotropin suppresses the EAE by inhibiting the T cell mediating immune response to MBP.

TABLE I

Effect of Neurotropin on DTH response to MBP.

Group	Treatment[1]	No. of rats	Ear thickness (mm)		Change in thickness[†] (mm)
			PBS[§]	MBP[§]	
1	Saline	7	0.54 ± 0.01	0.77 ± 0.02	0.23 ± 0.02
2	Neurotropin (10 mg/kg b.w.)	7	0.54 ± 0.01	0.68 ± 0.03	0.13 ± 0.02 (P<0.05)[‡]
3	Neurotropin (20 mg/kg b.w.)	7	0.56 ± 0.01	0.68 ± 0.01	0.12 ± 0.01 (P<0.01)[‡]

[1]Lewis rats were treated daily with saline or Neurotropin for 11 days after immunization with MBP/CFA.
[§]On day 10, Lewis rats were challenged with MBP or PBS (control) in the right or left ears, respectively. The thickness of each ears were measured 48 hr later.
[†]Difference in thickness between the MBP- and PBS-injected ears.
[‡]Significant difference from the control group.

The EAE of Lewis rats has been reported to be mediated by MBP-specific helper T cells. To further clarify the modes of the suppression by Neurotropin treatment, we examined the MBP-specific proliferative response of nylon T cells from rats immunized with MBP in CFA. As shown in Table 2, the MBP-specific proliferative response of rats treated with Neurotropin (20mg/kg b.w.) was significantly lower than that of saline treated rats. However, no difference was observed in the Con A-induced proliferative responses between saline and Neurotropin treated rats. These results indicated that the suppression of EAE by Neurotropin treatment seemed to be specific suppression.

TABLE II

Responses to MBP or Con A of nylon T cells from lymph node of treated rats[§]

Stimulator	[³H]-TdR uptake (cpm)		
	Saline[1]	Neurotropin[1]	
Medium	751 ± 128	535 ± 212	
MBP	12,072 ± 1,014	6,125 ± 807	(P<0.001)
Con A	25,535 ± 980	23,038 ± 608	(N.S)

[1]Lewis rats were treated daily with saline or Neurotropin (20mg/kg b.w) for 11 days after immunization with MBP/CFA.
[§]Nylon T cells were prepared from lymph node of Lewis rats 15 days after immunization and were cultured with MBP (1µg/ml) or Con A (2.5µg/ml) for 5 days or 3 days, respectively. The cultures were pulsed with 0.5µCi [³H]-Thymidine for last 6hr.

194

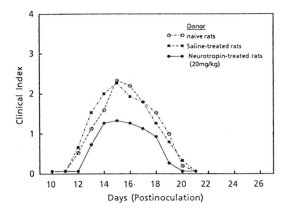

Fig.2. Suppression of EAE disease by cell transfer.

To clarify the mechanism by which Neurotropin suppresses the EAE, we tested for ability of lymph node cells from Lewis rat recovered from EAE to suppress the induction of EAE in recipient rats by using adoptive transfer experiments. As shown in Figure 2, there is no difference in the EAE induction between non-treated rats and the recipients of lymph node cells from saline treated rats. However, if donor rats were treated daily with Neurotropin for 11 days postimmunization, the adoptive transfer of lymph node cells from such donor rats suppressed the EAE in recipient rats. These results indicate that Neurotropin enhances the suppressive activity, leading to the inhibition of EAE.

REFERENCES
1. Naiki M, Imai Y, Nakanishi A. Hishinuma A, Osawa, T (1984) Effect on autoimmunity developed in (NZB/NZW)F1 mice of substance(s) extracted from inflammatory dermis of rabbits induced by inoculation of vaccinia virus. Clin. Immunol. 16, 506-516.

2. Naiki M, Suehiro S, Imai Y, Osawa, T (1989) Immunomodulatory effects of Neurotropin through the recovery of interleukin-2 production in autoimmune prone (NZB/NZW)F1 mice. Int. J. Immunopharmacol. in press

3. Paterson PY (1960) Transfer of allergic encephalomyelitis in rats by means of lymph node cells. J. Exp. Med. 111, 119-136.

4. Hickey WE, Gonatas NK, Kimura H, Wilson DB (1983) Identification and quantitation of T lymphocyte subsets found in the spinal cord of the Lewis rat during acute experimental allergic encephalomyelitis. J. Immunol. 131, 2805-2809.

5. Hinrichs DJ, Roberts CM, Waxman FJ (1981) Regulation of paralytic experimental allergic encephalomyelitis in rats: susceptibility to active and passive disease reinduction. J. Immunol. 126, 1857-1862.

6. Welch AM, Holda JH, Swanborg TH (1980) Regulation of experimental allergic encephalomyelitis II. Appearance of suppressor cells during the remission phase of the disease. J. Immunol. 125, 186-189.

© 1989 Elsevier Science Publishers B.V. (Biomedical Division)
Recent advances in multiple sclerosis therapy.
R.E. Gonsette, P. Delmotte, editors.

EFFECTS OF RETINOIC ACID ON PASSIVE EAE

MASSACESI L., SARLO F., CASTIGLI E., OLIVOTTO J., VERGELLI M.,
ABBAMONDI A.L.* AND AMADUCCI L.

Department of Neurology, University of Florence, Italy.
*Institute of Neurology, Catholic University, Rome, Italy.

INTRODUCTION

Experimental autoimmune encephalomyelitis (EAE) is a T cell-
mediated disease of the central nervous system (CNS) which can be
elicited by an injection of myelin basic protein (MBP) in
complete Freund's adjuvant (CFA). The disease can be passively
transferred to syngenic recipient animals by means of an adequate
number of spleen cells incubated in vitro with Concanavaline A
(ConA; 1).

Passive EAE allows a selective investigation of the efferent
phase of the immune response in the CNS, and avoids inoculation
with CFA which may alter immunological findings. Furthermore,
effects of treatment with immunosuppressive agents can be sought
at different stages of the immune response, and tentative
hypothesis can be made about their mechanism of action.

We previously described the suppressive activity of the
vitamin A derivative Retinoic Acid (RA) on active EAE induced in
Lewis rats (2). In this study we investigated the effects of
RA on EAE passive transfer.

MATERIALS AND METHODS

Donor Lewis rats were immunized by intradermal injection of
guinea pig MBP and sacrificed on day 12 after immunization
(a.i.).

Spleen cells were collected and cultured for 72 hours in vitro in presence of ConA. Syngenic naive recipients were then injected intraperitoneally with 40 x 10^6 cells.

Treatment with RA was performed at three different levels:

-1) a group of donor rats received 75 mg/kg/day of RA, in two oral administrations, from day 6 to day 11 a.i. . Control animals received the drug eccipient (corn oil) only.

-2) 10^{-6} M RA, in DMSO, was added in vitro to some of the spleen cell cultures; DMSO only was added to the control cultures.

-3) a group of recipient rats was administered with 75 mg/kg/day of RA, in two oral administrations, from day 1 to day 6 after cell transfer. Control rats were treated with corn oil only.

RESULTS AND DISCUSSION

Treatment of donor rats did not affect the transfer of EAE. In fact, spleen cells harvested from RA-suppressed EAE donors were able to induce the disease in the recipients, after a 72 hour culture in presence of ConA. Incidence and clinical course of the disease in the recipients were comparable to those obtained with cells from non-treated donors (Tab.1).

This observation suggests a merely functional and reversible lymphocyte suppression induced by RA, and indirectly excludes a cytotoxic activity. Other data from in vitro studies seem to confirm this hypothesis (see Massacesi et al., in this book).

10^{-6} M RA added in vitro to the spleen cell cultures markedly reduced ConA-induced lymphoproliferative response.

Such treatment powerfully suppressed the capacity of spleen cells from EAE rats to transfer the disease after a 72 hour ConA-stimulated culture. None of 12 recipient rats developed the disease, versus 7 out of 9 controls (Tab.1).

Treatment of 12 recipient rats preserved these animals from developing passive EAE. None showed clinical signs, while 7 out of 9 controls developed the disease by day 7 after cell transfer (Tab.1).

Histological evaluation was performed on the spinal cord of some of the recipients. Non-treated recipients showed typical perivascular cuffs, even in cases in which only mild clinical signs of EAE were present. No histological alteration was present in the spinal cords of RA treated rats.

Suppression of passive EAE by treatment of recipients suggests a prominent action of RA on the efferent phase of the immune response.

We previously reported suppression of actively induced EAE

EFFECTS OF RA ON EAE PASSIVE TRANSFER

TREATMENT			N. OF SICK RATS
DONORS	IN VITRO	RECIPIENTS	
RA*	DMSO	OIL	9/9
OIL	RA≢	OIL	0/12
OIL	DMSO	RA^	0/12
OIL	DMSO	OIL	7/9

*RA 75mg/kg/day from day 6 o day 11; ≢RA 10−6 M in DMSO
^ RA 75 mg/kg/day from day 1 after transfer

beginning treatment with RA only 3 days before the expected onset of the disease (2), i.e. when lymphocyte activation and clonal expansion have already been accomplished (3).

These data, once a cytotoxic effect of the drug is excluded, would account for a highly specific immunosuppressive activity of RA on previously activated and expanded lymphocyte clones.

An inhibiting in vitro activity of RA has been reported on MHC class II antigen expression (4) and gamma-interferon production (5).

Moreover, RA suppresses ConA-induced lymphoproliferative response in vitro (6), which is strictly Interleukine-dependent. Also in vivo, a specific interaction with one or more lymphokines might therefore be the most probable mechanism for a selective immunosuppression by RA.

<u>REFERENCES</u>

1. Panitch H.S. and McFarlin D.E., 1977, J.Immunol., 119:1134
2. Massacesi L., Abbamondi A.L., Castigli E., Sarlo F., Lolli F. and Amaducci L., 1987, J. Neurol. Sci., 80:55.
3. Castigli E., Massacesi L., Sarlo F., Abbamondi A.L., Vergelli M., and Amaducci L., 1988, in Abstracts of the Ninth European Immunology Meeting, Rome, 14-17 September 1988.
4. Rhodes J. and Stokes P., 1982, Imunology, 45:531.
5. Abb J., Abb H. and Deinhardt F., 1982, Int. J. Cancer, 30:307
6. Massacesi L., Sarlo F., Abbamondi A.L., Castigli E., Olivotto J. and Amaducci L., 1988, in Abstracts of the Ninth European Immunology Meeting, Rome, 14-17 September 1988.

© 1989 Elsevier Science Publishers B.V. (Biomedical Division)
Recent advances in multiple sclerosis therapy.
R.E. Gonsette, P. ·Delmotte, editors.

SUPPRESSION OF EXPERIMENTAL ALLERGIC ENCEPHALOMYELITIS BY AN
INHIBITORY T CELL FACTOR

AIMO A. SALMI, DOUGLAS R. GREEN, MATIAS RÖYTTÄ, LIN XIAN WU, MANDI
WANG, AND REID BISSONNETTE
Department of Medical Microbiology and Department of Immunology,
University of Alberta, Edmonton, Alberta, Canada T6G 2H7, and
Department of Pathology, University of Turku, SF-20520 Turku,
Finland

INTRODUCTION

Infiltration of the central nervous system (CNS) by immune cells
and demyelination are common pathological features of experimental
allergic encephalomyelitis (EAE) and multiple sclerosis (MS). As the
basic process of demyelination is similar in both diseases, EAE can
be used as an animal model of MS in therapeutic studies aimed at
reducing the immunological reactions and demyelination.

A major goal of experimental EAE therapy is to reduce the number
or functions of T cells which are central for the disease process.
Antibodies inhibiting T cell activation reduce the EAE onset (1-4)
and cyclosporin A which reduces T cell activation blocks EAE
induction (5). Immunosuppressive T cell lines have been isolated
from animals with EAE (6). Such cells may secrete a nonspecific
immunological inhibitor (7-8).

In this communication, we describe a T cell line secreting an
antigen non-specific suppressor factor, a single injection of which
inhibits induction of acute EAE in SJL mice.

MATERIAL AND METHODS
Animals.

Four to six weeks old SJL mice were purchased from Jackson
Laboratories (Bar Harbour, ME). Animals were housed in plastic cages
and given food pellets and water *ad libitum*. Virus-infected mice
were kept in separate but similar housing quarters.
Preparation of suppressive factor (SF).

Spleen T cells from mice 7 days after burn trauma (9) were fused
with BW5147 thymoma cells using polyethylene glycol. Hybrid cells
were selected in the presence of HAT (Gibco) and cloned by limiting
dilution. Clones producing factors inhibiting primary anti-SRBC
response *in vitro* were further characterized. A clone, P3E5, was

found to produce a large quantity of a SF inhibiting different T cell functions (data to be published). Supernatants from this cell line were collected after 72 h in culture, stored at -70 C and used to treat SJL mice.

Induction of EAE.

Lyophilized mouse spinal chord (MSCH) was suspended in sterile PBS at a concentration of 60 mg/ml and mixed with equal volume of incomplete Freund's adjuvant (IFA) supplemented with 4 mg/ml of M. tuberculosis and 0.5 mg/ml of M. butyricum. A total of 0.1 ml of this mixture was injected into 4 footpads of each animal on day 0. On days 1 and 3 after injection, 3×10^9 B. pertussis bacteria in 0.1 ml were injected i.v. into each animal. Mice were monitored and the signs of clinical EAE observed daily. For histological evaluation, anesthetized mice were perfused with 5% glutaraldehyde and brains and spinal cords removed for histology.

Treatment of mice with SF.

Total of 0.2 ml of different dilutions of SF was injected intravenously to groups of mice 5 days before (-5), the day of EAE induction (0) or 5 days afterwards (+5). Groups of mice were left untreated. The onset of clinical EAE was recorded.s

RESULTS

We have earlier established a T cell hybridoma (P3E5) by fusing spleen cells from a mouse 7 days after a thermal trauma with BW5147 thymoma cells (data to be published). This hybridoma produces a large quantity of a suppressive factor which has the following properties: 1) it inhibits T cell responses in vitro and in vivo; 2) its activity is destroyed by proteases, boiling, or low pH suggesting that it is protein in nature; 3) no interferon-gamma or tumor necrosis factor activity is detected in the tissue culture supernatants; 4) preliminary data indicate that the activity is eluted from an exclusion chromatography column in a fraction with a molecular weight of 25,000 to 30,000.

Supernatant of in vitro grown P3E5 cells was injected intravenously to SJL mice at different times before and after induction of EAE. One 0.2 ml single injection of undiluted supernatant between day 5 before and day 5 after EAE induction abolished or significantly reduced clinical EAE (TABLE I).

TABLE I

EFFECT OF P3E5 SUPERNATANT INJECTION ON THE CLINICAL EAE IN SJL MICE.

SF injected on day	No. of sick animal/total no. of animals (%)		
	Day 14	Day 20	Day 26
-5	0/10	0/10	0/10
0	0/20	3/20 (15%)	5/20 (25%)
+5	0/10	1/10 (10%)	1/10 (10%)
No SF injection	6/32(19%)	22/32(69%)	25/32(78%)

Groups of animals were also injected with a single injection of different dilutions of the supernatant on day -5 before the EAE induction (TABLE II).

TABLE II

EFFECT OF DIFFERENT DILUTIONS OF P3E5 SUPERNATANT ON EAE INDUCTION IN SJL MICE.

Dilution of SF	No. of sick animal/total no. of animals (%)		
	Day 14	Day 20	Day 26
Undiluted	0/10	0/10	0/10
1/10	0/10	0/10	1/10 (10%)
1/100	0/10	3/10 (30%)	6/10 (60%)
No SF injection	5/17(30%)	11/17(65%)	13/17(77%)

The results show that undiluted or 1/10 diluted P3E5 supernatant almost completely inhibited the onset of clinical EAE and that supernatant diluted 1/100 still significantly delayed the onset of EAE. A 1/300 dilution of the SF had no significant effect (not shown).

The effect of SF on EAE development was confirmed by histological examinations. In samples from animals treated with undiluted SF at days -5, 0 or +5, no increased cellular infiltration or demyelination was observed. No demyelination was seen in the spinal cords of animals injected with 1/10 diluted SF but when the SF was diluted 1/100, focal demyelination lesions and cellular infiltrates were seen.

DISCUSSION

We have described a potent suppressive factor secreted by a T cell hybridoma which is a fusion product of a thymoma cell line and spleen cells from mice 7 days after burn trauma. Although the factor has not yet been fully characterized, preliminary evidence suggests that it is not related to any known suppressive factors. As it is non-specific in nature and exerts its action on T cells, it has a potential for therapeutic immunosuppression in autoimmune diseases without known triggering antigen.

The effect of the factor on EAE development was dramatic in this work. Not only was the development of demyelination inhibited but the invasion of the CNS by immune cells was also prevented. The factor seems to be very potent as one single 0.2 ml injection of 1/10 diluted tissue culture supernatant prevented EAE induction and histpathological changes. These results suggest that the factor could be considered as a therapeutic agent for reduction of the damage by the local immunological reaction during the exacerbation of MS. Characterization of the factor and studies in a chronic form of EAE should be carried out before human studies are feasible.

ACKNOWLEDGEMENTS

Grant support by the MS Society of Canada, the Alberta Heritage Foundation for Medical Research, and the Medical Research Council of Canada is acknowledged.

REFERENCES
1. Sriram S, Topham DJ, Carroll L (1987) J Immunol 139:1485-1489
2. Waldor MK, Sriram S, Hardy R, Herzenberg LA, Herzenberg LA, Lanier L, Lim M, Steinman, L (1985) Science 227:415-417
3. Sriram S, Roberts CA (1986) J Immunol 136:4464-4469
4. Acha-Orbea H, Mitchell DJ, Timmermann L, Wraith DC, Tausch GS,Waldor MK, Zamvil SS, McDevitt HO, Steinman L (1988) Cell 54:263-273
5. Bolton C, Allsop G, Cuzner ML (1982) Clin Exp Immunol 47:127-132
6. Ellerman KE, Powers JM, Brostoff SW (1988) Nature 331:265-267
7. Beraud ES, Varrials S, Farnarier C, Bernard D (1982) Eur J Immunol 12:926-9xx
8. Brostoff ES, Ellerman K, Olee T, Powers J (1989) In: Kaplan JG, Green DR, Bleackley RC (eds) Cellular Basis of Immune Modulation. Alan R. Liss, New York, pp 395-398
9. Kupper TS, Green DR, Durum SK, Baker CC (1985) Surgery 98:199-204

© 1989 Elsevier Science Publishers B.V. (Biomedical Division)
Recent advances in multiple sclerosis therapy.
R.E. Gonsette, P. Delmotte, editors.

SUPPRESSING EFFECT OF SULFASALAZINE ON EXPERIMENTAL AUTO-
IMMUNE ENCEPHALOMYELITIS

MARIO PROSIEGEL, INGO NEU*, GERHARD RUHENSTROTH-BAUER**
Neurological Department, Fachklinik Enzensberg, 8958 Hopfen
am See, *Neurological Department, City Hospital Sindelfingen,
7032 Sindelfingen, **Max-Planck-Institute for Biochemistry,
8032 München-Martinsried (West Germany)

INTRODUCTION

In experimental autoimmune encephalomyelitis (EAE), the animal model of the early "encephalitic phase" (1) of multiple sclerosis (MS), an increased venular permeability precedes the invasion of autoaggressive T-lymphocytes and macrophages from the
blood into the parenchyma of the central nervous system (2).

As we have previously suggested, the sulfidopeptide leukotriene
C_4 (LTC$_4$), a 5-lipoxygenase product of the arachidonic acid metabolism and one of the most important mediators of vascular permeability, might be involved in the pathogenesis of MS (3). In
addition, we have recently found that pharmacological blocking of
LTC$_4$ with the dual cyclo-oxygenase and lipoxygenase inhibitor
BW755C suppresses EAE (4). Since BW755C is toxic and, therefore,
supplied for non-human experimental use only, we subsequently
studied the effect of sulfasalazine, a substance with a proved
leukotriene inhibiting effect, which has previously been described to exert beneficial effects in patients with inflammatory
bowel diseases and rheumatoid arthritis, respectively (5).

MATERIAL AND METHODS

For the induction of EAE, 40 female Hartley guinea pigs were
sensitized with 20μ g of bovine myelin basic protein, as described elsewhere (4). After sensitization, the animals were randomly
selected for two groups of 20 animals. Group A was treated with
200 mg/kg/day (800 mg suspended in 20 ml of 1% methylcellulose in
distilled water) of sulfasalazine (Pharmacia Uppsala, Sweden) and
group B with 1 ml of 1% methylcellulose in distilled water. The
substances were injected subcutaneously, starting at day 10 after
sensitization. One animal in group B died immediately after sensitization of an unspecified cause. The remaining 39 animals were
scored blind daily for clinical symptoms (no or only slight paresis, severe paresis and/or coma) and killed on day 21. For the

histology, one block of spinal cord and four blocks of brain were embedded in paraplast and stained with the haematoxilin-eosin and Kelemen methods. The five blocks from each animal were scored blind according to the presence and extent of inflammatory in-filtrates: absent = 0, very mild = 1, mild = 2, moderate = 3, severe = 4. Further details on both clinical and histological scores are described elsewhere (6). The significance of observed differences (2-tailed probability) was assessed with the Mann-Whitney U-test (histological score) and chi-square test (clinical outcome).

RESULTS

As shown in table 1, there was a significantly better clinical outcome and a significantly lower histological inflammation score in group A as compared to group B.

TABLE 1

EFFECT OF SULFASALAZINE ON CLINICAL PICTURE AND HISTOLOGICAL SCORE IN GUINEA PIGS WITH EXPERIMENTAL AUTOIMMUNE ENCEPHALO-MYELITIS

	Sulfasalazine	Controls	P Value
No. of animals with severe symptoms	3	9	0.0286
Histological Score (Means±SD)	7.5±6.5	15.4±7.0	0.0011

DISCUSSION

Since two different leukotriene inhibiting substances, BW755C and sulfasalazine, have now been proved to suppress EAE, clinical trials with sulfasalazine seem to be justified in patients with MS after their informed consent.

REFERENCES

1. Wekerle H, Melms A (1985) Allergologie 11: 469-475
2. Mc Donald WI (1988) The Natural History of the MS Lesion. Presented at the international Multiple Sclerosis Conference, Rome, September 14-17

3. Prosiegel M, Neu I, Wildfeuer A, et al (1987) Acta Neurol Scand 75: 361-363

4. Prosiegel M, Neu I, Wildfeuer A, et al (1989) Acta Neurol Scand 79: 223-226

5. Peskar BM, Dreyling KW, May B, et al (1987) Dig Dis Sci 32 (Suppl): 51-56

6. Scherer R, Simon J, Abd-el-Fattah, et al (1980) Immunol 40: 49-59

THE ROLE OF MAST CELLS IN DEMYELINATION

P.SEELDRAYERS, D. YASUI, H.L. WEINER AND D. JOHNSON
Center for Neurologic Diseases, Brigham and Women's Hospital, Boston,
MA 02115, U.S.A.

Mast cells were initially described as cells with prominent cytoplasmic granules staining metachromatically with cationic dyes. Another characteristic is that they bear high affinity surface receptors for IgE. Cross-linking of mast cell-associated IgE by the corresponding antigen leads to degranulation during which the contents of the granules are released to the exterior. These granules contain vasoactive amines such as serotonin and histamine, and neutral proteases. Chemoattractants are also synthetized in response to the degranulating stimulus and are released along with the granule contents. Mast cells are widespread throughout the body and are present in the peripheral nervous system (PNS), where they occupy strategic positions between blood vessels and myelin sheaths. Mast cells are also present in the central nervous system (CNS), again in perivascular locations, particularly the leptomeninges, the adjacent cortical area and the thalamus (1). It is of interest that, in both the CNS and the PNS, we have found a positive correlation between the density of nervous system mast cells and the susceptibility of various mouse and rat strains to develop experimental allergic encephalomyelitis (EAE) or experimental allergic neuritis (EAN) (2).

Mast cells have been shown to degranulate early in the development of EAN and the release of vasoactive amines by the degranulating mast cells has been linked to the appearance of perivascular and perineurial oedema (3,4). In addition, we have shown that incubation of mast cell degranulation supernatant with bovine PNS myelin leads to an extensive loss of P0 protein, suggesting that mast cell proteases could contribute to the demyelination in the inflammatory lesions in the PNS (5). Although the cause of mast cell degranulation in EAN is not known, we have found IgE positive cells in the sciatic nerves of EAN animals and not in the control animals, using a monoclonal antibody against the heavy chain of IgE. If this IgE were to play an active role in EAN, the most likely specificity of this cell associated IgE would be against P2, the main neuritogenic protein of the PNS myelin. As Lewis rats are known to have low titers of serum IgE, we have used a sensitive functional assay based on the

208

degranulation of rat basophil leukemia cells incubated successively with EAN serum and with the corresponding antigen (6). By this method, testing rat serum at day 0, 10 and 18 post inoculation with PNS myelin and complete Freund's adjuvant, we were able to demonstrate a progressive increase in the level of serum IgE, which we have shown is specific to the P2 protein. Similarly, we have found IgE positive cells in the CNS of rats with EAE and IgE antibodies against myelin basic protein in their serum.

To further assess the importance of mast cell degranulation in the initiation and the extension of the demyelinating lesions, we have treated EAN rats with nedocromil sodium (Fisons Pharmaceuticals, U.K.), an anti inflammatory drug with mast cell stabilizing properties, and found that treatment with nedocromil sodium 150mg/kg, three times daily starting on day 7 after disease induction, significantly decreased the incidence and reduced the severity of EAN (7). Preliminary experiments show that this drug at the same dose can also delay the onset and decrease the severity of EAE.

REFERENCES

1/ Olsson Y. (1968)   Mast cells in the nervous system   International Review of Cytology Bourne G.H., Danielli J.F. and Jeon K.W. (Eds), 24: 27-70

2/ Seeldrayers P.A., Yasui D., Levin L., Toms R., Johnson D. (1988) Studies of nervous system mast cells Trans. Am. Soc. For Neurochem. vol 19 (1), 55

3/ Powell H.C., Braheny S.L., Myers R.R., Rodriguez M. and Lampert P.W. (1983)   Early changes in experimental allergic neuritis.   Lab. Invest., 48: 332-338

4/ Brosnan C.F. and Tansey F.A. (1984) Delayed onset of experimental allergic neuritis in rats treated with Reserpine J. Neuropath. Exp. Neurol., 43: 84-93

5/ Johnson D., Seeldrayers P.A. and Weiner H.L. (1988) The role of mast cells in demyelination. 1. Myelin proteins are degraded by mast cell proteases and myelin basic protein and P2 can stimulate mast cell degranulation. Brain Res., 444: 195-198

6/ Conklyn M.J. and Showell H.J. (1987) Guinea pig IgE sensitizes rat basophil leukemia (RBL2H3) cells. 16th ann. meeting New England Pharmacol., Abstr. 23

7/ Seeldrayers P.A., Yasui D., Weiner H.L. and Johnson D. (1989) Treatment of experimental allergic neuritis with nedocromil sodium (J.Neuroimmunol. submitted for publication)

© 1989 Elsevier Science Publishers B.V. (Biomedical Division)
Recent advances in multiple sclerosis therapy.
R.E. Gonsette, P. Delmotte, editors.

211

CELL MEDIATED IMMUNE MECHANISMS IN MULTIPLE SCLEROSIS AND THE
IMPLICATIONS FOR TREATMENT

SAMANTHA OWEN, VIRGINIA CALDER, CAROLYN WATSON, ALAN DAVISON
Department of Neurochemistry, Institute of Neurology, Queen Square,
London WC1N 3BG, UK

INTRODUCTION

Using developing rodent CNS explants it has been claimed that
demyelinating activity present in the serum of some MS patients is
due to a toxic factor or to antibody directed against myelin or
oligodendrocytes. This activity is not specific to MS since
demyelination occurs with sera from healthy controls and other
neurological diseases. In addition peripheral blood T lymphocyte
(PBL) supernatants from MS relapse patients induces demyelination
in rat organ cultures. Supernatants from mitogen stimulated
healthy PBL's also showed demyelinating activity suggesting that
soluble factors produced by lymphocytes cause demyelination.

Interpretation of these experiments is complicated because endogenous macrophages and glia are present in tissue culture systems
and quantitative evaluation of the demyelination is difficult by
microscopy. To overcome these problems we have developed a biochemical method to quantitatively assess myelin degradation by serum
or peripheral blood mononuclear cells (PBMC). The assay measures
the release of 2'-3' cyclic nucleotide 3'-phosphodiesterase
(CNPase) from a human cell free myelin preparation. CNPase, the
main component of the Wolfgram protein fraction, has been shown to
be a reliable marker of myelin degradation. We have studied the
effect of serum or cells from MS patients at different stages of
disease activity, with other disease groups including the autoimmune inflammatory disease rheumatoid arthritis (RA).

MATERIALS AND METHODS

Patients. Blood was collected from 108 patients with clinically
probable MS. The group of other demyelinating diseases included
transverse myelitis and unidentified demyelinating disease,
none had oligoclonal IgG production in the CSF. The inflammatory
other neurlogical disease (OND) group included Guillian Barre syndrome, cerebrovascular disease and ventricular shunt. Non inflammatory OND cases included epilepsy, gait disorder, tumour, motor

neurone disease and cerebellar ataxia. None of the healthy volunteers or patients were on immunosuppressive therapy. In the RA
group 20 out of 31 patients were on some form of immunosuppressive
therapy.

Myelin degradation assay. Triplicate samples of human myelin were
incubated with serum (25% v/v) or PBMC in a ratio of 10μg myelin
protein : 2x10⁵ PBMC in 96 well plates for 24h at 37oC. Triplicate
samples of myelin alone were incubated as a control. The CNPase
activity of the myelin alone and myelin plus cells or serum pellet
was assayed fluorometrically as described in (1). Results are
expressed as % loss of CNPase activity of myelin when incubated
with cells or serum. Losses equivalent to or greater than 17% were
statistically significant ($p < 0.05$).

RESULTS

In contrast to the findings of previous authors only 2/35 sera
from MS patients showed significant degradation of myelin in vitro.
There was no correlation between serum or cellular demyelinating
activity (see RA results in Table 1).

TABLE 1

EFFECT OF SERUM AND PBMC ON MYELIN DEGRADATION IN VITRO

Clinical group	Serum or PBMC causing significant* CNPase loss from myelin	
	SERUM	PBMC
Multiple sclerosis	2/35 (6%)	40/108 (37%)
Other demyelinating diseases	0/5	3/8 (37.5%)
Other neurological diseases (non-inflammatory)	1/9 (11%)	0/11
Rheumatoid arthritis	1/12 (8%)	21/31 (67%)
Healthy controls	0/7	0/20

*% Loss CNPase from myelin >17% ($p < 0.05$).

The degradative activity of serum from other disease groups and
healthy controls was also negligible. It therefore seems that demyelinating factors previously detected in serum are acting directly
on the oligodendrocyte and not primarily on the myelin. However

significant losses of CNPase were seen with MS PBMC incubated with myelin, 37% of the 108 patients tested caused losses greater than 17% but this degradative activity did not correlate with disease status (Table 2). Similar results were seen with cells from patients with other demeylinating diseases. The OND groups and healthy controls showed no significant myelin degradation (Table 1).

TABLE 2

EFFECT OF MS PBMC ON MYELIN DEGRADATION IN VITRO

Clinical Status	PBMC samples causing significant* CNPase loss from myelin
Stable	8/17 (47%)
Active	6/11 (54.5%)
Relapse	8/17 (47%)
Progressive	18/63 (28.5%)

*$p < 0.05$ Students t-test

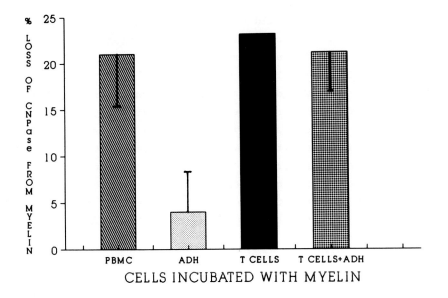

Fig.1. Myelin degradation by MS PBMC. $2x10^5$ PBMC, $2x10^4$ monocytes (ADH), $2x10^5$ T cells, or $2x10^4$ ADH plus $2x10^5$ T cells were incubated in triplicate with 10μg human myelin. Data as mean (±SD) for 4 relapsing remitting cases of MS. All losses significantly different from control myelin ($p < 0.05$) except for ADH cells alone.

In Figure 1 the effect of different cell populations from MS PBMC on myelin degradation in vitro is shown and suggests that T cells and or soluble factors produced by them may be able to cause myelin degradation in vitro.

In summary we show that PBMC from 38% of MS and 67% of RA patients caused in vitro myelin degradation. Thus the action of the cells or their products is not restricted to MS but is probably a non-specific cellular response shown by chronically stimulated T cells occuring in inflammatory autoimmune diseases.

DISCUSSION

In MS we propose that it is a centrally mediated disease where a myelin antigen is presented by astrocyte or microglia to resident lymphocytes within the brain parenchyma. Recruitment or peripheral inflammatory cells leads to further release of cytokines, macrophage activation and eventual localised demyelination with some demyelinating cells crossing the blood brain barrier. It is these circulating cells which are chronically stimulated that we think cause myelin degradation in vitro. In RA a similar initiation and progression of immune reactivity would occur in the synovial joints and not the CNS as with MS. There would be a circulation of T cells which are highly activated and which we detect in the blood that non-specifically degrade myelin in vitro.

If MS is a peripherally mediated disease, immunosuppressants such as azathioprine and cyclosporin A would be expected to be quite potent therapeutic agents, but previous clinical trials have shown there to be only mild benefit. However drugs which are known to cross the blood brain barrier such as methylprednisolone and cyclophosphamide are beneficial in shortening relapse rate suggesting that MS is a centrally mediated disease. We therefore suggest that there is a need to concentrate on developing low toxicity centrally acting immunosuppressants.

ACKNOWLEDGEMENTS
This work was supported by the MS Society of Great Britain and the Medical Research Council.

REFERENCES
1. Watson CM, Najbauer J, Owen SJ, Davison AN (1988) J. Neurochem. 50:1469-1477.

© 1989 Elsevier Science Publishers B.V. (Biomedical Division)
Recent advances in multiple sclerosis therapy.
R.E. Gonsette, P. Delmotte, editors.

THE GENETIC LINKAGE STRATEGY USING DNA MARKERS, AND ITS APPLI-
CATION TO FAMILIAL MULTIPLE SCLEROSIS, INHERITED ATAXIAS, AND
SPASTIC PARAPARESES

HELMUT ZANDER

Immunogenetics Laboratory, Kinderpoliklinik, University of Munich,
Pettenkoferstr. 8a, 8000 München 2, West Germany

INTRODUCTION

Unlike classic biochemical disease research, the genetic linkage strategy using DNA markers allows an approach toward the molecular understanding of enigmatic diseases without prior knowledge or assumptions concerning the biochemical nature of a defect.
The aim is to move from linked polymorphic markers to the very
true gene that causes the disease, or that confers susceptibility,
to sequence it, to delineate its product - i.e., to identify the
molecule that is involved in the pathogenesis -, to study the products function, and - ultimately - to modulate this function, thus
providing a molecular basis for prevention and therapy.

The approach is ambitious as well as laborious, but it is feasible and has a good chance of success.

The essential requirements, however, are (1) that genetic elements do exist in the pathogenesis of the disease, and (2), clinically, that multiple case families are available for study.

MATERIAL AND METHODS

In 1974 and 1975, questionnaires were mailed to 15.000 patient
members of the MS society and to 4.000 neurologists in West Germany, in order to ascertain multiple case families. In the first
phase it was decided to focus the study on sib-pair double case
families. In 1978 through 1982, all patients who could be motivat-
ed to participate in the study were visited at home, neurological-
ly reexamined by the author, and clinically documented. This effort involved 55.000 km of travel. All available hospital and con-
sultant records were reevaluated. Thus, 33 sib-pair double case
families with MS were available for study, with 28 families having
2 siblings with clinically definite disease. In five families, one
sib had definite MS and the other one probable or possible MS
according to the diagnostic criteria of Schumacher, 2nd revision.

216

Any careful neurologist studying multiple case families with MS
will meet with inherited ataxias and spastic parapareses. A series
of multiple case families which, upon careful clinical reexamina-
tion, were reclassified to suffer from inherited ataxias or spastic
parapareses rather than from MS has been excluded from the MS
sample. Their records were put on file for forthcoming DNA studies.

Conventional, i.e., non-DNA based laboratory analyses of the MS
families were performed for HLA-A,B,C,DR, and GLO markers located
on the short arm of chromosome 6,
- further, in cooperation with other research laboratories, for
the complement factor polymorphisms of C2, Bf, C4A, C4B, located
on the same chromosome within the HLA complex,
- for the complement factor polymorphisms of C3 and C6,
- for quantitative serum levels of the complement factors C2, C4,
and C3, since a hypocomplementemia of C2 had been postulated by
other authors to play a role in MS,
- for the IgG heavy chain markers Gm on chromosome 14, and for
the closely linked alpha 1-antitrypsin polymorphisms, and
- for three parameters of the natural killing(NK)/interferon(IFN)
system in vitro using nonadherent lymphocytes from peripheral
blood: (1) Spontaneous and (2) IFN-beta inducible NK activity, and
(3) production of IFN-alpha and IFN-gamma in response to viral and
nonviral stimuli.

RESULTS
The first 13 families of our sample - i.e., 26 patients all having clinically definite MS and 37 healthy siblings and parents -
were incorporated as the largest single contribution into the joint
analysis of the 8th International Histocompatibility Workshop, Los
Angeles, 1980 (8). This Workshop, analysing 53 multiple case pedi-
grees with MS, accepted a genetic linkage of at least one major
determinant for susceptibility to MS with HLA with a maximum lod
score of 3.93. Additional factors not linked with HLA were postulated but could not be identified (8).
In our entire sampling of 33 sib-pair double case families, HLA-
DR2 occurred in 24 out of 33 propositi, i.e., in 72.7% vs 25.2% in
healthy Caucasian controls. Genotypically, HLA-DR2 was present in
28 out of 66 propositus haplotypes (42.4% vs. 13.3% in controls).

With regard to the complement factor polymorphisms located
within the HLA complex, MS seemed to be more closely associated
with C4 A4,B2 than with HLA-DR2 (9,10). The other markers that
have been studied showed neither association nor linkage, or they
were not informative (9,10).

DISCUSSION

The HLA-D/DR loci on the short arm of chromosome 6 are the
only marker loci so far that have been unequivocally established
to include or to neighbor at least one gene that must be involved
in the pathogenesis of MS (8). Our observation of an even closer
association of MS with C4 A4,B2 than with HLA-DR2 remains to be
confirmed. C4 maps telomeric from HLA-D/DR. There is evidence for
an additional very close association of MS with an RFLP-defined
polymorphism in a non-coding region centromeric from HLA (4).
Markers for MS on other chromosomes include a T-cell receptor
V-alpha and C-alpha polymorphism (5).

In January 1984, at a Ciba House symposium in London, the participants felt that the one or more susceptibility genes for MS were
ready for focusing on by DNA biochemistry in a coordinated international effort. At this symposium, the 33 families from Germany
were offered for international cooperation. These 33 families were
considered a unique clinical and immunogenetically well-defined
basis for genetic linkage studies using DNA markers. But, clinical
support for doing the patient-related part of the work could not
be obtained.

High priority should be given to the study of polymorphisms in
non-coding, regulatory DNA sequences that could determine susceptibility to MS (4). Polymorphisms in regulatory DNA sequences
may influence the quantitative expression of HLA molecules and/or
the quantitative production of tumor necrosis factors (TNF) that
map within the HLA complex. Increased production of TNF by peripheral blood cells (2) - as well as elevated serum levels of soluble
interleukin-2 receptors (1) - have recently been found to precede
clinical relapses of MS. TNF is known to have a broad spectrum of
major effects on vascular endothelial cells (6). Thus, TNF is likely to play a key role in opening the blood-brain-barrier in MS. The
opening of this barrier is a crucial event in the development of
the early MS lesion. TNF is an essential mediator in murine cere-

218

bral malaria. Thus, mice susceptible to cerebral invasion of
malaria parasites could be protected by anti-TNF antibodies (3).
This observation elicits hope for MS patients. If such conjec-
tures as briefly outlined above can be substantiated for human
MS by basic studies, anti-TNF antibody should be tried for treatment and prevention of a bout.

ACKNOWLEDGEMENTS
   These studies have been supported by Deutsche Forschungsgemeinschaft, Za 59/1/2/3/5, by Habilitations-Stipendium Za 59/4, and
by Stiftung Volkswagenwerk, Akademiestipendium, Az. 11 2745.

REFERENCES
1. Adachi K et al (1989) Interleukin-2 receptor levels indicating
    relapse in multiple sclerosis. Lancet 1989 I:559-560
2. Beck J et al (1988) Increased production of interferon gamma
    and tumor necrosis factor precedes clinical manifestation in
    multiple sclerosis. Acta Neurol Scand 78:318-323
3. Grau GE et al (1987) Tumor necrosis factor as an essential
    mediator in murine cerebral malaria. Science 237:1210-1212
4. Heard RNS et al (1988) Detection of HLA class II restriction
    fragment length polymorphisms in multiple sclerosis.
    In: Cazzullo CL et al (eds) Virology and Immunology in
    Multiple Sclerosis. Springer Verlag, Berlin, pp 55-63
5. Oksenberg JR et al (1989) T-cell receptor V-alpha and C-alpha
    alleles associated with multiple sclerosis and myasthenia
    gravis. Proc Natl Acad Sci 86:988-992
6. Pober JS (1987) Effects of tumour necrosis factor and related
    cytokines on vascular endothelial cells. In: Bock G, Marsh J
    (eds) Tumour Necrosis Factor and Related Cytotoxins. Wiley,
    Chichester (Ciba Found Symp 131), pp 170-184
7. Steinman L et al (1981) In vivo effects of antibodies to immune
    response gene products: Prevention of experimental allergic
    encephalitis. Proc Natl Acad Sci 78:7111-7114
8. Tiwari JL et al (1985) Multiple sclerosis. In: Tiwari JL, Tera-
    saki PI (eds) HLA and Disease Associations. Springer Verlag,
    New York, pp 152-167
9. Zander H (1985) Clinical and immunogenetic data of 33 double
    case families with multiple sclerosis: A starting point for
    further analyses on the DNA level. In: Hommes O (ed) Multiple
    Sclerosis Research in Europe. MTP, Lancaster, pp 333-336
10. Zander H (1988) DNA and multiple sclerosis, inherited ataxias,
    and spastic parapareses. Adv Neurol 48:167-174

COMPUTERIZATION OF MS PATIENTS DATA:
AN EUROPEAN PROPOSAL

© 1989 Elsevier Science Publishers B.V. (Biomedical Division)
Recent advances in multiple sclerosis therapy.
R.E. Gonsette, P. Delmotte, editors.

COMPUTERIZATION OF MULTIPLE SCLEROSIS PATIENT DATA

CHRISTIAN CONFAVREUX*, ALBERT BIRON**, THIBAUT MOREAU*,

PHILIPPE MESSY**, JEAN-JACQUES VENTRE* and GILBERT AIMARD*

* Clinique de Neurologie, Hôpital Neurologique, and ** Département Informatique des Hospices Civils de Lyon, 59 boulevard Pinel, 69003 Lyon (France).

A COMMON MS DATABASING SYSTEM: WHY?

There is a clear need for a common databasing technique in Multiple Sclerosis (MS) with standardization in data collection, storage and retrieval. A common language promotes data and results sharing. Tracking of appropriate patients is made easier and faster for any research purpose, e.g. biological assays or therapeutic trials. We must keep in mind that, with the increasing number of neurologists, MS patients are referred to a number of centers which are not necessarily MS clinics or University Hospitals, at least during the first stages of the disease.

Several systems have been presented during the last years. Most of them have not successfully stood the test of time, often because they were too sophisticated and time consuming for a general use in the clinical wards. The Lyon MS database (LMSDTB) system is running continuously since 1976 and concerns, to date, more than 1200 patients. We present briefly here a modified version of this system which could serve as a basis of discussion for the anticipated common databasing system. This is the concise version (see below) of the system. The first step is, indeed, to reach a general agreement about the nature of the minimal clinical data to be collected for any MS patient and the way of collecting them.

A COMMON MS DATABASING SYSTEM: HOW?

System design and processing:

There are two different kinds of customers for such a system: physicians who deal with MS patients and are interested in their follow-up but, not necessarily, in personal research in this disease. They need a concise system easily allowing the collection and the retrieval of pertinent data. Others are involved in MS research and are ready to spend time enough to enter extensive data. They need an extensive system. For these

Fig. 1. First part of the LMSDTB system, concise version. It is devoted to patient identification, diagnostic confidence and disability chronology. Note this part is unique for any patient. It is updated when and where necessary.

Lyon MS database.

Code Number: |___|___|___|___|

PATIENT:
Name: |_____| given name: |_____|
Sex : |__| (M,F)
1st examination in the department: date: |___|___| (month, year)
Birth: date: |___|___|___| (day, month, year)
         place: France: county: |___| city: ....
                    abroad: |___|
Non caucasian: ☐   specify: ....
Other MS cases in the family: ☐   checked by a neurologist: |__| (no=0,yes=1,unknown=9)
MS onset residence: France: county: |___| city: ....
                        abroad: |___|
Present   address: |_____
_____| phone: |___|___|___|___|

PHYSICIAN: Name: |_____|
Address: |_____
_____| phone: |___|___|___|___|

DIAGNOSIS:

CLASSIFICATION:

Anatomic verification .. ☐
Space dissemination ...☐ ....date: |___|___| (month, year)
     Nevraxis: clinical ... ☐   SEP..☐   BAEP..☐   CT scan..☐   MRI..☐
     Optic nerve: clinical ... ☐   VEP..☐
Time dissemination .....☐ ....date: |___|___| (month, year)
Cerebro-Spinal Fluid ...☐ ....date: |___|___| (month, year)
          pleiocytosis ...... ☐   plasmocytosis ..... ☐
          increased IgG .... ☐   oligoclonal bands . ☐
"Wait and see" ....☐

PARACLINICAL EXAMS PERFORMED TO DATE:
     VEP ....☐   BAEP ....☐   SEP ....☐
     Myelography......☐   CT Scan ....☐
     Angiography.....................cerebral ....☐ ....spinal ......☐
     MRI ....cerebral ....☐ ....spinal ......☐
     Lumbar puncture ☐

RESIDUAL DISABILITY - DECEASE CHRONOLOGY:

(month, year)
03. Unable to run, unlimited walking .... |___|___|
04. Limited walking, > 1 000 m .... |___|___|
05. Limited walking, 500 - 1 000 m .... |___|___|
06. Limited walking, ± 100 m, cane(s)..................................... |___|___|
07. Home restricted, ambulation by walls or furniture assistance .... |___|___|
08. Wheelchair restricted, transfer > 0 .... |___|___|
09. Bed-ridden, transfer < 0 .... |___|___|
10. Decease .... |___|___|
          MS related .... ☐   MS unrelated.... ☐   specify: ....

reasons, it has been decided to prepare 2 versions of the system. These 2 versions are compatible. More concretely, the concise version is made of the minimal common data which are to be obtained from any patient. It is runnable on personal microcomputers of PC or MacIntosh type. Furthermore, it is connectable with a central computer, on which the extensive version must be runned owing to the size of the document.

Whatever the version, this system is flexible, i.e. compatible with any extension a customer could desire. These adaptations of the system can be temporary or lasting.

Chart design:

Several principles have been followed for the chart design:

- clarity, with no ambiguity in the proposed items or scales;

- convenient use and fast completion, compatible with current clinical activities;

- priority to symptoms in order to assure an uniform way of collecting data: during the course of the disease in a given patient, there are, inevitably, some periods without direct information and for which it must be relied on retrospective data;

- priority to analytic data: only uncorrected data are directly entered in the chart. Classifications about diagnostic confidence, clinical course, disease severity, topographic forms, ... for any given case are automatically generated by the computer from appropriate algorythms. This is time saving for the physician in charge of the updating of the system. An other advantage is that this way of processing allows any secondary modification in any classification without implicating original data: algorythms only, not the data, are then to be modified.

- attractivity: "secondary benefits" must automatically be provided by the system which thus becomes an efficient help for the clinician in the patient's survey. Beside the already quoted algorythms, the system is designed in order to automatically generate a "disease course diagram" for any patient (Figure 3).

THE TENTATIVE "LMSDTB" SYSTEM:

The document for each MS patient is made of 2 parts. The first part (Figure 1) is devoted to patient's identification, diagnostic confidence and non reversible disability chronology. Its size is fixed, i.e. each time new data are obtained in these fields, they are entered by modifying or completing the corresponding spaces of the document.

Fig. 2. Second part of the LMSDTB system, concise version. For any patient, one chart is used for each "disease event" and for each "current status" (see definitions in the text).

Lyon MS database.

EVENT CHART / CURRENT STATUS:

✦ Patient code number .... ⌊_⌊_⌊_⌊_⌋

✦ Data nature : "event chart" (=1)
"current status" (=2) ⌊_⌋

✦ Location in MS course: Date: ⌊_⌊_⌊_⌋ (day, month, year)

    Relapsing - remitting phase: ⌊_⌋ (no=0, yes=1)

        disease onset relapse (=1)
        subsequent relapse (=2)
        remission (=3)
        unreliable relapse chronology or counting (=4) ⌊_⌋ type: ⌊_⌋ (P,I,W,N)

    Chronic - progressive phase: ⌊_⌋ (no=0, yes=1)

        onset (=1)
        course (=2) ⌊_⌋ concurrent relapse: ⌊_⌋ (no=0, yes=1)

✦ Immunological treatments :

                                       starting   stopping

    Steroids .... ☐ .... ⌊_⌋ .... ⌊_⌋
    Azathioprine .... ☐ .... ⌊_⌋ .... ⌊_⌋
    Others (specify) .... ⌊___⌋ .... ⌊_⌋ .... ⌊_⌋

                          0=on the way,
                          1=<1 week,
                          2=1 week-1 month,
                          3=>1 month.

✦ Disability level ... ⌊___⌋ = maximum level observed during the given period in case of "event chart";
                         = current level in case of "current status".

                                    L U S S   BS   O M O
                                      E E S P O T F V B N T T
✦ Symptoms ....☐☐☐☐☐☐☐☐☐☐☐☐

                                    P C S S   BS   O M O
                                      Y E S P O T F V B N T T
✦ Signs .... ☐☐☐☐☐☐☐☐☐☐☐☐

Fig. 3. The automatically generated "disease course diagram" for a fictitious MS patient.

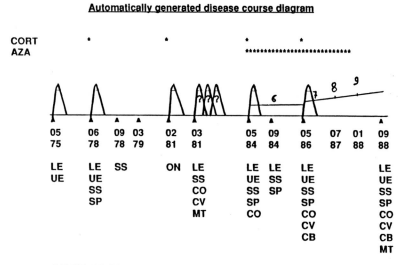

Automatically generated disease course diagram

(LE, UE, SS, SP, CO, CT, CF, CV, CB, ON, MT, OT).

The second part (Figure 2) has 2 purposes:

- describe any "disease event" (disease onset, relapses, progression onset) in terms of maximum disability level, symptoms, signs and concurrent treatments. The succession of "disease event charts" is central for the design of the "disease course diagram" (Figure 3);

- describe the "current status" of the patient each time the patient has been examined in the department. For the sake of convenience, effort has been made that disease events and current status are described on similar charts. The succession of "current status charts" can be used as consecutive neurological scores referred to time. The latest current status entered for a given patient provides the date of the last examination of this patient in the department.

In this second part, for any patient, one chart is completed for each disease event and each current status.

PERSPECTIVES:

The document which is presented here is the concise version of the LMSDTB system. Following the round-table devoted to "computerization of MS patient data" during the 5th ECTRIMS Congress, it has been sent to the more than 30 centers in Europe who were interested for testing it. They have been asked to return comments and suggestions about the system. Following this stage, the final program will be written. It may be anticipated it will be available for personal use by the beginning of 1990. In the meantime, any person interested for testing it or getting further informations about it may contact one of us (C.C.) at the above address.

ACKNOWLEDGEMENTS:

This work is supported by "Les Hospices Civils de Lyon" and by a grant from "La Ligue Française contre la Sclérose En Plaques" (LFSEP) and "L'Association pour la Recherche sur la Sclérose En Plaques" (ARSEP).

FREE COMMUNICATIONS

© 1989 Elsevier Science Publishers B.V. (Biomedical Division)
Recent advances in multiple sclerosis therapy.
R.E. Gonsette, P. Delmotte, editors.

ASSESSMENT OF THE NEUROLOGICAL IMPAIRMENT AND PROGRESSION IN MULTIPLE SCLEROSIS

WOJCIECH CENDROWSKI

The Neurological Out-Patients' Department, 00127 Warsaw, Sliska 5, Poland

The evaluation of neurological impairment and natural progression or the estimation of efficacy of therapeutical trials in multiple sclerosis /MS/ require quantitative and qualitative rating systems, Kurtzke /8/, Kuzma et al. /9/, Sheikh /14/. The assessment of neurological impairment comprises at least a twofold widely known system of defining disability /Disability Status Scale, DSS/ and of impairment itself /Functional Systems Scale, FSS/, Kurtzke /8/. The assessment of progression in MS is more difficult and complex because of variability of evolutive parameters. Progression in MS is a succession of quantities in which there is constant relation between each numerical score and the one of succeding it /3/. So-called progression year /7/, progression index /5, 13/, mean DSS score /2/ or severity grades /12/ have been put forward as estimates of the evolution of MS.

The purpose of this study is to assess the neurological impairment and natural progression using refined functional systems scale /RFSS/. An effort was made to compare the scores of this rating scale with grades at DSS in cross-sectional view or longitudinally over time.

CLINICAL MATERIAL AND METHOD

Clinical material. The study included 10 MS patients /6 women and 4 men/ in whom the disease was diagnosed after complete clinical examination. The diagnosis of remittent MW was made in 4 patients, remittent-progressive course in 4 patients and slowly progressive evolution in 2 patients. The assessment of neurological impairment was carried out at least twice by means of standard neurological examination, by RFSS and DSS. All patients were followed averagely over the period of 53.5 months.

Construction of rating scale. A refined functional systems scale /RFSS/ consisted of 4 fourfold item scales /pyramidal, cerebellar, superficial and deep sensory/, 1 double /visual/ and 9 sinle item scales /brain-stem, mental and bladder functions/ designed to quantify the results of the neurological examination. The scales varied from 1 /minimal or slight abnormality/ to 3 /severe deficit or loss of function/ except of pyramidal signs and visual acuity. All details of the RFSS were published by the author elsewhere /6/.

Rating of the neurological impairment. Steps on the scale were treated as real numbers and calculations of sums and means of scores were carried out. Intrarater reliability of RFSS used in this study was shown by three different evaluation methods. The methods were standard neurological examination, the difference between initial and consecutive score at RFSS, and the correlation between mean RFSS score and mean DSS degree.

The assessment of clinical progression. Numerical rating of clinical progression was attempted using mean annual RFSS score in 10 MS patients.

Statistical analysis. Pearson's correlation coefficient was used in the calculation of relationship between mean scores of scales /1/.

RESULTS

The initial score at RFSS ranged from 10 to 27 points /mean 16.6/ in 10 patients with clinically definite MS. Consecutive numerical estimate varied after averagely 53.5 months from 13 up to 32 /mean 22.9/. As group of MS patients worsened, they tended to worsen in some functional systems. The neurological impairment judged on rating scale was very slight in 2 patients /13 to 17 points/, slight in 5 /19 to 23/ and moderate in 3 /29 to 32 pts./. The difference between initial and final score /from -1 to -14/ reflected the severity of clinical deterioration. The Pearson's coefficient r between initial mean RFSS score and mean DSS degree was statistically significant / r = 0.808/. However, the comparison of mean scores at clinical follow-up failed to show such correlation / r = 0. 169/. The latter coefficient might depend on limited number of patients, relatively short period of follow-up or on other variables.

The assessment of clinical progression was carried out after almost 4 and half years in 10 MS patients. Mean annual RFSS score increased from 0.24 to 0.96 in 4 remittent patients. It suggested minimal or even decelerating clinical progression. In the remaining 6 patients either with remittent-progressive or slowly progressive course higher values from 1.2 up to 12.0

points seemed to reflect rather accelerating clinical progression. In some patients pyramidal and cerebellar signs have contributed more to the progression of the disease than other signs did. Pyramidal signs were scored too low, whereas in other patients acute retrobulbar neuritis or transient brain-stem signs were evaluated relatively too high. The latter scoring, including mean annual RFSS score, might give false impression of accelerated clinical progression.

DISCUSSION

With RFSS individual types of impairment can be followed over time in the same groups of patients or individuals for either dysfunction, natural history, rehabilitation or drug treatment purposes. However, this scale can not relate types of dysfunction to overall disability in different groups of patients. Therefore besides of the use of RFSS the employment of DSS and other scales is inevitable /8/.

The ideal scale for the assessment of the neurological impairment in MS has to be simple, accurate, valid, reliable and reproducible. Matthews /11/ has made fine remark that reliable rating scale in MS should split the difference of scores between minutiae and massive signs. One has to make choice between proper scoring of very subtle signs and too coarse abnormalities. Another problem is relatively low frequency of some neurological signs which should be omitted in the evaluation of the impairment. Forced crying or laughing, dysphasia, dysphagia, involuntary movements and others were not evaluated in the RFSS. The frequency of these signs does not exceed 15 % of necropsy proved series, Cendrowski et al. /4/. Cognitive impairment and sexual disturbances require separate and additional scales /15/.

Interrater reliability of RFSS was confirmed by results of two independent studies on the rehabilitation techniques and drug treatment in MS patients. There was satisfactory consistency between mean RFSS score and standard neurological examination in one study /10/, and between mean score at RFSS and FSS, DSS and IA /index of ambulation/ in another therapeutical survey on high doses of methylprednisolone /16/.

Whereas DSS was designed to quantify rather permanent motor deficit, RFSS tended to reflect numerically more varied and fluctuating signs. It is possible that both FSS and RFSS scores ex-

pressed mathematically not only the consequences of demyelination but also functional changes caused by oedema, inflammation
and reversible conduction blocks /15/.

In the assessment of clinical progression Fog /7/ used lo-
garithmic functions and Patzold /12/ stochastic analysis. These studies were based on orthogonal /normal/ polynomes /1st,
2nd and 3rd degree/ which approximated real progression of the
disease. It seems unlikely that mean annual RFSS score could
reflect properly genuine progression of MS. There is possibility that 2 remittent patients slightly declining steadily on
RFSS in this study could show decelerating progression according to Fog's analysis /7/. The mean annual RFSS score was therefore not appriopriate for the evaluation of progression in
MS patients.

REFERENCES
1. Bradford Hill A /1956/ Principles of medical statistics. The
Lancet Ltd, London
2. Broman T., Bergmann L, Andersen O /1972/ The terminology
used in our study for the determination of variables in the clinical course of MS and some preliminary registrations. Abstracts
of the Symposium on Multiple Sclerosis, Gothenburg
3. Cendrowski W /1968/ Post Hig Med Dosw 22 : 655 - 681
4. Cendrowski W. Wender M. Iwanowski L /1970/ J Chron Dis 22 :
797 - 803
5. Cendrowski W /1986/ Arch Suis Neurol Psychiat 137 : 5- 13
6. Cendrowski W /1971/ Neur Neurochir Pol 5 : 843 - 848
7. Fog T /1970/ Acta Neurol Scand suppl 47, 46 : 1 - 175
8. Kurtzke J /1983/ Neurology 33 : 1444 - 1452
9. Kuzma J Namerow N, Tourtellotte W /1969/ J Chron Dis 21 :
803 - 814
10. Kwolek A /1988/ A fixed period of active group treatment
in the process of continuous rehabilitation of patients with
MS. In : Grochmal S, Kwolek A /eds/ Rehabilitation of Multiple
Sclerosis. PTWK, Rzeszów, pp. 81 - 86
11. Matthews W, Acneson E, Batchelor J, Weller R /1985/ McAlpine's Multiple Sclerosis. Churchill Livingstone, Edinburgh
12. Patzold U /1985/ Multiple Sklerose. Verlauf und Therapie.
Thieme Verlag, Stuttgart

13. Poser S, Raun N, Poser W /1982/ Acta Neurol Scand 66 : 355 - 362

14. Sheikh K /1986/ Arch Phys Med Rehabil 67 : 245 - 249

15. Symposium on a Minimal Record of Disability for multiple sclerosis /1984/ Acta Neurol Scand suppl. 101, 70 : 1 - 217

16. Wajgt A, Szczechowski L, Marczewska E /1988/ Neur Neurochir Pol 22 : 188 - 194

© 1989 Elsevier Science Publishers B.V. (Biomedical Division)
Recent advances in multiple sclerosis therapy.
R.E. Gonsette, P. Delmotte, editors.

INFRACLINICAL EYE MOVEMENTS DISORDERS IN MULTIPLE SCLEROSIS

ALPINI D. CAPUTO D. HAEFELE E. MINI M.

Center for Multiple Sclerosis Institute "don C.Gnocchi",via Capecelatro 66,
Milan,Italy(20148)

INTRODUCTION

If the diagnosis of multiple sclerosis(MS)can be established on the basis of cli
nical information(8)any electrophysiological tests can only justified for investigation purposes,since even the most sensitive test is not specific.

But,if the neuroological evaluation raises the question of a possible MS,the
search for functional silent pathology should be in areas not already clinically involved.

The aim of this paper is to quantify eye movement disorders in patients(pt.)
with sensory findings or bladder or bowel problems,without any sign of ocularmotor alterations.

MATERIAL AND METHODS

We studied 37 pt.:23 females and 14 males,mean age 38 years.According to MacAlpine criteria they have been classified in clinically defined(30),probable(5)and
possible(2) MS.In this paper the classification is not important:pt.were selected according to the absence of clinically evident ocularmotor alterations.

Horizontal and vertical eye movements were recorded by monocular electrodes,
in DC.A computerized Nicolet Nystar electronystagmograph was employed.
Saccades were elicited e ther by random or fixed stimulation,respectevely 6–32°
and 20° in amplitude.In the horizontal plane they were recorded either by monocular or bitemporal electrodes.The following paramethers were evaluated:
velocity range;performance index(a velocity index)accuracy(in%)latency(in msec)
Smooth Pursuit was elicited as sigma-pursuit,by a sinusoidal wave 20° amplitude,
0.2 and 0.4 Hz.The following paramethers were evaluated : magnitude(maximum eye
velocity),total harmonic distorsion(THD),DC offset(an index of the simmetricity
of the movement);gain(ratio between target velocity and eye velocity,saccades
removed).

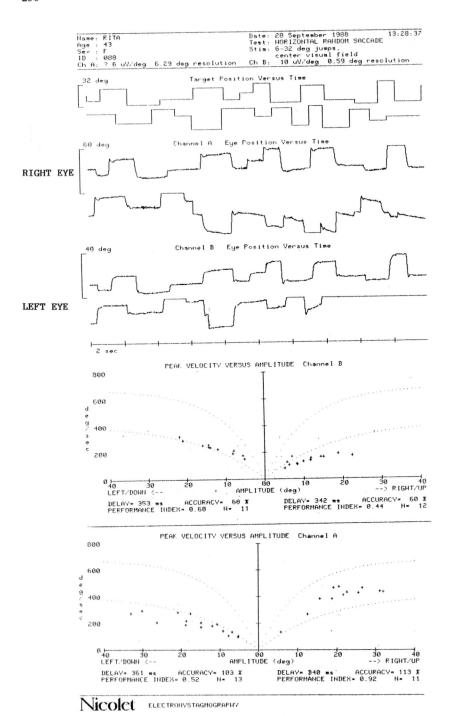

FIG. 1 :bilateral INO.Delay(Latency)is very increased,too.

RESULTS

In table I the percentages of infraclinical eye movements disorders.

11 pt.(30%) showed alterations of saccades either in the horizontal or in the vertical plane.Horizontal saccades are globally altered in 12 pt.(33%)and vertical saccades in the same number and percentage of pt.

In tab. II is shown this distribution.In tab. III is shown the distribution of paramethers alterations.A typical pattern of internuclear ophtalmoplegia(INO) was revealed in 4 pt.(11.1% of pt.;33.3% of pathological saccades).INO was bilateral in all 4 pt. :the adducting eye was hipometric and slower than the abducting eye.In Fig. 1 a typical bilateral,infraclinical,INO is shown.

13 pt.(36%) showed alterations of smooth pursuit either in the horizontal or in the vertical plane.Horizontal smooth pursuit are globally altered in 14 pt. (38.8%) while vertical movements are pathological in 44.4%(16 pt.).In Tab.IV the distribution of alterations is shown.

TAB. I 1:horizontal and vertical saccades;2:horizontal and vertical smooth pursuit 3:vert.saccdes;4:hor.saccades;5:hor.s.pursuit;6:vert.s.pursuit;7:INO(%on total pt.); 8:INO(% on pathological saccdes)

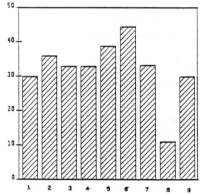

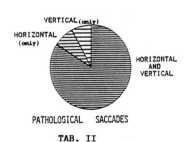

PATHOLOGICAL   SACCADES

TAB. II

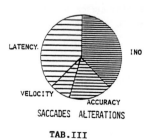

SACCADES ALTERATIONS

TAB.III

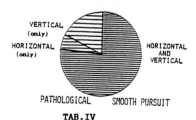

PATHOLOGICAL   SMOOTH PURSUIT

TAB.IV

Regarding paramethers,gain is frequentely decreased and THD(morphological para-
mether)is increased.DC offset modifications are less represented.

CONCLUSIONS

In this study eye movements are infraclinically altered in percentages from
30 to 44.4 %.If we compare tese data with other experiences reported in litera-
ture(1,2,4,6),we find that in our pt. sacc ades and smooth pursuit are less al-
terated.This is why our pt. are strictly selected on the basis of symptoms and
clinical signes:no pt. had ocularmotor troubles.In literature pt. are selected
on the basis of diagnostic staging.

Vertical tests are the most sensible and this is confirmed also in our previous
works.

It is important to underline that the evaluation of eye movements is a cornerstone of neurophisiological staging of MS and we propose EOG as a paraclinical
test just like multimodality evoked potentials.

REFERENCES

1. Alpini D,Berardi C,Milanese C(1987) Value of otoneurological tests for diagnostic staging of MS in :European Symposium on Epidemiology of MS,
   It.J.Neurl.Sc. Suppl.6:103–106/

2. Alpini D. Caputo D. Haefele E. Mini M.(1989)Otoneurological aspects of MS
   in :International MS Conference Rome september 1988–Free papers printed i,
   full;Monduzzi ed.,Bologna.

3.Barrè J.A,Reys L.(1924) Les trobles vestibulaires dans la S en P.Rev.Neurol.
   31:697–707.

4. Collard M. Conraux C(1980) L'electronystagmographie au cours de la S en P
   Ann.Otolaryng(Paris)97:467–481.

5. Gabersek V,Maton P,Salel D(1983) Etude comparative des alterations ENG dans
   la SenP et dans les neuroallergies.Ann.Otolaryng(Paris)100:193–201.

6. Mastaglia F.L,Black J.L,Collins D.W.K,(1979) Quantitative study of saccades
   and smooth pursuit eye movements in multiple sclerosis.Brain 102:817–825.

7. Reulen I.H.P,(1983)Eye movements disorders in multiple sclerosis and optic
   neuritis.Brain 106:121–132.

8. Toglia J(1987)Selection of electrophisiological tests in patients with suspec
   ted MS.It.J.Neurol.Sc. Suppl. 6:91–98.

© 1989 Elsevier Science Publishers B.V. (Biomedical Division)
Recent advances in multiple sclerosis therapy.
R.E. Gonsette, P. Delmotte, editors.

PHYSIOLOGICAL MEASUREMENT OF MUSCLE PERFORMANCE IN MULTIPLE SCLEROSIS.

R.J.S. JONES, D. L. PREECE, A. W. PREECE and J. L. GREEN

Biophysics Group, Radiotherapy & Oncology Unit, Horfield Road, Bristol BS2 8ED
(United Kingdom)

INTRODUCTION

Recent advances in functional electrical muscle stimulation (FES) for the
restoration of movement (standing, walking) have been made in paraplaegic
patients, but the feasibility of this approach in MS patients has yet to be
established. We are interested in the potential of neuromuscular stimulation
in a variety of contexts in the management of MS but there is very little
information on the range and stability of neuromuscular deficit in MS patients
with widely differing central lesions. We have therefore attempted to quantify
neuromuscular efficiency in MS patients using quantitative analyis of the
surface electromyograph (EMG) and tests of muscle strength and endurance.

Changes in motor unit recruitment can be studied during voluntary contraction
(1). We have employed fast, transputer based quantitative EMG analysis (2)
together with force measurement to test motor performance.

METHODS

Subjects are seated in a physiological measurement chair and recordings made
from tibialis anterior (TA) during maintained ankle dorsiflexion. To record
force, a strap placed over the front of the foot is attached via a pulley to a
force transducer mounted on the rear of the chair. Subjects are asked to
maintain maximum force for up to 1 minute using a digital force readout from
the transducer as feedback.

EMG Analysis

Surface EMG signals are recorded via an isolated amplifier using 8mm bipolar
silver/silver chloride electrodes placed 3 to 5 cm apart on the lateral aspect
of the proximal third of TA. The raw signal is stored on a PCV opus computer
which has a transputer and 8KHz, 12 bit A/D board installed. Menu run analysis
of the collected signal is described below.

Integrated EMG (iEMG)

The rectified integrated signal, which, in a surface recording, bears a
complex relationship to the sum of the motor unit action potentials (MUAPs)
modified by skin resistance and tissue impedence.

Signal Event Analysis

Analysis of the number of turns and zero crossings in the signal relates to the complexity of the interference pattern and hence, indirectly to motor recruitment levels (Nandedkar et al 1986). Turns, defined here as reversal of potential of the signal of more than 1% of the peak amplitude, and zero crossings, a change in polarity crossing a mid-point noise threshold are displayed separately.

<u>Signal Frequency Analysis</u>

Frequency domain analysis of the raw EMG signal is largely related to the contributions of the rise times and recovery phases of the complex signal. This, in turn, is related to the rise time of motor unit action potentials. The frequency/band power ratio (0 to 80 Hz : 96 to 320 Hz) representing 98% of all surface signal,provides a sensitive indication of frequency content at different times during the contraction.

To summarise, comparisons between EMG amplitude and polarity reversals would reveal primary muscle atrophy or motor unit regrouping (e.g. following reinnervation), iEMG and force indicate numbers of motor units active and the median signal frequency indicates presence or absence of primary or secondary myopathy involving changes in muscle excitation-contraction mechanisms.

PATIENTS

10 patients with definite MS, 3 male and 7 female ranging in age from 26 to 53 years were studied. Seven patients had walking difficulties, and one was confined to a wheelchair except for transfers. The other two patients, able to walk long distances, complained mainly of sensory problems. In this study we have assigned patients to categories of mild - able to walk >100m (2), moderate - able to walk 50m (4) or severe - able to walk <50m (4).

RESULTS

Fig. 1 shows results obtained from a control subject compared with those of patients with moderate and severe disability. Control subjects are able to maintain the contraction for 60 sec, with little loss of EMG signal and no change in force (Fig 1A).

In Fig 1B a patient with moderate disability was only able to maintain contraction for 40 seconds with the left leg and showed a rapid fall in force, iEMG and frequency of turns and zero crossings.

A severely affected patient (Fig.1C) was unable to maintain contraction for more than 15 seconds and showed accompanying rapid changes in levels of EMG. A rapid loss of motorunit activity was typical of all the patients with walking difficulties whether spastic or ataxic features predominate.

Asymmetry of records from right and left legs was pronounced and is well illustrated by the patient in Fig.1B, and in the severe patient where no adequate recordings could be obtained for the right leg, contraction time being too short.

The records obtained from the chair bound patient show extreme weakness and a low level of recruitment but an ability to maintain the contraction for 60 seconds. Recruitment and maintenance of contraction were essentially normal for this muscle in the two mild patients.

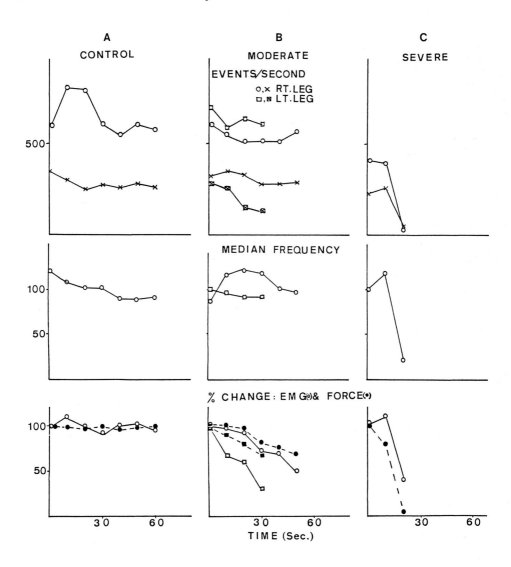

DISCUSSION

A striking feature of patients in both the moderate in the severe group was that initial levels of recruitment were relatively normal, falling after variable times as the ability to maintain force declined. Those whose symptoms did not affect the lower limbs showed near normal recruitment and maintenance of contraction.

These results suggest that failure to maintain contraction is due to loss of central drive with little or no alteration in muscle. The left right differences seen in most records suggest that attempts at functional stimulation would require very subtle control. We have found however (Emmery & Jones unpublished) that where differences between left and right legs are very great, unilateral functional stimulation can improve gait by supporting muscular activity in the weaker leg.

It has also been found (4) that neuromuscular stimulation aimed at improving range of movement in the lower limbs does improve gait and endurance. It remains to be seen whether muscle stimulation used in a rehabilitive context, or other treatment strategies, can alter the mechanisms which influence spinal motoneurones.

ACKNOWLEDGEMENTS

This work was supported by ARMS (Action for Research into Multiple Sclerosis).

REFERENCES

1. Milner-Brown, H.S., Mellenthin, M. & Miller, R.G. (1986) Arch.Phys.Med Rehabil. 67:530-535

2. Jones, R.J.S., Preece, D.L., Murfin (Green), J.L. & Preece, A.W. (1988) IEEE Engineering in Biology & Medicine 10:1607

3. Nandedkar, S.D., Sanders, D.B. & Stålberg, E.V. Muscle & Nerve 9:423-430.

4. Worthington, J. & De Souza, L. This publication.

© 1989 Elsevier Science Publishers B.V. (Biomedical Division)
Recent advances in multiple sclerosis therapy.
R.E. Gonsette, P. Delmotte, editors.

243

INTRATHECAL COMPLEMENT ACTIVATION IN INFLAMMATORY AND DEMYELINATING DISEASES
OF THE PERIPHERAL AND CENTRAL NERVOUS SYSTEM

HANS-PETER HARTUNG, BÄRBEL SCHÄFER, KURT HEININGER, GUIDO STOLL, KARLHEINZ
REINERS, AND KLAUS V. TOYKA
Department of Neurology, Heinrich-Heine-Universität Düsseldorf, Moorenstr.5,
D-4000 Düsseldorf, West Germany

INTRODUCTION

The complement system made up of some 20 proteins plays an important role in
natural host defence, participates in immunoregulation, and carries out decisive functions in the amplification and effector phases of immunoinflammatory
responses (1,2). Upon initiation of either the classical or alternative pathway of complement, split products are generated that act as ligands for receptors on immunocompetent cells, and terminal complement components are assembl-
ed into the membrane attack complex (3,4). Demonstration of increased concentrations of cleavage products such as C3a and C5a provides clear evidence of
activation of the complement system. In the present study we searched for complement activation in a number of inflammatory demyelinating conditions in
which complement-derived mediators could conceivably contribute to PNS or CNS
damage.

MATERIALS AND METHODS

Patient populations

34 patients suffered from acute Guillain-Barré syndrome according to the
diagnostic criteria of Asbury. 14 patients had a chronic progressive or
relapsing remitting chronic inflammatory demyelinating polyradiculoneuropathy
(CIDP) according to the clinical and electrophysiological criteria of McCombe
et al. 50 patients suffered an acute exacerbation of multiple sclerosis (definite disease according to Poser et al). 8 pateints were afflicted with

neisserial or Haemophilus meniningitis, 5 with tuberculous meningitis,
14 with viral encephalitis, and 5 with HIV encephalopathy without opportuni-
stic infections. 50 patients with noninflammatory , non-demyelinating
neurological diseases served as controls (OND).

Sample collection

Cerebrospinal fluid collected by lumbar puncture was frozen within 30 min.
of collection and stored at -70° C before assay. Venous blood was drawn
without a tourniquet into Vacutainer[R] tubes filled with EDTA. Plasma was
stored at -70° C until assay.

Radioimmunoassay for complement activation products

C3a desarg and C5a desarg were quantitated by radioimmunoassay according
to (5).

RESULTS

 In Guillain-Barrésyndrome CSF concentrations of C3a were elevated approximately tenfold when compared with those of OND patients (133 + 97 ng/ml vs.
17 + 6 ng/ml; means + S.D.) (cf. figure). CSF C5a was likewise elevated
(14 + 9 vs. 1 + 1 ng/ml). By contrast, plasma concentrations of both complement activation products were not significantly different in GBS compared
with OND patients. C3a and C5a concentrations in CSF were not correlated
with cell count, albumin or IgG indicating that peptide levels were not a
function of the blood-CSF barrier. There was further no apparent relationship of C3a and C5a concentrations in CSF and degree of clinical impairment.
However, serial intraindividual measurements showed a decline as the patients
made a recovery. CSF C3a and C5a were also elevated in patients with CIDP.
In MS patients, C3a and C5a levels in CSF were even more strikingly elevated
over those detectable in the CSF of OND patients with mean values of 402
and 19 ng/ml, respectively (cf. figure). Again, plasma concentrations
were no different from controls. CSF anaphylatoxin concentrations in
these MS patients were correlated to intrathecal IgG synthesis as reflected
by the IgG index of Delpech.

245

Highest C3a (up to 1300 ng/ml) concentrations were measured in patients with
bacterial non-tuberculous meningitis due to Neisseria meningitidis or Haemophilus. In tuberculous meningitis C3a concnetrations in CSF were raised
over 200 ng/ml. In contrast, neither patients with viral encephalitis nor
with HIV encephalopathy were noted to have increased anaphylatoxin levels
in their CSF.

Figure: CSF C3a concentrations in acute MS and GBS

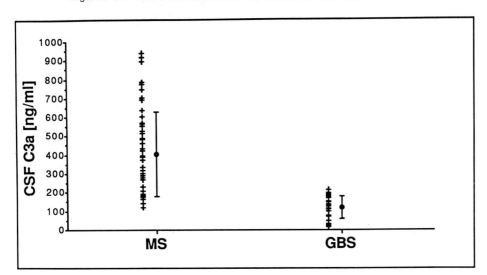

DISCUSSION

 Our results indicate an involvement of complement in the pathogenesis of
the Guillain-Barré syndrome, CIDP, and MS. They corroborate previous findings
on intrathecal C9 consumption and membrane attack complex formation in MS
(6,7). Further evidence that complement contributes to tissue damage in demyelinating disease of the CNS is the immunolocalization of the membrane attack
complex to MS plaques in association with endothelial cells (8) and the demonstration that complement depletion by cobra venom factor markedly reduces
severity of the animal model experimental allergic encephalomyelitis (9).

Likewise, our findings in GBS and CIDP patients emphasize the important role of humoral factors in the pathogenesis of immune-mediated neuropathies (for review, cf. 10). Activated complement components act as chemoattractants, augment phagocytosis, enhance vascular permeability, promote oedema, and stimulate the release of additional proinflammatory mediators from leukocytes. The membrane attack complex opens transmembrane pores permitting influx of electrolytes and proteases that could consequently damage the myelin sheath and impede proper neural conduction. How is complement activation initiated in demyelinating diseases of the PNS and CNS? Apart from antibodies a 56 kDa protein of central myelin and the PO protein of peripheral myelin can directly activate the complement cascade (11). In bacterial inflammatory disorders activation of the complement system is achieved through the alternative pathway.

In conclusion, the presence of increased concentrations of complement split products in the CSF of patients with inflammatory demyelinating diseases of the PNS and CNS implicates complement in the pathogenesis of these disorders. Pharmacological intervention to block complement-mediated amplification of immunoinflammatory responses may prove of therapeutic values.

REFERENCES

1. Rother K, Till GO (eds.) (1988) The complement system. Springer, Berlin, pp 1-535

2. Brown EJ, Joiner KA, Frank MM (1982) In: Paul WE (ed.) Fundamental Immunology. Raven, New York, pp 645-668

3. Hartung HP, Hadding U (1983) Synthesis of complement by macrophages and modulation of their functions through complement activation. Springer Semin Immunopathol 6: 283-326

4. Müller-Eberhard HJ (1984) The membrane attack complex. Springer Semin Immunopathol 7: 93-142

5. Wagner JL, Hugli TE (1984) Radioimmunoassay for anaphylatoxins: a sensitive method for determining complement activation products in biological fluids. Anal Biochem 136: 75-88

6. Compston DAS, Morgan BP, Olesky D, Fifield R, Campbell AK (1986) Cerebrospinal fluid C9 in demyelinating disease. Neurology 36: 1503-1506

7. Sanders ME, Koski CL, Robbins D, Shin ML, Frank MM, Joiner KA (1986) Activated terminal complement in cerebrospinal fluid in Guillain-Barré syndrome and multiple sclerosis. J Immunol 136: 4456-4459

8. Compston DAS, Morgan BP, Campbell AK, Wilkins P, Cole G, Thomas ND, Jasani B (1989) Immunocytochemical localization of the terminal complement complex in multiple sclerosis. Neuropathol Appl Neurobiol (in press)

9. Linington C, Morgan BP, Scolding NJ, Wilkins P, Piddlestone S, Compston DAS (1989) The role of complement in the pathogenesis of experimental allergic encephalomyelitis. Brain 112 (in press)

10. Hartung HP, Heininger K, Schäfer B, Fierz W, Toyka KV (1988) Immune mechanisms in inflammatory polyneuropathy. Ann NY Acad Sci 540: 122-161

11. Hartung HP, Heininger K (1989) Non-specific mechanisms of inflammation and tissue damage in MS. Res Immunol 140 : 226-232

© 1989 Elsevier Science Publishers B.V. (Biomedical Division)
Recent advances in multiple sclerosis therapy.
R.E. Gonsette, P. Delmotte, editors.

THE INFLUENCE OF CYCLOPHOSPHAMIDE VERSUS METHYLPREDNISOLONE THERAPY ON BLOOD LYMPHOCYTE SUBPOPULATIONS IN MULTIPLE SCLEROSIS

ANDRZEJ WAJGT, LECH SZCZECHOWSKI, ELŻBIETA MARCZEWSKA, LARYSA STRZYŻEWSKA

Department Neurology, Medical School, Katowice /Poland/

INTRODUCTION

The aim of presented study is: 1/ an analysis of the influence of cyclophosphamide /CY/ + prednisone therapeutic regimen on blood lymphocytes profile and Th and Ts subsets in chronic progressive multiple sclerosis /MS/, 2/ comparative analysis of mega-dose methylprednisolone /ME/ therapy supplemented with prednisone on blood lymphocytes profile in relapsing MS, and 3/ comparative analysis of lymphocytes profile in both MS groups versus normal healthy control

MATERIAL AND METHODS

Patients with clinically definite MS were selected to 2 therapeutic regimens: group 1 was subjected to CY + prednisone therapy. 4000 mg of CY was given intravenously over 10 days and supplemented with 775 mg of prednisone over next 20 days. This cases were characterized by relapsing-remitting course and Kurtzke disability score 4 to 6. Group 2 was subjected to Solu-Medrol + predniso ne therapy in time of relapse. 7500 mg of ME was given intaravenously over 10 days and supplemented with 775 mg of prednisone. This group was characterized by relapsing course and Kurtzke disability score 3 to 5.

Blood lymphocytes analysis was performed immediately before treatment, on 10th day of treatment /i.e. at the end of CY or ME administration/, on 30th day of therapy /i.e. at the end of prednisone administration/ and 3 months after beginning of CY + prednisone therapy. CD4 and CD8 cells were specified by indirect immunofluorescence by the method of Vargas-Cortes /1/.

Results were analysed by t-Students s test for data and paired data and by Wilcoxon s test.

RESULTS

Table 1 shows blood lymphocytes profile in chronic progressive MS /group 1/ and in MS group 2 characterized by relapsing-remitting course in comparison to healthy control group. Significantly lower number and percentage of CD4 lymphocytes was noticed in both MS groups in comparison to healthy control group. In MS group 2 tested in the time of relapse, CD8 cells percentage was significantly higher and Th/Ts ratio lower than in healthy control.

Table 2 shows blood lymphocytes profile in the course of ME + prednisone medication. On 10th day of therapy, i.e. at the end of ME administration transient increase of total WBC was observed. Total lymphocytes number, CD4 and CD8 cells number and percentage, and Th/Ts ratio did not differ in comparison to the values from before therapy. On 30th day of therapy, i.e. at the end of prednisone supplementation a significant increase was noticed

TABLE I
WBC AND LYMPHOCYTES COUNT AND PERCENTAGE, AND T_H AND T_S SUBSET
IN MS GROUP I AND GROUP II BEFORE THERAPY IN COMPARISON
TO HEALTHY CONTROL GROUP.

		Group I	Group II	Group C	Significance between I : C II :C	
WBC	x	6868,3	6102,3	6721,0	-	-
	SD	1443,7	2036,2	1876,0		
Lymph. %	x	30,7	32 ,1	34,9	-	-
	SD	7,7	11 ,8	9,6		
Lymph. count	x	2099,2	1990,7	2236,0	-	-
	SD	608,9	821,3	655,5		
T_H %	x	22,4	25,0	34,7	0,01	0,05
	SD	11,1	8,0	12,3		
T_H count	x	470,3	473,7	790,2	0,01	0,05
	SD	258,2	284,8	348,0		
T_S %	x	14,9	21,2	17,4	-	0,05
	SD	6,5	4,6	4,4		
T_S count	x	338,2	424,4	395,1	-	-
	SD	182,5	193,5	182,2	-	
T_H : T_S	x	1,6	1,1	2,0	-	0,01
	SD	1,3	0,3	0,7		

Group I - MS chronic progressive course.
Group II MS relapsing remmiting course.
Group C   Control healthy group.

in total lymphocytes number /P 0,05/, in CD4 cells number /P 0,05/
and in CD8 cells number /P 0,05/ in comparison to the values from
before therapy. Increase in CD4 cells number and percentage on
30th day of therapy was significant at P 0,01 in comparison to the
values noted on 10th day of therapy.

   Table 3 shows the influence of CY + prednisone therapy on blood
lymphocytes profile in chronic progressive MS. On 10th day of therapy, i.e. at the end of CY administration a significant decline
was observed in total lymphocytes count and percentage /P 0,001/,
and also in CD4 cells count /P 0,01/ and CD8 cells count /P 0,05/.
On 30th day of therapy, i.e. at the end of prednisone supplementation, we have noticed a restoration of total lymphocytes number
and CD4 and CD8 cells subset. However, 3 months after beginning
of therapy total lymphocytes number and percentage was lower at
P 0,05 in comparison to the values from before therapy. CD4 cells
count and percentage was lower at P 0,01. On the contrary, CD8
cells subset was normal. We conclude that restoration of CD8 subset precedes CD4 subset restoration.

TABLE II
THE INFLUENCE OF SOLU - MEDROL AND PREDNISONE MEDICATION ON WBC
AND BLOOD LYMPHOCYTES NUMBER AND PERCENTAGE, AND ON T_H AND T_S
SUBSET IN MS CHARACTERIZED BY REMMITTING COURSE.

		Before therapy	10 th day of therapy	30th day of therapy	Significance between : 1 : 2	1 : 3	2 : 3
WBC	x	6102,3	14337,7	7000,0	0,001	–	0,001
	SD	2036,2	4102,0	1671,6			
Lymph. %	x	32,1	13,9	31,2	0,001	–	0,001
	SD	11,8	6,4	10,0			
Lymph. count	x	1990,7	1810 ,0	2337,6	–	0,05	–
	SD	821,3	1033 ,4	674,1			
T_H %	x	25,0	18 ,7	29,9	–	–	0,01
	SD	8,0	10 ,0	8,8			
T_H count	x	473,7	401 ,1	740,9	–	0,05	0,01
	SD	284,8	459 ,3	420,1			
T_S %	x	21,2	21 ,8	25,9	–	–	–
	SD	4,6	14, 4	5,4			
T_S	x	424,4	491, 5	598,6	–	0,05	–
	SD	193,5	703, 3	188,0			
$T_H : T_S$	x	1,1	0, 8	1,1	–	–	0,05

DISCUSSION

We have reported in this studies statistically significant deficit in Th cells number and percentage in active MS, even before
therapy. Should it be lowering of CD4 2H4+ suppression-inducer
subset responsible for our results? In that case our results are
in concert with recent observations concerning a complicated cellular basis for the deficit of immune suppression in MS /2,3,4,5,
6,7/. Cellular basis for suppression deficit in MS is evidently
very sifisticated and comprises a number of T and non-T cell subsets, among others Ts subset, NK cells, but also T4 2H4+ suppression-inducer subset. Deficiency of this particular subset was recently discovered in active disease in positive correlation with
suppression deficit, as was estimated in functional; in vitro studies / IgG production evoked by PWM, deficit of Con A activated
immune suppression/.

As one could predict, high dose CY therapy in chronic progressive MS resulted in a significant decline in total blood lymphocytes number and percentage, and in CD4 and CD8 subsets. Restoration of CD4 subset was delayed in comparison to CD8 subset restoration. 2 months after therapy CD4 cells number was still signifi·
cantly lower than at the beginning of medication. Contrary to
that, CD8 subset was normal.

Mega-dose ME medication did not reduce total blood lymphocytes,
neither CD4 nor CD8 population, and did not cause any significant changes in CD4 or CD8 ratio. However, at the end of therapy
a significant increase of total blood lymphocytes, and CD4 and
CD8 subsets was observed as a kind of a rebound phenomenon.

TABLE III
THE INFLUENCE OF CYCLOPHOSPHAMIDE AND PREDNISONE MEDICATION
ON WBC AND BLOOD LYMPHOCYTES NUMBER AND PERCENTAGE,AND ON
T_H AND T_S SUBSET IN CHRONIC PROGRESSIVE MS.

		Before therapy	10th day of therapy	30 th day of therapy	3 months from beginning of therapy	Significance between : 1:2	1:3	1:4	2:3	3:4
WBC	x	6968,3	6586,0	8508,7	7016,8	-	0,01	-	0,05	0,05
	SD	1443,7	3339,4	2113,6	1493,9					
Lymph. %	x	30,7	18,5	22,0	22,1	0,001	0,01	0,05	-	-
	SD	7,7	7,5	10,1	2,5					
Lymph. count	x	2099,2	1157,5	1899,7	1525,0	0,001	-	0,05	0,01	-
	SD	608,9	684,9	993,9	426,6					
T_H %	x	22,4	22,1	23,4	16,7	-	-	0,01	-	-
	SD	11,1	10,9	8,9	13,5					
T_H count	x	470,4	291,1	435,9	236,4	0,01	-	0,01	-	-
	SD	258,2	214,5	298,8	217,4					
T_S %	x	14,9	15,4	17,3	15,2	-	-	-	-	-
	SD	6,5	8,7	9,7	8,5					
T_S count	x	338,2	206,6	383,9	380,1	0,05	-	-	0,05	-
	SD	182,5	170,6	325,7	346,0					
$T_H : T_S$	x	1,6	1,9	1,6	1,2	-	-	-	-	-
	SD	1,3	1,8	1,0	1,4					

REFERENCES
1. Vargas-Cortes M, Hellstrom U, Perlmann P /1983/ J Immunol Meth 63:87-99
2. Morimoto C, Hafler DA, Weiner HL, Letvin NL, Hagan M, Daley J, Schlossman SF /1987/ N Engl J Med 316/2/:67-72
3. Mickey MR, Ellison GW, Fahey JL, Moody DJ, Myers LW /1987/ Arch Neurol 44/4/:371-375
4. Cafaro A, Spadaro M, Pandolfi F, Tilia G, Scarselli E, Liberati F, Aiuti F /1987/ Riv Neurol 57/3/:159-162
5. Gonsette RE, Defalque A, Demonty L /1987/ Riv Neurol 57:181-184
6. Oger J, Kastrukoff L, O´Gorman M, Paty DW /1986/ J Neuroimmunol 12/1/:37-48
7. Antel JP, Bania MB, Reder A, Cashman N /1986/ J Immunol 137/1/:137-141

© 1989 Elsevier Science Publishers B.V. (Biomedical Division)
Recent advances in multiple sclerosis therapy.
R.E. Gonsette, P. Delmotte, editors.

ANTI-MYELIN BASIC PROTEIN ANTIBODY SECRETING CELLS IN CSF AND BLOOD OVER
COURSE OF MULTIPLE SCLEROSIS AND IN CONTROLS

HANS LINK, SHAHID BAIG, JIANG YU-PING, OVE OLSSON, BO HÖJEBERG, VASILIOS
KOSTULAS AND TOMAS OLSSON
Department of Neurology, Karolinska Institutet, Huddinge University
Hospital, S-141 86 Huddinge, Stockholm, Sweden

We have previously reported on evaluation of the B cell response in MS by
enumeration of numbers of cells in CSF and peripheral blood (PB) secreting
immunoglobulins (Ig) and antibodies (ab) of different isotypes (1-3).
Rationales for this approach include that it gives information about
localization of the B cell response; it also reflects B cell response at
time of lumbar puncture, while determinations of circulating ab reflect a
process that may have occurred days or weeks ago; the approach is highly
sensitive and may yield positive results when tests for corresponding
circulating Ig or ab are negative (1-5); concentrations of Ig and ab in
body fluids are influenced by several factors including ab binding to
target structures, accelerated metabolism of auto-ab and, in CSF, by
blood-brain barrier function.

Because myelin basic protein (MBP) has been focused upon as possible
target for immune attack in MS, we have now determined numbers of anti-MBP
ab producing cells in CSF and PB from MS patients. For reference, patients
with other inflammatory neurological diseases (OIND) and subjects with
muscular tension headache (TH) were examined. To evaluate fluctuations in
numbers of ab secreting cells over the course of disease, subgroups of
patients with MS and OIND were followed by two consecutive examinations.
Our results indicate that most patients with MS have a B cell response
directed against MBP, which seems to be more pronounced early during the
course of disease. This response is restricted to IgG isotype and preferentially compartmentalized to CSF. It is, however, not specific for MS
since it can also be demonstrated in OIND, although at lower frequency and
level, and rarely in TH.

MATERIALS AND METHODS

CSF and PB were obtained from 57 patients with clinically definite MS who
had not been treated with immunomodulatory drugs. 25 of the patients were
examined during exacerbation and 27 during remission, while 5 had primary

254

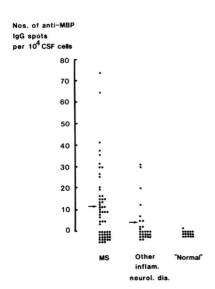

Fig. 1. Numbers of cells secreting anti-MBP IgG ab per 10^4 isolated CSF-L from patients with MS, other inflammatory neurological diseases, and tension headache ("normal").

TABLE I

NUMBERS OF ANTI-MBP IgG SECRETING CELLS PER 10^4 CSF-L IN MS AND OTHER INFLAMMATORY NEUROLOGICAL DISEASES (OIND)

DIAGNOSIS		Nos. of anti-MBP IgG spots		Nos. of IgG spots	
		CSF	Blood	CSF	Blood
MS	Range	0-74	0-1	14-522	1-11
	Mean	12		106	3
	No. pos/No. exam	34/57 (61%)	4/57 (7%)	53/53	57/57
OIND	Range	0-31	0-1	9-280	0-89
	Mean	4		61	10
	No. pos/No. exam	10/27 (37%)	2/27 (7%)	27/27	26/27
Tension headache	Range	0-5	0	2-24	0-6
	Mean			14	3
	No. pos/No. exam	1/16 (6%)	0/16	8/8	15/16

chronic progressive MS. Their age was 22-67 years (mean 40). 43 of the patients had no or slight disability, while the remaining 14 were moderately or severely disabled. Duration of MS varied from 0.5 to 32 years (mean 8). 37 of the patients (65%) had mononuclear pleocytosis (>5 per mm^3) in CSF, 40 (70%) had elevated IgG index, and all had oligoclonal IgG bands demonstrable by agarose isoelectric focusing of unconcentrated CSF followed by protein transfer to nitrocellulose membrane, immunolabelling, biotin-avidin amplification and peroxidase staining (6). From 19 of the MS patients, 2 consecutive specimens were obtained 3-14 months (mean 8) apart. - 27 patients had OIND (17 had acute aseptic meningitis (AM), 4 chronic AM, 3 acute encephalitis or myelitis, and 3 had treated neurosyphilis). - 16 subjects had TH and normal neurological and laboratory studies including CSF examination for cells, CSF/serum albumin, IgG index and oligoclonal bands.

The method which we used for determination of numbers of cells producing anti-MBP ab, and of cells secreting Ig of different isotypes, has been described in detail in a previous report from ECTRIMS (3). This assay utilizes microtitre plates where the bottom of the wells are replaced by a nitrocellulose filter, which is coated with MBP for enumeration of cells secreting anti-MBP ab, or with heavy chain specific anti-human IgG, IgA or IgM to determine numbers of cells secreting IgG, IgA or IgM. Aliquots containing 4-16 x 10^3 CSF cells (CSF-L) or 10^5 blood cells (PBL) are applied per well, and plates are incubated overnight at $37^{\circ}C$ with 5% CO_2. The cells are then discarded and after extensive washing, immunolabelling, avidin-biotin amplification and peroxidase staining discloses brown plaques which correspond to individual cells which have secreted anti-MBP ab or Ig of different isotypes. Plaques are counted in light-microscopy, and values obtained are reported per 10^4 CSF-L or PBL.

RESULTS

Among the 57 patients with MS, 34 (61%) had in CSF cells secreting anti-MBP IgG ab, with a mean value of 12 per 10^4 CSF-L (Fig. 1 and Table 1). Anti-MBP IgG antibody secreting cells were also found in 11 of 27 patients (37%) with OIND (mean $4/10^4$ CSF-L). One of the 16 subjects with TH had 5 anti-MBP Ig ab secreting cells per 10^4 CSF-L.

This anti-MBP IgG ab response was preferentially compartmentalized to CSF, since only 4 (7%) of the 57 MS patients, 2 (7%) of the patients with

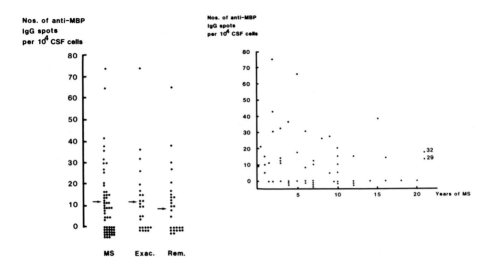

Fig. 2. Numbers of cells secreting anti-MBP IgG ab per 10^4 isolated CSF-L from 57 patients with MS, subdivided as to examination during exacerbation (25 patients) or remission (27) (to the left), and in relation to duration of disease (to the right).

TABLE II

NUMBERS OF ANTI-MBP IgG ANTIBODY PRODUCING CELLS PER 10^4 MONONUCLEAR CELLS IN CSF FROM PATIENTS WITH MS AND OTHER INFLAMMATORY NEUROLOGICAL DISEASE (OIND) EXAMINED TWICE OVER COURSE OF DISEASE

Diagnosis		Sample 1	Sample 2
MS[1]	Range	0–74	0–42
	Mean	18	13
	No. pos/No. exam	12/19	16/19
OIND	Range	0–31	0–6
	Mean	3	1
	No. pos/No. exam	4/15	4/15

[1]Interval between obtaining samples 1 and 2 in MS was 3–14 months (mean 8)

OIND, and none of those with TH had corresponding cells in PB, despite the fact that 10^5 PBL were applied per well in the assay. The number of anti-MBP IgG ab secreting cells did not exceed $1/10^4$ PBL in any of the positive cases.

Among 7 patients with MS examined for anti-MBP IgA ab spots, none was positive in CSF or PB, while 1 of 15 MS patients studied for anti-MBP IgM ab secreting cells was positive in CSF (1 per 10^4 CSF-L) and another one in PB (0.1 per 10^4 PBL).

We found a tendency of higher numbers of anti-MBP IgG ab secreting cells in CSF from MS patients examined curing exacerbations and in those with a duration of MS of at most 6 years(Fig. 2). Studies on larger groups of patients are necessary to confirm these observations.

19 of the MS patients were examined for anti-MBP IgG ab secreting cells at two occasions, 3-14 (mean 8) months apart. 12 of them had ab secreting cells in the first CSF sample, and 16 in the second (Table 2). Altogether, 17 patients (90%) had anti-MBP IgG ab secreting cells in CSF at least at one occasion. 15 patients with OIND were also examined twice. Two patients (1 with acute AM, and 1 with encephalitis) had ab secreting cells at both occasions, and 4 (2 with acute AM, 1 chronic AM, and 1 myelitis) at one occasion. Altogether, 6 of the patients (35%) had anti-MBP IgG ab secreting cells in CSF at least at one occasion.

DISCUSSION

Using an assay which makes possible the detection of individual cells producing anti-MBP ab, we have shown that a majority of patients with MS have such cells in CSF. We consider that our results from the immunospot assay reflect secretion of ab and Ig, since we obtained negative results when we tested about 30 MS patients with histones as antigen control, and immunospot formation was suppressed by inhibition of secretion with mon-ensin, and of protein synthesis with cycloheximide (data not shown). We also found that a minimum of 4000 cells per well is necessary for safe estimation of ab or Ig secreting cells.

Intrathecal production of anti-MBP IgG ab may reflect myelin breakdown. Alternatively, this auto-ab production has importance for the pathogenesis of MS. Our data do not discriminate between these two possibilities which, however, are not mutually exclusive. Anti-MBP ab may participate in ab-dependent cell-mediated demyelination, that is in opsonization for macrophage attack on myelin. There are clues for such a mechanisms since, morphologically, macrophages possessing coated pits have been observed in close relation to myelin, indicative of receptor-mediated endocytosis (7). Complement-mediated lysis is another possibility.

In OIND, anti-MBP IgG ab secreting cells are less frequent in CSF and present at lower numbers when comapred to MS. Larger numbers of patients need to be examined to evaluate whether any of the conditions represented among OIND is more frequently accompanied by this intrathecal auto-ab response. We have recently reported that subjects with TH regularly have Ig secreting cells in CSF (5). Anti-MBP ab seem, however, not to belong to the repertoire of ab characteristic for these subjects.

In conclusion, most patients with MS have in CSF cells secreting anti-MBP IgG ab. Such cells are less frequently detected in PB and then present in low numbers, thus reflecting sequestration of this B cell response to CSF and CNS. Anti-MBP ab secreting cells can be detected in OIND, but less frequently and at lower number. As a consequence of the substantial number of anti-MBP ab secreting cells present in MS CSF, this auto-aggressive immune response may - in an autoimmune-prone individual - play a role in the pathogenesis of neurological disease.

REFERENCES

1. Henriksson A, Kam-Hansen S, Andersson R (1981) J Neurimmunol 1:299-309
2. Henriksson A, Kam-Hansen S, Link H (1985) Clin Exp Immunol 62:176-184
3. Link H, Baig S, Olsson T, Lolli F (1988) In: Confavreux C, Aimard G, Devic M (eds) Trends in European Multiple Sclerosis Research. Excerpta Medica, Amsterdam, pp 173-181
4. Olsson T, Henriksson A, Link H (1985) J Neuroimmunol 9:293-305
5. Link H, Baig S, Jiang Y-P, Olsson O, Höjeberg B, Kostulas V, Olsson T (1989) Res Immunol 140:219-226
6. Olsson T, Kostulas V, Link H (1984) Clin Chem 30:1246-1249
7. Prineas JW, Graham JS (1981) Ann Neurol 10:22-31.

© 1989 Elsevier Science Publishers B.V. (Biomedical Division)
Recent advances in multiple sclerosis therapy.
R.E. Gonsette, P. Delmotte, editors.

MAGNETIC RESONANCE IN MULTIPLE SCLEROSIS TWINS.

C.H. Polman (1), B.M.J. UitdeHaag (1), J. Valk (2), J.C. Koetsier (1) and
C.J. Lucas (3).

From the Departments of Neurology (1) and Neuroradiology (2) of the Free
University Hospital, Amsterdam, The Netherlands and the Central Laboratory
of the Netherlands Red Cross Blood Transfusion Service (3), Amsterdam, The
Netherlands.

SUMMARY

Magnetic Resonance Imaging (MRI) examinations were performed in a series
of 7 twin sets (4 monozygotic and 3 dizygotic) and one triplet set who
were clinically discordant for multiple sclerosis (MS). MRI abnormalities
were detected in a number of the unaffected members of the monozygotic
twin pairs. The possible implications of our findings for the present view
on the aetiology of MS are discussed.

INTRODUCTION

Recent population-based studies in multiple sclerosis (MS) twins have
demonstrated concordance rates to be significantly higher in monozygotic
than in dizygotic pairs (1,2). This finding suggests a major genetic
component to play a role in the susceptibility of MS. Because of the
possibility of subclinical disease the analysis of concordance rates on
clinical grounds only might be misleading. For this reason Magnetic
Resonance Imaging (MRI) was performed in our series consisting of 1 set of
monozygotic triplets, 4 sets of monozygotic twin pairs and 3 sets of
dizygotic twin pairs, all clinically discordant for MS.

METHODS

The twin pairs and the set of triplets who volunteered for the MRI
examinations were part of a larger panel of twin pairs which had been
identified by public appeal. The zygosity diagnosis in all pairs was
established by extended blood and serum group determinations. Cerebral MRI
was performed with a 0.6 Tesla superconductive magnet. Proton density, T2W
and T1W spin-echo and inversion-recovery series were obtained in all
candidates.

RESULTS

As demonstrated in Table 1, MRI was abnormal in 7 out of the 8 MS patients. In these patients areas of prolonged T1 and T2 times were detected in the cerebral white matter. MRI abnormalities with the same features as in the patients with definite MS were identified in 3 out of 4 unaffected monozygotic twins and in none of 3 unaffected dizygotic twins. In one of the unaffected dizygotic twins (7b in Table 1) two small lesions were detected but they were not localized in white matter. All MRI examinations in the monozygotic triplet were reported to be normal. An example of a monozygotic twin pair in whom both patient and non-patient had white matter abnormalities on MR Imaging is given in Figure 1 (1a:patient, 1b: non-patient).

TABLE 1

PAIR	ZYGOSITY	CLINICAL MS	WHITE MATTER MR-ABNORMALITIES
1a	MZ	+	+
1b		−	+
2a	MZ	+	+
2b		−	+
3a	MZ	+	+
3b		−	−
4a	MZ	+	+
4b		−	+
5a	DZ	+	+
5b		−	−
6a	DZ	+	+
6b		−	−
7a	DZ	+	+
7b		−	−
8a		+	−
8b	MZ	−	−
8c		−	−

Fig 1a

Fig 1b

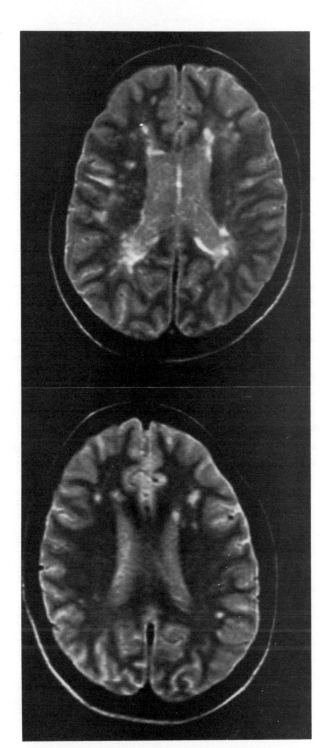

DISCUSSION

Our study clearly demonstrates in the first place the presence of white matter abnormalities in asymptomatic twins of patients with MS and in the second place suggests that these abnormalities are more frequent in asymptomatic monozygotic than in asymptomatic dizygotic twins.

Of course it is very important to discuss the meaning of these findings. The presence of MRI lesions in periventricular white matter in apparently healthy individuals, especially when over the age of 60 years, was demonstrated by Ormerod et al. (3). Although the origin of these changes is uncertain, it is suggested that they could be a consequence of cerebral involvement in vascular disease. All our patients, however, were below this age and did not have any clinical signs of cerebrovascular disease or systemic vascular disease.

The difference in concordance rates between monozygotic and dizygotic twins could not be accounted for by differences in age or age at onset of the disease, since these parameters were essentially the same in both groups.

In our view it is, at this time, not justified to assume that asymptomatic twins with MRI abnormalities have subclinical MS or will develop clinical MS. However, if longitudinal follow-up of these patients should demonstrate that these persons do develop clinical signs of MS, our findings of the percentage of MRI concordance rates being much greater in monozygotic twins than in dizygotic twins, would be in agreement with previous studies demonstrating much higher clinical concordance rates in monozygotic twins, which is probably indicative of a major genetic component playing a role in the susceptibility to MS.

REFERENCES

1. Ebers GC, Bulman DE, Sadovnick AD et al (1986) A population-based study of multiple sclerosis twins. N Engl J Med 315:1638–1642.

2. Kinnunen E, Koskenvuo M, Kaprio J and Aho K (1987) Multiple sclerosis in a nationwide series of twins. Neurology 37:1627–1629.

3. Ormerod IEC, Miller DH, McDonald WI et al (1987) The role of NMR imaging in the assessment of multiple sclerosis and isolated neurological lesions. Brain 110:1579–1616.

© 1989 Elsevier Science Publishers B.V. (Biomedical Division)
Recent advances in multiple sclerosis therapy.
R.E. Gonsette, P. Delmotte, editors.

263

NMR MICRO-IMAGING OF EXPERIMENTAL ALLERGIC ENCEPHALOMYELITIS

Greet V. PEERSMAN[1], Frank L. VAN DE VYVER[1], Ursula LUBKE[2], Dirk K. LANENS[1],

Erwin P. BELLON[1], Jan GHEUENS[2], Jean Jacques MARTIN[2], Roger DOMMISSE[1].

[1] Research Group for Biomedical NMR and [2] Department of Neurology
University of Antwerp (U.I.A.), Universiteitsplein 1, B-2610 Wilrijk, Belgium.

INTRODUCTION

Nuclear magnetic resonance (NMR) imaging is widely used in the diagnosis and follow-up of multiple sclerosis (MS). NMR characteristics of MS lesions are variable and correspond to different signal intensities of the lesions seen on NMR images. It is not yet well known which NMR characteristics correspond to which neuropathological feature of the lesion *(edema, inflammation, demyelination, remyelination, gliosis)*.

The present study involves an animal model of MS to establish the neuropathological correlation of abnormal NMR signals.

MATERIALS AND METHODS

We induced chronic recurrent-experimental allergic encephalomyelitis (CR-EAE) in 33 strain-13 guinea pigs, currently the best animal model for MS in terms of clinical and pathological features[1]. We also induced acute EAE in 39 Hartley-guinea pigs, for comparison with the chronic disease[2]. The disease was induced by a single subcutaneous inoculation of isologous spinal cord in complete Freund's adjuvant, for both strains under particular conditions. The animals were weighted daily and examined clinically.

The NMR-instrument (Biospec, Bruker) operated at a field of 1.89 Tesla and had an internal bore diameter of 30 cm. Gradient strength was 1G/cm. The internal diameter of the RF coil was 8 cm. The imaging protocol is shown in Table I. Because of technical limitations we only imaged the brain in-vivo.

TABLE I

IMAGING PROTOCOL

Matrix	128 x 128
In-plane resolution	0.3 mm x 0.3 mm
Slice thickness	1.7 mm
Number of averages	8
Spin echo sequence	
Repetition time (TR)	3000 msec
Echo times (TE)	40 msec
	100 msec

For morphological study, the animal was perfused with 4 % paraformaldehyde through the heart.

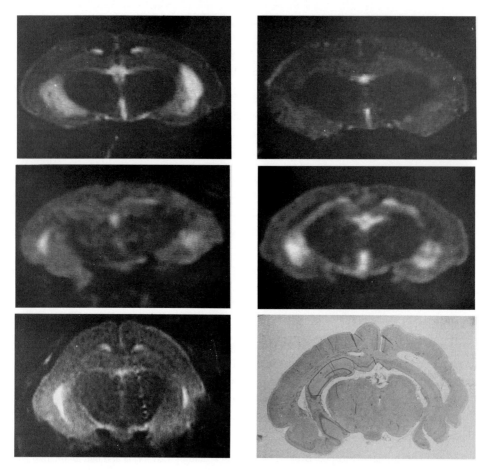

Fig 1A A T2-weighted image (3000/100) of a strain 13-guinea pig with chronic recurrent EAE, demonstrating large periventricular hyperintensities. The clinical sign at the time of imaging was hindlimb weakness.

Fig 1B Comparison image of a control animal. Approximately the same region as in Fig 1A; the same imaging parameters were used.

Fig 2A A T2-weighted image (3000/100) of a strain 13-guinea pig with chronic recurrent EAE, but no clinical signs at the time of imaging. Notice the small periventricular hyperintense rim in the left temporal area.

Fig 2B The same animal as in Fig 2A, was imaged again, six weeks later. There are more extensive periventricular hyperintense areas, indicating that lesions vary in function of time.

Fig 3A T2-weighted image (3000/100) of a Hartley-guinea pig with acute EAE, showing periventricular hyperintensities. This animal showed no clinical signs at the time of imaging.

Fig 3B A corresponding light microscopic section *(cresyl violet)*, showed scattered inflammatory foci. Compared to Fig 3A, only histological lesions of a certain extent can be seen on the NMR image. Periventricular lesions were detectable by the irregular shape of the hyperintense periventricular areas.

Following dissection, the brain and spinal cord were postfixed in a 10 % formalin solution and were processed for light microscopic study. Special care was taken to make the transverse sections exactly from the areas corresponding to the NMR images. The sections were stained with cresyl violet and an immunohistological staining using polyclonal antibodies against myelin basic protein.

NMR images as well as microscopic sections of 5 normal animals were made as control.

RESULTS

Clinical data

The clinical findings are shown in Table II. In general the first clinical signs were more severe in acute EAE than in chronic recurrent EAE.

TABLE II

DIFFERENCES IN CLINICAL COURSE IN ACUTE EAE AND CR-EAE

ACUTE EAE	CR-EAE
Incubation period : 9 - 43 days	Incubation period : 11 - 114 days
85 % developed clinical signs	88 % developed clinical signs
severe first clinical signs	moderate first clinical signs
progression to PPL, FW, IN, AM	progression to PPA, some PPL, IN
monophasic	chronic relapsing

TABLE III

FIRST CLINICAL SIGNS

	Acute EAE	CR-EAE
AG	27 %	10 %
HW	37 %	69 %
PPA	15 %	14 %
PPL	21 %	7 %

AG = abnormal gait; AM = automutilation; FW = forelimb weakness; HW =hindlimb weakness; IN = incontinence; PPL = paraplegia; PPA = paraparesis

NMR imaging results

In chronic recurrent EAE, the T2-weighted images (3000/100) and sometimes also the proton density images (3000/40) showed abnormal signal intensities, whereas in acute EAE only T2-weighted images showed abnormalities. The T2-weighted images showed periventricular hyperintensities *(Fig 1A)*, varying in extent as a function of time *(Fig 2A+B)*.

Control images did not show the above mentioned abnormalities *(Fig 1B)*.

Correlation NMR imaging — Histopathology

The microscopic sections showed infiltrates and perivascular cuffs scattered in   the cortex, the subcortical area, the white matter and the ventricle area *(Fig 3B)*. Sometimes, confluent perivascular

266

infiltrates were present. In general, the infiltrates consisted of microglia, macrophages and lymphocytes. In all cases, there was minimal demyelination in the inflammatory areas and around perivascular cuffs. Some macrophages with myelin basic protein-positive content occurred, but destruction of myelin was in fact very rare. Microscopic sections of normal animals did not show abnormalities. Only histological lesions of a certain extent could be seen on the NMR-image *(Fig 3A+B)*. The microscopic sections were much thinner than the corresponding NMR-sections. Therefore, one NMR image was always compared to several microscopic sections.

Although it was difficult to distinguish between the CSF and the periventricular lesions, the presence of lesions was detectable by the irregular shape of the hyperintense periventricular areas *(Fig 3A)*.

CONCLUSIONS

1. The NMR characteristics are variable: No lesions are seen on T1-weighted images. The T2-weighted images and sometimes also the proton density images showed hyperintensive areas.

2. Only histologic lesions of a certain extent can be seen on NMR images. However, edema is more apparent on NMR images than on histologic sections. This may also account for the discrepancy between the NMR images and the histopathologic findings.

3. There is no clear distinction between the CSF and the periventricular lesions.

To further define NMR imaging in demyelinating disease, NMR micro-imaging of spinal EAE in-vivo is currently performed. In view of our in-vitro study[3], we believe that the correlation will be better.

REFERENCES

1. Raine CS, Snyder DH, Valsamis MP, Stone SH (1974). *Chronic experimental allergic encephalomyelitis in inbred guinea pigs*. An ultrastructural study. Lab Invest 31:369-380.

2. Wisniewski HM, Keith HB (1977). *Chronic relapsing experimental allergic encephalomyelitis : an experimental model of multiple sclerosis*. Ann Neurol 1:144-148.

3. Peersman GV, Van de Vyver FL, Lohman JE, Lübke U, Gheuens J, Bellon E, Connelly A, Martin JJ (1988). *High resolution nuclear magnetic resonance imaging of the spinal cord in experimental demyelinating disease*. Acta Neuropathol 76:628-632.

© 1989 Elsevier Science Publishers B.V. (Biomedical Division)
Recent advances in multiple sclerosis therapy.
R.E. Gonsette, P. Delmotte, editors.

VASCULARIZATION OF THE PERIVENTRICULAR DEMYELINATION AREAS IN MULTIPLE SCLEROSIS

RAYMOND VAN DEN BERGH
Department of Neurology and Neurosurgery
Catholic University of Leuven
Leuven, Belgium.

The periventricular white matter has a very particular blood supply, that could play a role in the predilection of this area to demyelination in multiple sclerosis. Its typical vascularization, with ventriculofugal arterioles and ventriculopetal venulas and with a very striking angioarchitecture, is described.

NEUROPATHOLOGICAL DATA

The periventricular white matter of the area of the cornu anterius and the pars centralis has the most typical characteristics. Its territory is situated in the corner between the corona radiata and the radiatio corporis callosi. It was termed "Wetterwinkel" (i.e." thundercorner") by G. Steiner (1). Other predilection sites are : the area situated lateral to the cornu inferius and the cornu posterius, the corpus callosum, the peri-aqueductal gray and the fourth ventricle floor.

Besides the macroscopical predilection areas of demyelination, attention should be paid to the particular relationship between MS lesions and the central nervous vascular system. It has generally been accepted that MS plaques originate in the perivascular and more specifically on the perivenous areas.

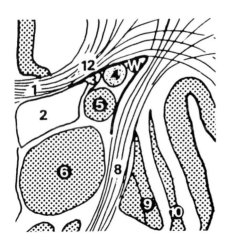

Fig 1
Periventricular area at the level of the Pars centralis ventriculi lateralis. W. Steiners's "Wetterwinkel" (Thundercorner) 1. Corpus callosum; 2. Pars centralis; 3. Stratum subependymale. 4. Fasciculus subcallosus; 5. Nucleus caudatus; 6. Thalamus; 7.Corona radiata;8. Capsula interna; 9. Nucleus lentiformis; 10. Claustrum; 12. Radiatio corporis callosi.

NEURO-IMAGING DATA

In past decennia, neuroradiological techniques, in particular tomographical and progressive pneumo-encephalography, were able to demonstrate some typical pathological aspects of MS such as ventricular enlargement, cortical atrophy and global cerebellar atrophy. The development of computerized axial tomography (CAT-scan) and nuclear magnetic resonance (NMR) however enabled a direct visualization of MS-plaques. L.A. Cala and F.L. Mastaglia (2) were the first to describe in 1976 low-density areas in the cerebral white substance of MS-patients by means of CAT-scanning procedures. In 1981 J.R. Young et al. (3) reported their experience with NMR- imaging of MS-lesions. Areas of hypo-intensity were discovered on T1- weighted images, hyperintensity was seen with T2-weighting.

W.J. Mc Donald (4) investigated the nature of the pathological NMR-images by scanning formaline-fixed MS brains and cutting them afterwards in accordance with the scan slices. A perfect conformity was encountered, thus establishing convincing evidence for the correlation of NMR-indentified abnormalities in MS with demyelination plaques.

VASCULARIZATION OF THE PERIVENTRICULAR DEMYELINATION AREAS

The ventricufugal arteries

The periventricular predilection sites of MS plaques grossly correspond with the territory of the ventriculofugal arterial system, that has been described by the same author (5,6,7,8,9).

At the cornu anterius and the pars centralis, the ventriculofugal arteries represent terminal branches of the outer rami striati laterales, derived from the arteria cerebri media. They have a maximal lenght of 15 millimeter and terminate in the immediate vicinity of the ventriculopetal arteries that converge from the periphery. A threedimensional periventricular demarcation zone exists between both vascular systems.

At the cella media, the cornu inferius and the cornu posterius, the ventriculofugal arteries are predominantly terminal ramifications of the arteria chorioidea posterior and the arteria cerebri posterior.

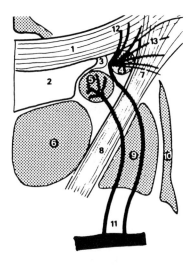

Fig . 2

Ventriculofugal arte-
ries
1. Corpus callosum 2. Pars
centralis ventriculi lateralis; 3. Stratum subependymale; 4. Fasciculus subcallosus; 5. Corpus nuclei
caudati;   6. Thalamus;
7. Corona radiata; 8. Capsula   interna;   9. Nucleus
lentiformis; 10. Claustrum;
11. Rami striati laterales;
12. Radiatio corporis callosi;   13. Ventriculofugal
arterioles;

The ventriculopetal veins

As the venous drainage of the deep parenchyma is for the most part orientated
towards the ventricle, this structure is surrounded by a crown of radiary veins.
This ventriculopetal veins collect in subependymal veins, that join the venae
cerebri internae and the venae basales.   They are connected by transcerebral
anastomoses   with   the   corticopetal   veins   and   have   large   perivascular
Virchow-Robin spaces, that join the subarachnoid space.   Together with the
ventriculofugal arterioles,the ventriculopetal veins constitute a very dense
vascular   fan,   situated   more   or   less   within   Steiner's   Wetterwinkel,   a
predilection site of demyelination.

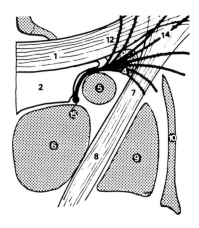

Fig. 3 : Ventriculopetal
veins
1. Corpus callosum;2. Pars
centralis   ventriculi   lateralis; 3. Stratum subependymale; 4. Fasciculus
subcallosus;5. Corpus nuclei   caudati;
6. Thalamus;7. Corona   radiata;8. Capsula   interna;
9.   Nucleus   lentiformis;
10.Claustrum;   11. Rami
striati   laterales;
12. Radiatio corporis callosi; 13. Ventriculofugal
arterioles.
14. Ventriculopetal   ve-
nulas;   15. Vena
thalamostriata.

270

CONCLUSION

The vascularization of the periventricular white matter presents particular characteristics that might be involved in the location, the shape and the extension of the most important demyelination areas in multiple sclerosis. The ventriculofugal arterial supply might be more precarious, rendering nutrition and metabolism more vulnerable. The ventriculopetal veins, with their perivascular spaces, play probably an important role as well, taking into account the active participation of veins and venulas in the demyelination process.

REFERENCES

1. Steiner G (1952) Acute plaques in multiple sclerosis, their pathogenic significance and the role of spirochaetes as etiological factor. J Neuropath Exp Neurol ,11, 343 - 372

2. Cala L A and Mastaglia F L (1976) Computerized axial tomography in multiple sclerosis. Lancet, 1, 689 - 705

3. Young J R, Hall A S, Pallis C A, Legg N J, Bydder G M and Steiner R E (1981) Nuclear magnetic resonance imaging of the brain in multiple sclerosis. Lancet, 11, 1063 - 1066

4. Mc Donald W J (1988) The role of NMR imaging in the assessment of Multiple Sclerosis. Clin Neurol and Neurosurg, 90, 3 - 9

5. Van den Bergh R (1960) De subcorticale angioarchitectuur van het menselijk telencephalon. Thesis, Leuven, Arscia, Brussel

6. Van den Bergh R (1961) La vascularisation artérielle intracérébrale. Acta neurol et psychiat belg, 61, 1013 - 1023

7. Van den Bergh R (1962) Les caractères fondamentaux de l'angioarchitecture sous-corticale du télencéphale humain. World Neurol, 7, 546 - 560

8. Van den Bergh R (1969) Centrifugal elements in the vascular pattern of the deep intracerebral blood sypply. Angiology, 20, 88 - 94

9. Van den Bergh R (1969) The periventricular intracerebral blood supply. Research on the cerebral circulation, Third international Salzburg Conference, Charles C Thomas, Springfield Illinois

© 1989 Elsevier Science Publishers B.V. (Biomedical Division)
Recent advances in multiple sclerosis therapy.
R.E. Gonsette, P. Delmotte, editors.

A CLUSTER OF MULTIPLE SCLEROSIS CASES IN CENTRAL BRITTANY. HLA MARKERS AND EVALUATION OF CONSANGUINITY IN THE POPULATION

G. EDAN*, M. MADIGAND*, M. MERIENNE*, G. MOREL*, O. SABOURAUD*,

D. SALMON**, G. SEMANA***, R. FAUCHET***

*Department of Neurology RENNES - ** C.N.T.S. PARIS - *** C R T S RENNES -
FRANCE

INTRODUCTION

In 1977, we conducted a survey of multiple sclerosis (M.S.) cases in the french province Brittany. We established the overall prevalence of multiple sclerosis at 25 per 100 000 inhabitants. Distribution of MS cases was very uneven, showing four circumscribed high prevalence zones with more than 45 per 100 000 and where we found clusters of M.S. cases.

Between 1982 and 1985, we conducted the present study in order to try to ascertain whether the existence of such clusters of MS cases could be explained by genetic factors, using two ways : the major histocompatibility complex markers, the frequency of intermarriage.

MATERIAL AND METHODS

1 - Major histocompatibility markers

Among the four zones of high prevalence, we choose to examine the one nearest to our laboratory, exempt from migratory movement over the last 100 years. Analysing this zone, ward by ward, it became obvious that 5 wards were responsible for the increased prevalence. For a total of 12 680 inhabitants, our survey revealed 8 cases of M.S. We concentrated the study on the age range between 20 to 50 years in which most M.S. cases are observed.

We compared this studied population to M.S. Brittany population and to a sample population of 1 000 healthy unrelated individuals coming from all over Brittany, designated as general Brittany population.

Class I (HLA A,B) and class II antigens (HLA DR) were determined using the microlymphocytotoxicity technique with a panel of 131 allo antisera. Phenotypic frequencies were calculated ; gene frequencies were established according to the formula $P = 1 - V1 - F$ where F is the antigen frequency. Results of this studied population were compared to those of control population using the X^2 test.

272

2 - Evaluation of consanguinity

As in Brittany 99% of the marriages were performed by the catholic chearch, we used church's registrars recording of special authorisations for interkin marriages beetween 1896 and 1945. These authorisations included marriages beetween 4th degree cousins. So we were able to compare the interkinship coefficient beetween the population of high MS prevalence, the surrounding population of low MS prevalence and the population of the department. By definition the interkinship coefficient is close to the consanguinity coefficient.

RESULTS

1 - Major histocompatibility markers (table 1)

A quite large sampling (about 25%) of the population accepted to take part in the study. Our results are summarized on table 1. Only the significant differences are here presented. These differences were highly significant as we used for the statistic analysis the corrected probability, taking into account the number of comparisons made for each antigen. In MS Brittany population, we found an increased percentage of B7 an DR2, compared with the Brittany control population. In the high prevalence zone, we observed an increased percentage of B7, B8, DR4 and a decreased percentage of B5, compared with the Brittany control population.

TABLE I

COMPARISON OF THE ANTIGENE FREQUENCY BEETWEN THE STUDIED POPULATION [HIGH PREVALENCE ZONE] AND THE M.S. POPULATION WITH THE BRITTANY CONTROL POPULATION

Antigen	Brittany control population [n - 1 000]	High MS prevalence zone [n - 750]	M.S. population [n - 122]
B 5	13.2	8.8**	NS
B 7	27.3	34.2*	38*
B 8	23.2	27.4*	NS
DR2	34.3	NS	50*
DR4	21.1	32.4**	NS

NS : non significant
* - $p < 10^{-2}$
** - $p < 10^{-3}$

2 – Evaluation of consanguinity (table 2)

From 1896 to 1945, there was an increase in the mean interkinship coefficient which was stronger and longer lasting in the high prevalence area. From 1926 to 1945, the consanguinity coefficient in the high prevalence area was much higher than the one of the departement.

TABLE 2

COMPARISON OF THE INTERKINSHIP COEFFICIENT BEETWEEN THE HIGH PREVALENCE AREA, THE NEIGHTOURING LOW PREVALENCE AREA AND THE SURROUNDING DEPARTMENT

	High prevalence wards		Low prevalence wards		Department
	Nb of marriages	interkinship coefficient	Nb of marriages	interkinship coefficient	interkinship coefficient
1896 – 1905	925	$37 \ 10^{-4}$	628	$15 \ 10^{-4}$	
1906 – 1915	788	$38 \ 10^{-4}$	502	$22 \ 10^{-4}$	
1916 – 1925	906	$48 \ 10^{-4}$	645	$31 \ 10^{-4}$	
1926 – 1935	796	$32 \ 10^{-4}$	573	$12 \ 10^{-4}$	$16 \ 10^{-4}$
1936 – 1945	561	$17 \ 10^{-4}$	411	$4 \ 10^{-4}$	$10 \ 10^{-4}$

CONCLUSION

Under the reserve of non randomized sampling of individuals for the HLA marker study, our findings yield a double argument in favor of a genetic factor influencing MS susceptibility : the HLA phenotype pattern and the increased consanguinity coefficient. The particularities of HLA polymorphism observed in the studied population are more likely the consequence of the intermarriage habits which characterised this population from 1896 to 1945. The non coincidence in our findings between B7 (over represented in the high prevalence population) and DR2 (over represented in MS, but not in the high prevalence population) does not specially argue in favor of a chromosome 6 gene affecting MS susceptibility.

© 1989 Elsevier Science Publishers B.V. (Biomedical Division)
Recent advances in multiple sclerosis therapy.
R.E. Gonsette, P. Delmotte, editors.

P2 PROTEIN IN THE CEREBROSPINAL FLUID IN MULTIPLE SCLEROSIS

*J. COLOVER, *AMBEREEN QURESHI, **PROF. CATHERINE F.C. MACPHERSON,
***L.S. ILLIS

*Dept. of Immunology, Rayne Institute, St. Thomas' Hospital, London SE1 7EH,
England; **Dept. of Psychiatry, University Hospital, London, Ontario, Canada
and ***Dept. of Neurosciences, Southampton General Hospital, Southampton,
Hants. England

INTRODUCTION

It is believed that there are 4 basic proteins present in human myelin and
that the P2 protein is the smallest. It was originally found in peripheral
nerve but later an identical protein was found in the CNS myelin (1,2) and
also it was found to inhibit EAE (experimental allergic encephalomyelitis).
Its occurrence in different zones of the CNS was found to vary in different
species. It was then found (3) that a monoclonal antibody to myelin stained
both the myelin and breakdown products of myelin in paraffin sections of
guinea pigs, whose spinal cords showed demyelination in animals that had
acute EAE induced by sensitization to myelin basic protein (MBP) after
pretreatment with muramyl dipeptide (MDP) and ovalbumin (OA) followed by a
second injection of OA (3). This monoclonal antibody was prepared by Prof.
B. Cohen of the ICRF and in blot tests did not react with MBP from a number
of species. However, it did react with bovine P2 protein prepared by Prof.
R.A.C. Hughes. In view of this it was decided to assay P2 protein in human
CSF in MS and other conditions using both this monoclonal antibody and also
polyclonal antibody to bovine P2 prepared in rabbits, using an enzyme linked
immunosorbent assay (ELISA) which could be read by an automatic
spectrophotometer.

MATERIALS AND METHODS

The spinal fluids were obtained from 2 main sources: emergency and acute
admissions to St. Thomas' Hospital (60) and from Dr. L. S. Illis, Dept. of
Neurosciences, Southampton Hospital. Those from St. Thomas' Hospital were
stored at -20°C in plastic screw capped containers but those from Southampton
(33) were kept at -20° in siliconised glass containers. The volume of fluid

TABLE I

P2 LEVEL IN CSF AND DIAGNOSIS
        (93 samples)

Diagnosis	High Positive	Low Positive	Undetectable (Negative)
MS	14 (93%)	8 (30%)	12 (23%)
Non MS	*1 (7%)	18 (70%)	40 (77%)
Total	15	26	52

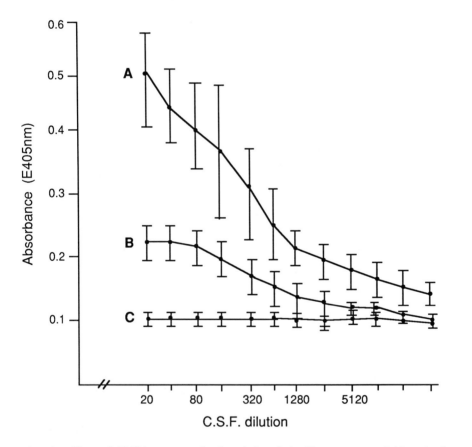

Fig. 1. Shows 3 ELISA curves, A, B and C. A is the average of 10 spinal fluids, highpositive. B is the average of 10 spinal fluids, low positive. C is the average of 20 negative or undetectable fluids. Standard deviations for each dilution point are shown as vertical points at each point.

used was 100 μl, but since it was found that a 1/20 solution of CSF could be used, only 10 μl were necessary. The assay was performed on plastic plates. The fluid was diluted with carbonate buffer and serial dilutions from 1/20 to 1/40960 were assayed. Each flat bottomed well had 100 μl of diluted CSF. The rabbit antibody was diluted to 1/300 and after washing, goat anti rabbit antibody linked to alkaline phosphatase was applied and then p-nitrophenyl phosphate was used as the indicator. The O.D. of the reaction product was determined by a Multiscan Titertek apparatus under standard conditions. The absorbance was plotted against the dilution of CSF using a standard series of dilutions. It was found that at dilutions of less than 1/20 the curve often turned down and therefore readings at such low dilutions were considered unreliable. Repeated estimations on the same fluid gave consistant results. Storing the fluid in a plastic container at -20°C for up to 6 months showed no significant variation in the curve. The first 40 fluids (Fig. 1) showed that the curves fell into 3 categories which were easily recognizable. 20 fluids fell into the undetectable range, the readings were horizontal lines (curve C, see Fig. 1, the average of the 20 fluids). The standard deviation for each point is shown as a vertical line. The next curve (curve B, Fig. 1) was low positive and had a low but definite slope or angle and is the average of 10 such fluids. The O.D. is higher than on curve C. Curve A, Fig. 1, the average of 10 fluids, high positives, has a steeper slope and the 1st reading is about O.D. 0.5. In all these curves the points lie on an easily recognizable line. All the plates included control wells without CSF or without antibody and in all plates a standard solution of bovine P2 was included as a check on the activity of the P2 antibody. The polyclonal antibody was far more sensitive than the monoclonal antibody and so it became the standard assay. Known amounts of P2 were assayed for comparison and these showed the high positive curve was produced by 125 μg/l of P2. The low positive curve was produced by 16 μg/l of P2. Some inhibitory tests were done as a means of cross checking the findings. The first batch of CSFs done were mainly from St. Thomas' Hospital and numbered 53. Then another 7 were added and also a further 33 from Southampton, which were assessed blind. These had 2 high positives - both untreated cases of MS. The test could not be performed on serum. On fluids from patients with subarachnoid haemorrhage the xanthochromic pigment interfered with the O.D. 93 fluids are shown in Table 1 and the results obtained. In the cohort of 33 fluids from Southampton, 6 included patients with MS (multiple sclerosis) who had been treated with steroids.

DISCUSSION

The overall proportion of MS or provisional MS (this included suspected and probable MS) was about 1 in 3. All patients with 2 or 3 exceptions, had organic neurological diseases. There were 15 high level positives, 14 came into the MS category. Only 1 did not have MS and that was a patient with lymphoma, which might have had demyelination. Of the low positives, 30% came into the MS category. The negative or undetectable fluids contained 24% of MS cases. This figure is higher than in the first 53 cases where it was 14%. It is believed that a number of cases of MS under treatment with steroids has increased this figure. The P2 in the high positive levels (125 $\mu g/l$) is much higher than published or reputed for MBP in the CSF. The assay for MBP is usually a radioimmunoassay on undiluted fluid and is a single estimation. It is therefore somewhat questionable that the figures are wholly reliable. This may be due to MBP reacting with plastic containers. It certainly is a subject that requires more basic and corraborative observation.

Regarding the diagnosis of the other CSF fluids examined, these included Borrelia, Guillain-Barre disease, viral and bacterial meningitis, vascular disease, tumours, lupus, syphilis, etc. There was no direct or inverse relationship of P2 to the level of protein or IgG in those fluids which had this information available. There was no relationship between duration of disease or number of lesions in those cases where this was known. No longitudinal studies have yet been undertaken. The level of P2 protein in relation to course progress and other features of MS requires further study.

SUMMARY AND CONCLUSIONS

93 CSFs from patients with neurological conditions have been assayed for P2 levels by means of an indirect ELISA. 15 were found to have high levels (125 $\mu g/l$). Of these, 14 had been diagnosed as MS or provisional MS.

The levels of P2 found were much higher than reported levels of MBP.

A cohort of 33 spinal fluids from Southampton were assayed blind. 2 had high levels of P2 and both were from untreated patients with MS.

Some MS patients had low positive or undetectable levels but some had been on steroids.

The level of P2 protein in the CSF in MS requires further investigation in relation to course, treatment and prognosis.

279

ACKNOWLEDGEMENTS

We wish to thank ARMS (Action for Research into Multiple Sclerosis) for assistance to two of us (J C and A Q).

REFERENCES

1.   MacPherson C F C, Armstrong H, Tan O (1976) J Immunol 16: 227-231

2.   Deibler G E, Driscoll B F, Kies M W (1978) J Neurochem 40: 47-54

3.   Colover J, Qureshi A (1988) In: Confavreaux C, Aimard G, Devic M (eds) Trends in European Multiple Sclerosis Research.   International Congress Series, 772, pp 229-234

© 1989 Elsevier Science Publishers B.V. (Biomedical Division)
Recent advances in multiple sclerosis therapy.
R.E. Gonsette, P. Delmotte, editors.

AUTORADIOGRAPHIC DETECTION OF MULTIPLE SCLEROSIS PLAQUES WITH AN ω3 (PERIPHERAL TYPE BENZODIAZEPINE) BINDING SITE RADIOLIGAND

J.-J. HAUW*, P. CORNU**, A. DUBOIS***, V. SAZDOVITCH*,
J. BENAVIDES***, E. MAC KENZIE *** and B. SCATTON***

Laboratoire de Neuropathologie R. Escourolle*, Service de Neurochirurgie
(Pr J. Philippon)**, Hôpital de La Salpêtrière, 47 Bd de l'Hôpital, 75651 Paris Cedex 13
and Synthelabo Recherches (LERS), Biology Department***, 31 Av. P.Vaillant
Couturier, 92220, Bagneux, France.

Two main classes of binding sites for benzodiazepines have been described for anxiolytic/hypnotic compounds: the central types, or ω_1 and ω_2 sites and the so-called peripheral type or ω_3 site (1). The significance and effector mechanisms of ω_3 sites are not known. In the immune system, the ω_3 sites are mainly associated with cells of the monocyte- macrophage lineage and also with T cells (2). In the central nervous system, these sites are present at low levels in the normal brain. They are essentially absent from neurons but are abundant in glial cells, such as astrocytes and ependymal cells. Omega $_3$ site levels are higher in the gray matter than in the white matter. The choroid plexus also displays high densities of ω_3 sites (3,4). The density of these sites increase after experimental brain injury likely as a result of macrophage invasion, astroglial hypertrophy and proliferation which are the consequences of any central nervous system injury and degeneration. In experimental infarction, the labelling of ω_3 sites has been shown to constitute a reliable marker for imaging the extent of brain damage (4).

In Multiple Sclerosis (MS), the presence of monocyte-macrophages and microglial cells in active plaques is a constant feature. They are numerous at the border of active lesions where they constitute, with other cell types such as lymphocytes and oligodendrocytes, the so-called glial wall. Monocyte-macrophages and microglial cells are thought to be directly involved in the process of demyelination. Some macrophages laden with myelin degradation products are also seen in the center of the plaque, often located in the perivascular cuffs. In addition, astrocytic gliosis occurs in the center of the plaques. As all these cell types are richly endowed with ω_3 sites, we have investigated the feasibility of using ω_3 site autoradiography to detect the demyelination plaques in the brain of post-mortem cases of Multiple Sclerosis.

MATERIAL AND METHODS

Patients :

Three cases of definite Multiple Sclerosis (women 32-39 year-old) were used.

Tissue processing :

Postmortem brain samples were frozen in isopentane and processed for $\omega 3$ site autoradiography as described elsewhere (2,3,4,5). Briefly, both reversible (^{3}H PK 11195) and photoaffinity (^{3}H PK 14105) $\omega 3$ radioligands were used to assess the gross and microscopic localization of these binding sites in sections of control and multiple sclerosis brain . Irreversible labelling of $\omega 3$ sites and various histoenzymo-logical, immunocytochemical staining were performed on serial sections.

RESULTS

In the demyelination plaques of sections of patients who died with MS, there was a 10 fold increase in $\omega 3$ site density as compared to control white matter. A good correlation was observed between the topography of increased binding and the areas of demyelination as assessed by the Loyez stain. The density of $\omega 3$ sites was much higher in the periphery of active plaques, whereas their center displayed lower binding levels (5). Emulsion autoradiography of irreversibly bound ^{3} H PK 14105, revealed an association of $\omega 3$ sites with cells with a very high acid phosphatase and non specific esterase activity stained by Leu M3 and Leu M5 . These results suggest a predominent localisation of these sites on macrophages. (6)

DISCUSSION

The increase in the density of $\omega 3$ sites in MS plaques which is maximum at the active edge is likely to be related to the presence at this level of macrophages and activated glial cells. This is supported by the fact that $\omega 3$ site-associated autoradio-graphic grains were mainly associed with cells that in adjacent sections were identified as macrophages and astrocytes (by histochemical and immunohisto-chemical procedures). A similar cellular localisation of $\omega 3$ sites has been observed in other experimental (ischaemic and excitotoxic) and human neuropatho logical ischaemic and tumoral lesions. Double labelling experiments ($\omega 3$ sites and specific cell markers) are in progress to definitely identify the cell type (to which $\omega 3$ sites are associated) in MS plaques.

The available posit on (^{11}C-PK 11195) and gamma- ray (^{125}I-PK 11195) emiting ligands (7,8) may render possible the in vivo detection of $\omega 3$ sites and help to the diagnosis and study of Multiple Sclerosis. More specifically, it could be an in vivo marker of the activity of the disease.

ACKNOWLEDGEMENTS

This work was helped by Association Claude Bernard and Association de Recherche pour la Sclérose en Plaques.

REFERENCES:

1. Langer SZ, Arbilla S (1988) Imidazopyridines as a tool for the characterization of benzodiazepine receptors: a proposal for a pharmacolo gical classification as omega receptor. Pharmacol. Biochem. Behav. 29: 763-766

2. Benavidès J, Dubois A, Dennis T, Hamel E, Scatton B. J. ω_3 (Peripheral type benzodiazepine binding) Site distribution in the rat immune sytem: an autoradiographic study with the photoaffinity ligand (^{3}H) PK14105. Pharmacol. Exp. 1989, 249:1-7.

3. Benavidès J, Savaki HE, Malgouris C, Laplace C, Daniel M, Begassat F, Desban M, Uzan A, Dubroeucq MC, Renault C, Guérémy C, Le Fur G (1984) Autoradiographic localization of peripheral benzodiazepine binding sites in the cat brain with [^{3}H]PK 11195. Brain Res. Bull. 13: 69-77.

4. Dubois A, Benavidès J, Peny B, Duverger D, Fage D, Gotti B, MacKenzie E, Scatton B (1988) Imaging of primary and remote ischaemic and excitotoxic brain lesions. An autoradiographic study of peripheral type benzodiazepine binding sites in the rat and cat. Brain Res. 445: 77-90.

5. Benavidès J, Cornu P, Dennis T, Dubois A, Hauw J-J, MacKenzie E, Sazdovitch V, Scatton B (1988) Imaging of human brain lesions with an ω_3 site radioligand. Ann. Neurol. 24: 708-712.

6. Cornu P, Hauw J-J Benavidès J, Dennis T, Dubois A, MacKenzie E, Sazdovitch V, Scatton B (1988) Localization of ω_3 sites in Multiple sclerosis brain. submitted.

7. Charbonneau P, Syrota A, Crouzel C, Prennat C, Crouzel M (1986) Peripheral-type benzodiazepine receptors in the living heart characterized by positon emission tomography. Circulation 73: 476-483.

8. Ciliax BJ, Starosta-Rubinstein S, Wieland DM, Van Dort ME, Gildersleeve DL, Penney JB, Young AB. In vivo imaging of rat C6 glioma by [^{125}I]-iodinated benzodiazepines and isoquinoleines. Soc Neurosc. Abstr XIII, 263.5 (1987).

© 1989 Elsevier Science Publishers B.V. (Biomedical Division)
Recent advances in multiple sclerosis therapy.
R.E. Gonsette, P. Delmotte, editors.

285

[31]-P NMR SPECTROSCOPY IN MULTIPLE SCLEROSIS

E.L. MOOYAART[1], R.L. KAMMAN[1], M.C. HOOGSTRATEN[2], E.J. 'S-GRAVENMADE[2], J.M. MINDERHOUD[2]

1) Department of Magnetic Resonance 2) Department of Neurology, University Hospital, P.O. Box 30.001, 9700 RB Groningen (The Netherlands)

In vivo [31]-P NMR spectroscopy was performed using a 1.5 Tesla Philips Gyroscan in 10 multiple sclerosis (MS) patients and 12 healthy controls. After routine imaging of the brain a volume of interest for spectroscopy was chosen and ^{31}P NMR spectra were recorded. The seize of the volume was at least 80 cc with a maximum of 260 cc. The ^{31}P spectrum was obtained using a repetition time of 3000 msec.

At this moment (March 1989) the peak-heights of β-ATP, phosphocreatine (PCr), in organic phosphate (Pi), phosphomonoesters (PME) and phosphodiesters (PDE) and expressed as the relative percentage of their sum, e.g. were used to compare the spectra of MS patients and controls without clinical signs and with a normal MRI-scan.

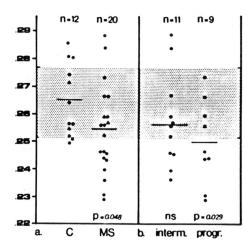

Fig. 1a: Relative peak-heights of phosphodiesters in 12 healthy persons and 20 MS patients.
Fig. 1b: Idem, in 11 out of 20 MS patients with an intermittent course of the disease, and in 9 out of 20 MS patients with a primary or secondary progressive course. Hatched: mean ± sd of the control group. Statistics: Mann-Whitney test, two-sided.

The relative peak-heights of Pi, β-AT,P PME and PCr in spectra of MS patients did not differ from those of similar metabolites in the healthy controls.

The relative peak heights of PDE, however, were lower in MS patients (p=.048) than in the controls, particularly in those with a primary or secondary progressive course of the disease (p=.029) (fig. 1). The decrease of the PDE peak correlated with the "delta progression rate" in these chronic progressive patients (r=-.73; p<0.05)(fig. 2). The "delta progression rate" is the mean yearly increase of EDSS during the progressive period, either primary or secondary. The changes of the spectra were not related to age, sex, duration of the disease or the total clinical handicap of the patient.

In 8 patients and 4 controls spectra from two hemispheres were obtained separately. There seems to be no relation between the intensity of the lesions as detected by MRI and the abnormalities as observed by spectroscopy.

It is too early to give a full interpretation of these results.

	all MS patients		patients with progression rate	
duration MS	.16	ns	.07	ns
duration progression	–		−.42	ns
progression rate	.02	ns	.03	ns
delta progression rate	–		−.73	<005
EDSS	.21	ns	.03	ns
	n.20		n.9	

Fig. 2: Correlation with the relative peak-height of phosphodiesters in all MS patients and in the group of 9 primary or secondary progressive cases of MS.

POSTERS

© 1989 Elsevier Science Publishers B.V. (Biomedical Division)
Recent advances in multiple sclerosis therapy.
R.E. Gonsette, P. Delmotte, editors.

ARE SMOOTH PURSUIT EYE MOVEMENTS(SPEM)ALTERATIONS DEPENDING ON PATTERN STIMU-
LATION ?

ALPINI D.[1] MARFORIO S.[2] CAPUTO D.[3] HAEFELE E.[3] GHEZZI A.[2] ZAFFARONI M.[2] MINI M.[3]
[1] ENG Lab H. Busto Arsizio [2] MS Center H. Gallarate [3] MS Center Institute   don Gnocchi

INTRODUCTION

Eye movements alterations are frequent during the course of multiple sclerosis
(MS).Smooth pursuit eye movements(SPEM) are especially involved at every stage
of the disease.SPEM have been studied by a number of investigators using different pattern stimulations.The aim of this paper is to evaluate if SPEM alterations are depending on methodology of examination.

MATERIAL AND METHODS

We studied horizontal and vertical SPEM by the mean of a LED bar(sigma-SPEM),
using electronystagmography(ENG),by monocular right and left horizontal and
right vertical electrodes.

Three groups of patients have been evaluated:

A) 25 pt. by triangular wave(to-and-fro stimulation)at 10-20-30°/sec and 20°
 in amplitude.Eye movements were recorded by a traditional electronystagmograph
(Beckman,with contemporary recording of velocity and target).

B)40 pt. by random single ramp stimulation at $\pm$ 20° in amplitude and 10-20-30°
/sec in velocity.The same electronystagmograph was employed.

C)36 pt. by sinusoidal wave;maximum velocity 20°;0.2 and 0.4 Hz. A computerized
Nicolet Nystar electronystagmograph was used.

All patients were classified(according to MacAlpine criteria)clinically defined
multiple sclerosis.None of them showed clinical evidence of ocularmotor altera-
tions.The three groups of pt.may be considered comparable in a clinical point
of view.

RESULTS

Group A-Triangular wave: 10 pt.(40%) normal SPEM;10(40%) pathological SPEM in
both planes;2(9%) pathological only horizontal SPEM;3pt(11%)pathological only
vertical SPEM.Globally,horizontal SPEM were altered in 48% and vertical SPEM
in 52%.

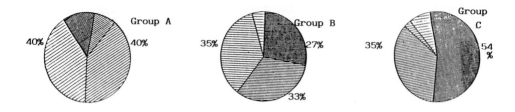

Group B-Ramp smooth pursuit: in 33%(13)SPEM were normal;in 27%(11pt.)SPEM were alterated in both planes;in 5%(2 pt.)SPEM were alterated only in the horizontal plane and in35%(14 pt.)they were alterated only in the vertical plane.Globally,horizontal SPEM were pathological in 32% while vertical SPEM were pathological in 62%.

Group C-Sinusoidal wave: SPEM were normal in 20 pt.(54%);alterated in both planes in 13 pt.(35%);in the horizontal plane in 1 pt.(2%);only in the vertical plane in 3 pt.(9%).Globally,horizontal SPEM were alterated in 37% and vertical SPEM in 44%.

CONCLUSIONS

Percentages of pathological SPEM are lower than in other papers of internatio nal literature. In this study pt. were selected according a symptomatologic criterium:none of them had clinical evidence of ocularmotor disorder.We think this as a good explanation of low pathological SPEM results.

The frequerce of alterations are quite similar into the three groups of pt.Vertical SPEM are generally more involved than horizontal SPEM.Single ramp stimulation is the most alterated ,in the vertical plane(the difference with the other two stimulations is significative at 0.05).

If the SPEM test is performed and evaluated by a well trained and expert neuro-otologist,traditional electronystagmograph is as accurate as a computerized one.

REFERENCES

1. Bahill A.T,Iandolo M.J,Troost B.T(1980)Smooth pursuit eye movements in respon se to unpredictable target waveforms.Vision Res 20:923-931

2. Mastaglia F.L,Black J.L,Collins D.K.W(1979)Quantitative studies of saccades and smooth pursuit eye movements in multiple sclerosis.Brain 102:817-825.

3. Schalen L(1980) Quantification of tracking eye movements in normal subjects. Acta Otolaryng.(Stochk)90:404-413

© 1989 Elsevier Science Publishers B.V. (Biomedical Division)
Recent advances in multiple sclerosis therapy.
R.E. Gonsette, P. Delmotte, editors.

INTERLEUKIN-2 (IL-2) REGULATES LECTIN-INDUCED SUPPRESSOR CELL ACTIVITY IN PATIENTS WITH MULTIPLE SCLEROSIS (MS)

EMMANUEL ANASTASOPOULOS, GEORGE J.RECLOS, PAULA ARSENIS, ANNA KATSIYIANNIS, NICK MATIKAS*, CONSTANTIN N. BAXEVANIS and MICHAIL PAPAMICHAIL.

Dept. Immunology,Hellenic Anticancer Institute,171 Alexandras Ave,11522

Athens,and   *Dept.Neurology,Evangelismos Hospital,Athens.

INTRODUCTION

A consistent immunologic finding in patients with active MS is a loss

of functional suppression and a decrease in IL-2 production (1,2).In this

report we demonstrate a correlation between these two immune defects: the

levels of IL-2 produced by activated peripheral blood T cells determine the

extend of ConA-induced suppressor cell activity.

MATERIALS AND METHODS

Patients. Patients with progressive MS were in an active phase of their

disease as defined by a decline in at least one grade on the Kurtzke

disability scale (3).

Generation of IL-2. T cells were cultured with ConA (5-10µg/ml) for 48h at

37oC,5% CO_2 in air.Culture supernatant (sups) were then collected and stored

at -35oC untill tested in the CTLL assay (4).

ConA suppressor assay. T cells were cultured for 2 days with ConA(see

above); these cells were then trated with mitomycin C (1) and used as test

cells in mixing experiments with allogeneic responder cells (R-cells) and

ConA (1).

RESULTS

T cells from MS patients cultured with ConA produced lower levels of

IL-2 and suppressed considerably weaker,compared to normal donors, the proliferative response of allogeneic R-cells to ConA.

TABLE I

THE LEVELS OF IL-2 PRODUCED BY ACTIVATED T CELLS DETERMINE THE EXTENT OF ConA-INDUCED SUPPRESSOR CELL ACTIVITY*

Individuals tested	CTLL proliferation	R-cell proliferation to ConA**
MS patients (n=19)	6032 ± 2415	97471 ± 18793 (16.3)***
Healthy donors (n=22)	14793 ± 3897	24258 ± 7935 (79.2)

* T cells were cultured for 48h with ConA and the culture sups were collected and tested in the CTLL-assay for IL-2 activity.The cultured T cells were then tested as test cells for suppressor cell activity.Data are expressed as mean cpm+SD from pooled values.
** R-cells plus ConA without test cells: 116478cpm.
*** Indicates the calculated percent suppression (in parentheses).

ACKNOWLEDGEMENTS

This work was supported by a grant from the Greek Ministry of Research and Technology to C.N.Baxevanis.

REFERENCES

1. Antel J P et al.,(1986) J Immunol 137:137.

2. Merill J M et al.,(1984) J Immunol 133:1931.

3. Kurtzke J F (1956) Arch Neurol Psychiat 76:175.

4. Chouaib S et al.,(1985) J Immunol 134:940.

© 1989 Elsevier Science Publishers B.V. (Biomedical Division)
Recent advances in multiple sclerosis therapy.
R.E. Gonsette, P. Delmotte, editors.

REGULATION OF DEFICIENT INTERLEUKIN-2 (IL-2) PRODUCTION IN PATIENTS WITH MULTIPLE SCLEROSIS (MS) BY PROTHYMOSIN α (ProTα).

CONSTANTIN N.BAXEVANIS, EMMANUEL ANASTASOPOULOS,
GEORGE J.RECLOS, PAULA ARSENIS, ANNA KATSIYIANNIS,
NICK MATIKAS* and MICHAIL PAPAMICHAIL.

Dept. Immunology, Hellenic Anticancer Insitute, 171 Alexandras Ave,11522

Athens and *Dept. Neurology, Evangelismos Hospital, Athens.

INTRODUCTION

IL-2 is produced by activated T lymphocytes and play an important role in immunoregulation (1).The production of IL-2 by peripheral blood T lymphocytes is reduced in patients with MS undergoing an exacerbation (2).In this report we demonstrate that ProTα,a powerful immunopotentiator in vitro (3),enhances the production of IL-2 by peripheral blood T lymphocytes in MS patients.

MATERIAL AND METHODS

Patients. Sixteen patients with active MS entered this study.

Generation of IL-2. T cells (4×10^6/ml) were cultured with PHA (10μg/ml) for 48h in the absence or presence of ProTα (1μg/ml) at 37oC,5% CO_2 in air. Culture supernatants (sups) were then collected and stored at -35oC until tested.

Assay for IL-2 activity. 100μl containing 8×10^3 CTLL cells (2) were cultured in triplicate in microwells with 100μl of the sample to be tested or recombinant IL-2 (rIL-2) for 24h at 37oC,5% CO_2 in air.

RESULTS

T lymphocytes from patients with active MS when cultured for 2 days
with PHA produced reduced levels of IL-2 compared to normal individuals.This
defect in IL-2 production was restored to almost normal levels when ProTα
was included in the cultures.Since IL-2 production by T cells is important
for optimal immunoregulation,we suggest that ProTα might contribute to the
restoration of dysregulation in MS.

TABLE I

THE EFFECTS OF ProTα ON IL-2 PRODUCTION BY MS T LYMPHOCYTES

Individual tested	ProTα in PHA cultures	CTLL proliferation*
MS patients	-	4252 + 1848
(n = 16)	+	12435 + 2286
Normal Donors	-	15982 + 3218
(n = 18)	+	20413 + 4016

* Mean cpm values ± SD from the pooled data.CTLL proliferation (a)
in the absence of PHA culture sups:372+16cpm,(b) in the presence of
rIL-2 (100U/ml):63278±3522cpm.

ACKNOWLEDGEMENTS

This work was supported with a grant from the Greek Ministry of
Research and Technology to C.N.Baxevanis.

REFERENCES

1. Palacios R (1983) Immunol Rev 63:73.

2. Merill J M et al.,(1984) J Immunol 133:1931.

3. Baxevanis C N et al.,(1988) Immunoparmacology 15:73.

© 1989 Elsevier Science Publishers B.V. (Biomedical Division)
Recent advances in multiple sclerosis therapy.
R.E. Gonsette, P. Delmotte, editors.

REGULATION OF DEFICIENT T CELL RESPONSES IN PATIENTS WITH MULTIPLE SCLEROSIS (MS) BY PROTHYMOSIN α (ProTα)

CONSTANTIN N. BAXEVANIS, EMMANUEL ANASTASOPOULOS, PAULA ARSENIS, ANNA KATSIYIANNIS, NICK MATIKAS*, and M. PAPAMICHAIL

Dept. Immunology, Hellenic Anticancer Institute, 171 Alexandras Ave, 11522 Athens, and *Dept. Neurology, Evangelismos Hospital, Athens.

INTRODUCTION

Class II MHC antigens (Ia, DR) are expressed by macrophages/monocytes and play an important role in immunoregulation (1). We have recently reported an abnormal low DR expression on MS monocytes that correlates with impaired responses in the autologous mixed lympocyte reaction (auto MLR) in these patients (1). In this report we demonstrate that ProTα, a powerful immunopotentiator in vitro (3), restores to normal levels the deficient auto MLR in MS patients by increasing DR expression on the MS stimulatory monocytes.

MATERIAL AND METHODS

Patients. Twenty-nine patients with active MS entered this study.

Cell cultures. T cells and monocytes were isolated as previously described. Monocytes before testing were incubated for 2 days without (non-treated) or with ProTα (treated). ProTα was tried up to 2 µg/ml in steps of 200 ng/ml. AutoMLR cultures were set up as described elsewhere (2).

Cell binding assay. This assay detecting the binding of radiolabelled (Na125I) L243 monoclonal antibody in DR expressed by monocytes has been described on details elsewhere (2).

RESULTS

Treated MS monocytes were demonstrated to express increased levels of DR and to stimulate higher T cell responses in the autoMLR compared to non-treated or to freshly isolated (non-cultured) autologous monocytes. This is the first demonstration suggesting a link between decreased expression of DR on monocytes and cellular immune defects in MS.

TABLE I

THE EFFECTS OF ProTα ON DR EXPRESSION BY MS MONOCYTES. CORRELATION WITH AUTO MLR RESPONSES

Monocytes tested	Binding of anti-DR (^{125}I cpm x 10^{-3})		AutoMLR** (^{3}H cpm x 10^{-3})	
	MS*	Normal*	MS*	Normal*
Treated	10.8 ± 3.9	15.7 ± 4.5	21.5 ± 0.7	29.8 ± 10.8
Non-treated	2.5 ± 1.0	5.2 ± 1.7	4.3 ± 1.5	12.3 ± 3.9
Fresh	4.3 ± 1.5	11.9 ± 4.0	7.2 ± 2.5	21.5 ± 7.8

*   Mean values ± SD from pooled data (29 MS patients and 20 normal were tested).
**   Freshly isolated responder T cells were used.

AKNOWLEDGEMENTS

This work was supported with a grant from the Greek Ministry of Research and Technology to C.N.B.

REFERENCES

1. Unanue ER (1981) Adv. Immunol 31:1

2. Baxevanis CN, et al, (1989) J Immunol   (In press)

3. Baxevanis CN, et al, (1988) Immunopharmacology 15:73.

© 1989 Elsevier Science Publishers B.V. (Biomedical Division)
Recent advances in multiple sclerosis therapy.
R.E. Gonsette, P. Delmotte, editors.

REGULATION OF SUPPRESSOR CELL ACTIVITY IN PATIENTS WITH MULTIPLE SCLEROSIS (MS) BY MHC CLASS II GENE PRODUCTS

CONSTANTIN N. BAXEVANIS, EMMANUEL ANASTASOPOULOS, PAULA ARSENIS, ANNA KATSIYIANNIS, NICK MATIKAS*, and MICHAIL PAPAMICHAIL

Dept. Immunology, Hellenic Anticancer Institute, 171 Alexandras Ave, 11522 Athens, and *Dept. Neurology, Evangelismos Hospital, Athens.

INTRODUCTION

A consistent finding in patients with active MS has been the inability of the immune system to induce suppression (1). In this report we demonstrate that this defect is due to the reduced expression of DR molecules by the lectin-activated T cells. In addition we demonstrate that the levels of DR on expressed by MS monocytes dictate both the expression of DR autologous T cells in cultures with ConA and the extend of the induced suppression.

MATERIAL AND METHODS

Patients. All patients had clinical evidence of progressive MS for at least 3 years with a kurtzke disability rating between 3 and 7.

Cell cultures. DR+ T cells were detected in 6d cultures with 10% autologous monocytes and ConA as described elsewhere (2) ConA suppressor assay was performed as described by Antel et al (1).

Radioimmune assay. Determination of DR molecules on monocytes and T cells was performed using a radiolabelled anti-DR mAb (L243) and isotype matched but antigen irrelevant control mAb as previously described (3).

RESULTS

T cells from MS patients cultured with autologous monocytes [expressing low levels of DR(3)] and ConA expressed lower DR molecules and suppressed considerably weaker the proliferative response of allogeneic responder cells to ConA.

TABLE I

THE LEVELS OF DR EXPRESSED BY MONOCYTES DICTATE THE EXTEND OF ConA-INDUCED SUPPRESSION

Donors	DR on monocytes (^{125}I cpm × 10^{-3})	DR on activated T cells* (^{125}I cpm × 10^{-3})		% Suppression
MS	13 ± 5	T + Mo + ConA	6 ± 2	21 ± 9
(n = 14)		T + a-DR + Mo + ConA	2 ± 1	3 ± 1
Normals	28 ± 9	T + Mo + ConA	15 ± 4	76 ± 12
(n = 12)		T + a-DR + Mo + ConA	5 ± 2	24 ± 8

* Tcells were cultured with autologous monocytes (Mo) and ConA with or without anti-DR mAb. DR estimation on Mo was performed at the initiation of cultures. After culture the isolated viable Tcells were tested for DR expression and for suppressive activity (treated with mitomycin C).

AKNOWLEDGEMENTS

This work was supported by a grant from the Greek Ministry of Research and Technology to C.N.B.

REFERENCES

1. Antel JP, Bania B, Reder A, Cashman N (1986) J Immunol 137:137

2. Moriya N, Sanjoh K, Yokoyama S, Hayashi T (1987) J Immunol 139:3281

3. Baxevanis CN, et al, (9189) J Neuroimmunol (In press).

© 1989 Elsevier Science Publishers B.V. (Biomedical Division)
Recent advances in multiple sclerosis therapy.
R.E. Gonsette, P. Delmotte, editors.

PREVENTION OF SUBACUTE EXPERIMENTAL ALLERGIC ENCEPHALOMYELITIS IN GUINEA-PIGS
WITH DESFERRIOXAMINE, ISOPRINOSINE AND MITOXANTRONE

M. BISTEAU, G. DEVOS, J.M. BRUCHER and R.E. GONSETTE

Department of Neuropathology, Cliniques Universitaires St Luc, Avenue Mounier
52, B 1200 Brussels, Belgium

INDUCTION OF EAE

Immature Hartley Guinea pigs (250 g) are challenged with 0.3 ml of a saline
(1 ml) and complete Freund's adjuvant (2 ml) emulsion containing isogeneic
Guinea pig spinal cord tissue (1 g) and Mycobacterium tuberculosis (40 mg).
Three doses of 0.1 ml (amounting to 3 x 25 mg spinal cord tissue) are injected
respectively in the hind legs and in the nuchal area. Animals are weighed and
assessed daily for neurological signs. Most animals develop a subacute form of
EAE starting between day 9 and 13 after injection. Once started, the motor
deficit increases in severity until death which occurs on day 25 as a mean.
When moribund, Guinea pigs are killed and the brain and spinal cord are fixed
in buffered formaldehyde. Paraffine sections are stained with hematoxylin-
eosin and luxol fast blue.

SUPPRESSION OF EAE

DESFERRIOXAMINE (500 mg/ml) was administered via an osmotic pump (reservoir :
2 ml) implanted subcutaneously for 7 days at a continuous rate of 10 µl/h (120
mg/day). The drug was given either from day 1 to 7 or from day 7 to 14 (10
treated / 10 controls in each series).

ISOPRINOSINE was administered intraperitoneally from day 1 to 15 at doses of
100 mg/Kg/day or 500 mg/Kg/day (10 treated / 10 controls in each series).

MITOXANTRONE was administered intraperitoneally at a dose of 0.5 mg/Kg or
0.25 mg/Kg according to different time schedules.

RESULTS

Days of death and of onset of symptoms for treated animals and controls were analyzed using a BMDP statistical software (University of California, 1983) P1L programme (Kaplan-Meier analysis).

DESFERRIOXAMINE : continuous administration via the osmotic pump immediately after inoculation moderately delays both death and onset of symptoms. Administration after day 7 has no suppressive effect. As a matter of fact, effects on EAE with desferrioxamine in Guinea pigs are definitely less marked than those reported in rats.

ISOPRINOSINE : effects of Isoprinosine on EAE appear to be dose-related. Doses of 100 mg/Kg/day do not protect animals and make EAE even worse. With doses of 500 mg/Kg/day the mean and median survival time is higher in treated animals but there is no effect on the onset of symptoms.

MITOXANTRONE : daily administration of 0.5 mg/Kg Mitoxantrone yielded a complete suppression in nearly all animals. Very mild pathological changes were observed. Intermittent administration has no efficacy unless using higher doses (1 mg/Kg). Of note is that pathological changes are reduced even in non-clinically responding animals. In opposition to the findings in mice, Guinea pigs died from toxic effects (ascitis and/or infections) with effective doses.

CONCLUSIONS

Mitoxantrone is by far the most potent agent in preventing EAE. Both pathological and clinical changes are markedly reduced. This substance has proved safer in cancer therapy already and appears to be a good candidate in rapidly progressing MS patients.

Desferrioxamine and Isoprinosine are much less effective but have a very low toxicity and could be candidates in the early stages of the disease.

ACKNOWLEDGEMENTS

The advices of E. Gonsette for statistical evaluation are acknowledged. Investigation supported by funding from the Belgian Research Group.

© 1989 Elsevier Science Publishers B.V. (Biomedical Division)
Recent advances in multiple sclerosis therapy.
R.E. Gonsette, P. Delmotte, editors.

CLINICALLY DEFINITE MULTIPLE SCLEROSIS IN A ZAIRIAN WOMAN OF MIXED RACE

D. BOUCQUEY, C.J.M. SINDIC, C. LATERRE

St-Luc Hospital, Neurology Department, Avenue Hippocrate 10, Brussels, Belgium

INTRODUCTION

Multiple sclerosis (MS) is an unusual condition among tropical and sub-
tropical populations, especially in Central Africa. As far as we know, clinically definite MS has not yet been reported in Bantu people. We report here
the case of a Zaïrian woman of mixed race for whom we believe that a diagnosis
of clinically definite MS may be appropriate.

CASE REPORT

This 44-year-old woman has always lived in the province of Shaba, Zaïre.
Her father was Jewish and her mother Bantu. She never knew her father. She
was married and had 7 children in good health. Past medical history revealed
only a pre-diabetic state. Her neurological disease began in 1983 by transient paresthesiae first involving the right foot and then the left. She
experienced also a characteristic Lhermitte's sign wich has been present
intermittently since. In April 1987, she complained of numbness and hypaesthesia in the left limbs and face. Simultaneously, she suffered from episodes of blurred vision. Nobody in her family or surroundings had similar
medical problems. In October 1987, neurological examination revealed a slight
left hemiparesis. The gait was unsteady. Muscle stretch reflexes were slightly increased in the right arm and the left leg. Extensor plantar responses
were observed bilaterally. The finger-to-nose testing was disturbed on the
left side. Sensitive examination showed tactile hypaesthesia of the left side
and right leg. Pin-prick sensation was normal except for the right hemiface.
Left corneal hypaesthesia was noted but the cranial nerves were otherwise
intact. General examination was unremarkable.

Blood analysis disclosed a normal haemogram, the absence of systemic
inflammation (ESR 16 mm/h, CRP < 0.5 mg/dl, no anti-DNA and anti-ENA autoantibodies). Anti-HIV-1 and 2 and anti HTLV-1 antibodies (Bio Tech, Du Pont)
were not detected. Syphilitic serology was negative. CSF analysis revealed
$19/mm^3$ lymphocytes without malignant cells. Glucose level was 105 mg/dl and
the protein content 40 mg/dl. IgG oligoclonal bands restricted to the CSF
were detected by an immunoblotting method after agarose isoelectric focusing
(Figure). Evoked potentials disclosed abnormal responses in visual and somes-
thethic pathways. Brain MRI showed multiple hyperintense signals of the
periventricular white matter on proton-density-weighted images (Figure).

302

DISCUSSION

MS is considered to be a place-related disorder. Although sparse cases of demyelinating disease have been reported in Central Africa[1-3], MS remains an unusual condition in these regions. However, a slowly progressive neurological disorder, known as tropical spastic paraparesis, has been linked to HTLV-1 retrovirus infection[4]. MRI of these patients may reveal areas of increased signal intensity and evoked potentials may show alterations of the visual or brainstem responses as in MS. In this case, HTLV-1 serology was negative and biological data did not support a diagnosis of vasculitis. This patient therefore fulfilled recommended criteria for MS diagnosis[5]. To explain this unique occurrence of MS, one has to take into account a genetic susceptibility transmitted from her father. However, environmental agent(s) wich induce the disease should be more ubiquitous than thought until now.

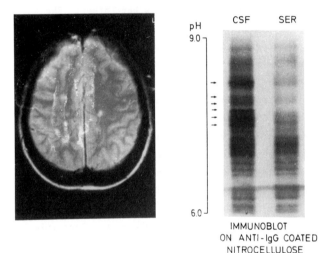

Figure : left panel : high signal lesions in the periventricular white matter on proton density weighted images. Right panel : IgG oligo- clonal bands restricted to the CSF (arrows) detected by an immunoblotting method.

REFERENCES

1. Foster RM, Harries Jr (1970) Br Med J 3 : 628

2. Collomb H, Dumas M, Lemercier G, Girard PL (1970) Afr J Med Sci 1 : 257-266

3. Kurtzke JF (1980) Neurology 30 : 61-79

4. Osame M, Matsumoto M, Usuku K et al Ann Neurol 21 : 117-122

5. Poser CM, Paty DW, Scheinberg L et al (1983) Ann Neurol 13 : 227-231

© 1989 Elsevier Science Publishers B.V. (Biomedical Division)
Recent advances in multiple sclerosis therapy.
R.E. Gonsette, P. Delmotte, editors.

EVOLUTION OF COGNITIVE DYSFUNCTION IN MULTIPLE SCLEROSIS: A COMPARISON WITH VASCULAR DEMENTIA AND ALZHEIMER'S DISEASE.

L. BRACCO, M.P. AMATO, M. BALDERESCHI, C. GIORGI, A. LIPPI, L. FRATIGLIONI, D. INZITARI AND L. AMADUCCI.
Departement of Neurology, University of Florence, Florence, Italy.

AIMS OF THE STUDY, MATERIALS AND METHODS

This study is devoted to define the neuropsychological profile of patients with Multiple Sclerosis (MS) and to establish if pattern and evolution of their cognitive deficit conform to the typical feature of subcortical dementias, as suggested by some authors (1). For this purpose we administered an extensive neuropsychological battery to 23 hospital controls affected by diseases of the PNS; 32 patients with clinically definite MS according to Poser's criteria; 10 patients suffering from probable Alzheimer's Disease (AD) according to the NINCDS-ADRDA criteria and 45 patients presenting Cerebro-Vascular-Disease (CVD) diagnosed on the basis of Hachinski's score $>$ 7, focal neurological signs and white matter hypodensity on CT scan. Each subject was investigated at basal examination and two years later as far as Information (Inf), Orientation (Casor), Mental Ability (Casma), Concentration (Conc), Personal and Remote Memory (Pmem, Rmem), Short Term Memory (Digit), Acquisition and 10'-Delayed Recall of a Short Story (BAB acq, BAB 10'), Acquisition, 10'- and 24hours- Delayed Recall of Five Items and Paired Words (FI acq, FI 10', FI 24h, PW acq, PW 10', PW 24h), Spatial Memory (Corsi), Verbal Comprehension (Token Test, TT) and Constructive Capacities (Copying Drawing, CD) were concerned. Test scores were adjusted according to age and educational level and converted in "z" scores to obtain neuropsychological profiles. All the subjects were classified as "no" or "mildly" mentally impaired using some battery tests that showed to stage with high accuracy the overall mental impairment degree (2).

RESULTS AND CONCLUSIONS.

All the controls, 17 MS (4 M, 13 F; mean age 32.5 years, SD 7.8) and 29 CVD (24 M, 5 F; mean age 64.1, SD 6.4) were mentally health. All AD (4 M, 6 F; mean age 61.1, SD 7.2), 15 CVD (10 M, 5 F; mean age 64.1, SD 9) and 15 MS (6 M, 9 F; mean age 44.7, SD 7.2) presented mild mental impairment. Their performances were significantly worse than controls and no demented MS and CVD patients in all tests but Digit Forward and Personal Memory. AD, CVD and MS mildly demented patients displayed similar neuropsychological profiles (Fig.1).

FIG 1   NEUROPSYCOLOGICAL PROFILES IN CONTROLS, AD, CVD, AND MS

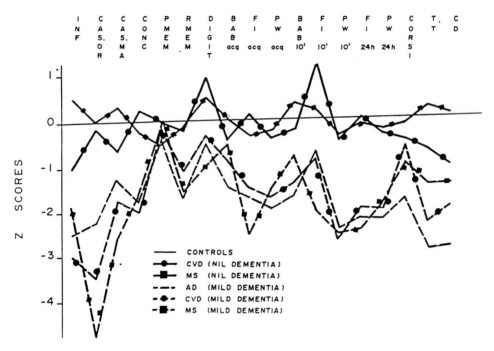

In particular, no significant difference was detected in scores of tests exploring specific cognitive functions such as concentration, prose memory, verbal comprehension, constructive capacities. Specific features of the neuropsychological pattern of cortical dementia, such as impairment of language and praxia, were displayed by AD as well as by CVD and MS patients, while concentration impairment, considered characteristic of subcortical dementias, was present with the same severity in the three groups. The two-years follow up identified three different trends of evolution: no control showed signs of mental impairment; the 15 MS patients remained at the same degree of dementia showing only a trend towards a decrement in most cognitive functions, 4 CVD patients became moderately impaired while the whole AD sample progressed from mild to moderate dementia. Therefore, we suggest that the progression of mental impairment is slower in MS and CVD than in AD and that the different neuropsychological pattern evidentiated in cortical vs. subcortical dementias could be due to the different stages of the disease rather than to real specific neuropsychological profiles.

REFERENCES

Huber SJ, Shuttleworth EC, Paulson GW, Bellchambers MJ and Clapp LE (1986) Arch Neurol 43: 392-394.

Bracco L, Tiezzi A; LippiA; Amaducci L. (1986) Inter J Ger Psych 1: 99-106.

© 1989 Elsevier Science Publishers B.V. (Biomedical Division)
Recent advances in multiple sclerosis therapy.
R.E. Gonsette, P. Delmotte, editors.

CHAIN OF EVENTS LEADING TO DEMYELINATION

J. COLOVER*, D.S. SKUNDRIC** AND B.V. ZLOKOVIC**

*Department of Immunology, Rayne Institute, United Medical and Dental
Schools, St. Thomas' Hospital, London SE1 7EH, England and **Institute of
Physiology and Pathophysiology and Histology, Medical Faculty, University of
Belgrade, Yugoslavia

INTRODUCTION
    Although a number of studies have been performed on changes in Blood
Brain Barrier permeability in multiple sclerosis (M.S.) using MRI techniques
and gadolinium, the precise nature and relation of such changes to the onset
of histological features in demyelination are not known and such precise
information has not been obtained by studies on humans. We have studied an
animal model to obtain this information. In guinea pigs pretreated with
muramyl dipeptide and ovalbumin followed 4 weeks later by I.P. ovalbumin and
then sensitized to myelin basic protein (MBP), extensive demyelination occurs
(1) and has been studied in the earlier stages before histological changes
and clinical features become apparent. Also the guinea pig is very suitable
for such studies as the cerebral circulations on the two sides are
independent and it is possible to perfuse one half of the brain independently
from the other by carotid perfusion. There is no circle of Willis to allow
cross circulation.

MATERIALS AND METHODS
    Guinea pigs were subjected to the demyelinating protocol previously
outlined (1) and then at set intervals (Fig. 1), the carotid vessels on
either side were perfused using a pump at constant pressure for 10 minutes.
The perfusion fluid was made up of a synthetic plasma and the oxygenation was
done by means of sheep red cells. To this perfusion medium was added
^{125}I-IgG or normal IgG or D-(^{3}H) mannitol according to the method of Zlokovic
et al (2) where the method is described in detail. Standard size blocks of
brain tissue were then assayed for the labelled IgG or mannitol from
different areas of the brain. Also immunocytohistology was done on sections
using antibody to IgG. Samples of cisternal fluid were examined for albumin
and IgG simultaneously with samples of serum and the results expressed as

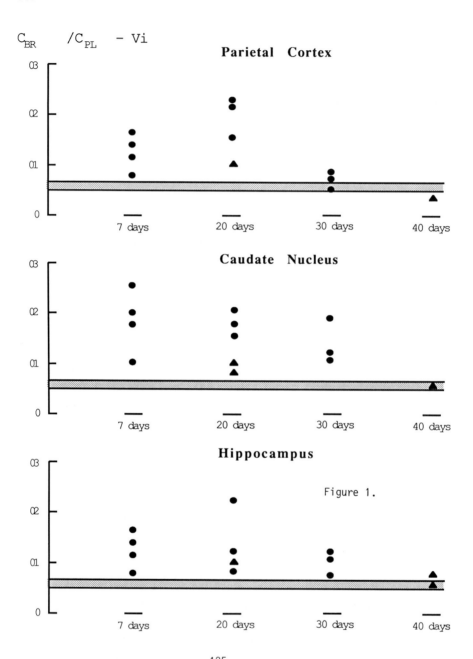

Fig. 1. Shows cerebral uptake of ^{125}I-IgG in different areas of the brain. Each round dot = 5 animals. Triangles are single animals. Shaded areas are levels in normal animals.

CSF/serum albumin and IgG quotients. Many animals developed signs of EAE.
Normal animals were similarly perfused as controls (3).

RESULTS AND DISCUSSION

Changes in the brain and CSF are shown in Figs. 1 and 2. These show
that within 7 days of the injection of MBP there was considerable uptake in 3
areas of the brain parietal cortex, caudate nucleus and hippocampus of IgG.
This subsided at 30 days and was normal at 40 days. Radiolabelled mannitol
was absorbed more erratically. Immunocytohistology after normal IgG
perfusion showed that the uptake of IgG was into the endothelium of the
cerebral vessels and that this IgG also diffused out into the perivascular
regions. Previous histological studies did not show any recognizable
histological changes at 7 days and it would appear that this specific change
in permeability and IgG uptake is the earliest recognizable change in the
brain. Fig. 2 shows that the albumin quotient in the CSF shows a steady rise
up to 40 days and that the IgG quotient shows a transient rise between 21-32
days after the MBP and then begins to fall and is much less. The CSF and the
neural tissue thus behave quite differently.

SUMMARY

A form of EAE characterized by acute demyelination has been studied
using well controlled perfusion techniques in which the brains of guinea pigs
at different stages were perfused by an artificial blood medium to which was
added radiolabelled IgG, or mannitol. Standard blocks of brain tissue from 3
different areas were assayed for the radiolabelled IgG or mannitol.
Immunocytohistological studies were done on sections. Also the CSF/serum
quotients for albumin and IgG were measured in the CSF.

The results showed that there is a specific transport system for IgG
into the endothelium of the cerebral vessels and that the IgG migrates into
the perivascular areas within 7 days after the myelin basic protein is
injected, prior to the development of histological changes. Mannitol was
taken up much less uniformly. The capacity to take up the IgG was lost at
about 40 days. In the CSF there was a steady increase in the albumin
quotient up to 40 days. The rise in IgG quotient was much less and maximal
at 21 to 32 days .

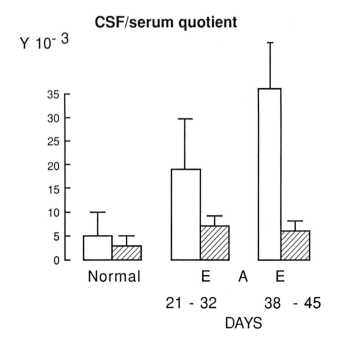

CSF/serum quotient

Y 10⁻³

Fig. 2. Cerebrospinal fluid quotients of albumin (clear rectangles) and IgG (shaded rectangles) . Days after sensitization.

ACKNOWLEDGEMENTS

     J.C. is pleased to acknowledge assistance from ARMS (Action for Research into Multiple Sclerosis). We also wish to thank the British Council, The Wellcome Trust and the Republicki Zavod za Medjundrodnu Saradnuju SR Srbije for support.

REFERENCES

1.   Colover J. (1980). Brit. J. Exp. Path. 61: 390-400.

2.   Zlokovic B.V., Begley D.J., Djuricic B.M. and Mitrovic D.M. (1986).   J. Neurochem. 46: 1444-1451.

3.   Zlokovic B.V., Skundric D.S., Segal M.B., Colover J. , Jankov R.M., Pejnovic N., Lackovic V., Mackic J., Davson H., Dumonde D.C. and Rakic L.J. (1989). Metabolic Brain Disease (in the press).

© 1989 Elsevier Science Publishers B.V. (Biomedical Division)
Recent advances in multiple sclerosis therapy.
R.E. Gonsette, P. Delmotte, editors.

309

MAGNETIC STIMULATION OF MOTOR CORTEX IN MS: CORRELATIONS WITH CLINICAL, SEP
AND BRAIN MRI FINDINGS.

GIANCARLO COMI, GIUSEPPE GALARDI, MASSIMO FILIPPI, MARIA GRAZIA NATALI SORA,
TIZIANA LOCATELLI, VITTORIO MARTINELLI, CHIARA LIA, ANNA VISCIANI.
Multiple Sclerosis Center, Scientific Institute H.S. Raffaele, University of
Milan, Via Olgettina 48, 20132 Milan (Italy).

INTRODUCTION

Magnetic stimulation allows to measure the conduction time in the descending
motor pathways, applying single magnetic stimuli over the scalp and spinal column.

In this study we performed both cortical and spinal magnetic stimulation in a
group of MS patients in order to assess the frequency of Motor Evoked Potential
(MEP) abnormalities and to evaluate the correlations with clinical signs of
pyramidal involvement, brain Magnetic Resonance Imaging (MRI) and Somatosensory
Evoked Potential (SEP) findings.

PATIENTS AND METHODS

We investigated 42 MS patients (14 male and 28 female) aged between 16 and 66
yrs (mean age: 37.1 yrs). The mean duration of the disease was 6.9 yrs. According
to McDonald and Halliday's criteria we classified 27 patients as definite, 6 as
probable and 9 as suspected MS.

Magnetic stimulation was performed with a Dantec equipment at motor cortex
(coil positioned at the vertex), at cervical (C5-C6) and the lumbar column (L4-L5)
levels. Recording sites were the abductor pollicis brevis for the upper limb and
the adductor hallucis for the lower limb. Cortical, cervical and lumbar MEP
latencies, upper and lower limb Central Motor Conduction Time (CMCT) and CMCT
side to side difference were evaluated bilaterally in all patients. The parameters
were considered abnormal if exceeding the mean value + 3 SD of normal controls.

MRI and SEPs were performed as previously described (1).

RESULTS

We observed a significant increase of both upper and lower limb CMCT in MS
patients versus normal subjects (Table I).

MEPs were abnormal in 83% of MS patients (94% of definite and probable and 44%
of suspected cases). Upper and lower limb MEPs were delayed in 56% and 61% of
patients respectively. 69% of our patients had clinical involvement of motor

pathways: 57% of these patients had also abnormal CMCT, while 13% of patients with delayed CMCT had no pyramidal signs. SEPs were abnormal in 71% of the patients (58% had clinical sensory signs). Both SEPs and MEPs were abnormal in 35% and in 46% of patients for upper and lower limb respectively; while 23% for upper and 16% for lower limb had only delayed CMCT. MRI was abnormal in 78% of the patients; 12% of patients with normal MRI had delayed CMCT.

TABLE I MEAN VALUES OF MEPs IN MS PATIENTS AND NORMAL CONTROLS

Upper limb	MS	Controls	t-Student
cortical MEP latency	24.51	20.07	p<0.001
cervical MEP latency	13.95	13.50	N.S.
CMCT	10.56	6.58	p<0.001
side to side difference	1.92	0.38	p<0.001
Lower limb			
cortical MEP latency	46.87	40.18	p<0.001
lumbar MEP latency	25.01	24.35	N.S.
CMCT	22.16	15.81	p<0.001
side to side difference	3.30	0.50	p<0.005

DISCUSSION

Central motor conduction was more frequently abnormal than SEPs and MRI in our group of MS cases. These data agree with previous reports (2,3). In some patients MEP abnormalities were unilateral or restricted to upper or, more frequently, to lower limbs; these findings can be justified by the patchy distribution of MS plaques. We found a good correlation in about 3/4 of patients between MEPs and clinical and MRI findings and in about 1/2 of patients between MEPs and SEPs. As far as MEPs and pyramidal signs relationship is concerned, magnetic stimulation demonstrated subclinical central motor involvement in 13% of the cases.

In conclusion we consider advisable in the assessment of MS patients the bilateral evaluation of central motor pathways in addition to evoked potentials and MRI examination.

REFERENCES

1. Comi G et al. (1989) J Neurol 236: 4-8

2. Berardelli et al. (1988) J Neurol Neurosurg Psych 51: 677-683

3. Ingram DA et al. (1988) J Neurol Neurosurg Psych 51: 487-494

CYTOGENETIC EVALUATION IN MULTIPLE SCLEROSIS

*E. D'ALESSANDRO, *M. DI COLA, *C. LIGAS, *M.L. LO RE, *C.VACCARELLA,°F.D'ANDREA, °C. MARINI and M.°PRENCIPE.

*Cattedra di Genetica Medica, °Cattedra di Neurologia, Università degli Studi di L'Aquila, I-67100, ITALIA.

INTRODUCTION

Genetic factors seem to be involved in the aethiology of Multiple Sclerosis (MS). Cytogenetic studies (1,2) have shown an higher incidence of aspecific chromosomal changes and spontaneous Sister Chromatid Exchanges (SCEs) in MS patients, but no significant structural abnormalities have yet been found. In previous reports (3, 4) we failed to find a significative frequency of spontaneous SCEs and aspecific aberrations in patients studied in different clinical phases, however cytogenetic analysis showed same sporadic abnormal chromosomes.

MATERIALS AND RESULTS

The present study was performed on 48 patients (32 females, 16 males) with relapsing remitting form in 34 cases and remitting progressive in 14. All MS cases were sporadic, with negative family history and had none been ascertained as being in contact with environmental mutagens. In 50% of the patients we found at least one metaphase with one or more chromosomal abnormality, including X chromosome aneuploidy (14.6%). The abnormal chromosomes are supernumerary and only a few of them have been identified. Structural aberrations, translocations or deletions of chromosome 3, with breakpoints in q23 and q21-23, occurs in 20.8% of our patients

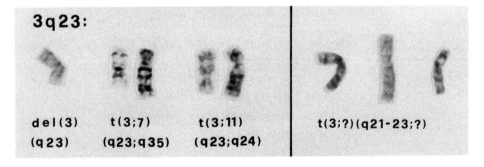

3q23:

| del(3) | t(3;7) | t(3;11) | t(3;?)(q21-23;?) |
| (q23) | (q23;q35) | (q23;q24) | |

Fig. 1 . Structural aberrations involving chromosome 3.

312

in three cases these rearrangements involve chromosomes 7, 8 and 11 with breakpoints in q35, q24 and q24 respectively. The premature centromere division (PCD) of X chromosome has been identified (12.5%). In seven cases (14.6%) two metaphases of the same patient show an identical abnormality. The rate of SCEs/cell has been also evaluated. There was not statistically significant difference of SCE rate for MS patients (7.09+/-1.50) and our normal population (6.71+/-1.45) p=0.1 . Therapy does not seem to modify our findings: the comparison between treated and untreated subjects did not show significant differences for chromosomal changes or SCE's rate (p=0.7). Chromosomal aberrations are present in 44.1% of patients with remitting form of MS and in 64.3% of patients with remitting progressive form. Nevertheless a statistically significant difference was found analysing the frequency of relapse in cases with remitting form of the disease (p=0.04).

DISCUSSION

This work confirms our previous results which pointed out a sporadic gain of some abnormal chromosomes. Therefore, these findings appear to be nonrandom, but we cannot consider them chromosomal markers although an identical abnormality was found in two metaphases of the same patient (could this be a clonal formation ?). We would like to emphasize the involvement of chromosome 3. These aberrations could be explained as other sporadic rearrangements involving chromosomes 7 and 14 (5), but they are present more than once in patients with the same pathology (20.8%). Moreover we would like to underline the presence of PCD,X. We found PCD, X in supernumerary elements and the aneuploid X chromosome, as probable expression of the same phenomenon, in 22.9% of our patients. This phenomenon has been previously associated with striking aneuploidy in human malignancies, in deficiency states and autoimmune disorders (6). Clinical cytogenetic correlations showed the greatest incidence of chromosomal changes in the remitting progressive form and in the progressive form with high frequency of relapse.
In conclusion our results suggest a possible nonrandom DNA damage associated with a more "active" disease.

REFERENCES

1. Träder J.M. et al. (1985) Fortschr Neurol Psychiat,53,134-137.
2. Senecal-Quevillon M. et al. (1986) Mutat Res,110,141-146.
3. D'Alessandro E. et al. (1987) Riv Neurol,57(2),107-110.
4. D'Alessandro E. et al. (1988) Excerpta Medica, Amsterdam, p70.
5. Scheres J.M.J.C. et al. (1986) Cancer Genet Cytogenet,19,151-158.
6. Bülher E.M. et al. (1987) Ann Genet, 30(2),75-79.

© 1989 Elsevier Science Publishers B.V. (Biomedical Division)
Recent advances in multiple sclerosis therapy.
R.E. Gonsette, P. Delmotte, editors.

313

SERUM FACTORS INTERACTING WITH T CELL RECEPTORS

F D'ANDREA° C MARINI° P PELLEGRINI°° A BERGHELLA°° D ADORNO°° M PRENCIPE°
° Clinica Neurologica Università di L'Aquila °° Istituto CNR di Tipizzazione
Tissutale L'Aquila - ITALY

INTRODUCTION

The reduction of T8+ lymphocytes during the exacerbating phase of Multiple

Sclerosis, has been reported by many authors (Bach 1980, Reinherz 1980). It

has been suggested that autoantibodies or other factors may modulate the

density or conformation of T8 lymphocyte antigens (Antel 1982, Paty 1983,

Reder 1984). Aim of this study is to verify the presence of immunomodulating

factors in serum of MS patients.

MATERIAL AND METHODS

T lymphocyte subset count and serum collection were performed on 226 blood

samples from control subjects, 157 from MS patients on remission phase and 48

from MS patients on acute phase. Each blood sample was incubated with three

different type of sera: 1) from control subjects (Ctrl-s) 2) from MS patients

on remission phase (RP-s) 3) from MS patients on acute phase (AP-s). After the

first incubation, blood samples were submitted to a subsequent incubation with

the three different type of sera. T-cell subsets count was performed by an

indirect immunofluorescence assay using monoclonal antibodies (Ortho

Diagnostic) to human T suppressor/citotoxic cell (OKT8) surface antigens.

Positively stained cells were counted using a fluorescence microscope.

Incubation of PBMC with sera: equal volumes (500 ul) of PBMC at 5x10 /ml

concentration and serum were incubated "in vitro" for 30 min. at 37° in

triplicate. Cells were then washed twice in a large volume of HBSS. An aliquot

of this suspension was used for T cell subset count, the remainder cells at

5x10 /ml concentration were further incubated with same or other sera. Data

analysis was performed by using analysis of variance (ANOVA).

RESULTS

Results of first incubation are showed in Table 1. T8+ cells of controls and

of MS patients on remission showed a significant decrease after incubation

with AP-s (P 0.001, ANOVA). On the contrary no modification was observed when the cells were incubated with Ctrl-s and RP-s. T8+ cells of MS patients on acute phase showed a significant increase after incubation with RP-s (P 0.001) while no modification were observed with AP-s and Ctrl-s.

TABLE 1: RESULTS OF FIRST INCUBATION

Source of T8 cells	Basal Values	INCUBATION		
		+ Ctrl-sera	+ RP-sera	+ AP-sera
Controls	33.8+/-2.3	32.9+/-1.5	34.0+/-2.0	24.0+/-2.5
Remission phase	33.3+/-2.1	33.0+/-2.0	33.8+/-1.9	24.0+/-1.8
Acute phase	23.9+/-3.1	23.9+/-1.7	34.5+/-2.6	22.9+/-2.1

Results of second incubation are showed in Table 2. T8+ cells of controls and of MS patient on remission phase, submitted to a subsequent incubation with RP-s showed a return to normal values (P 0.001). No modification was observed when the second incubation was performed with Ctrl-s and RP-s. On the other hand T8+ cells of MS patients on acute phase were restored to low values after incubation with AP-s (P 0.001) while no modification was observed with Ctrl-s and RP-s.

TABLE 2: RESULTS OF SECOND INCUBATION

Source of T8 cells	Values after 1°incubation	INCUBATION		
		+ Ctrl-sera	+ RP-sera	+ AP-sera
Controls +A-sera	23.1+/-2.7	23.1+/-2.4	34.5+/-1.8	22.5+/-2.6
Remission phase +A-sera	23.0+/-1.8	22.9+/-1.6	33.1+/-2.0	22.0+/-1.9
Acute phase + R-sera	33.9+/-2.0	33.7+/-2.0	33.5+/-2.3	23.3+/-2.2

COMMENT

These data suggest that MS patients sera have two different factors: the former is able to mask the T8 surface antigens and is present in acute phase of the disease, the latter is able to remove the masking effect and is present in remission phase of the disease. A possible explanation of our results may be that after a brief exposure to masking factor a proportion of cells with T8 antigen are unable to bind T8 moAb. It can be due to the binding of this factor either to T8 antigen or to a molecule present on the cell surface that is able to sterically mask the T8 antigen.

REFERENCES

1. Bach M A, Phan-Dhin-Toy E et al (1980) Lancet 2: 1221–1223

2. Reinherz E L, Weiner H L et al (1980) N Engl J Med 303: 125–129

3. Antel J P, Oger J F (1982) Proc Natl Acad Sci USA 79: 3330–3334

4. Paty D W, Kaustroff L et al (1983) Ann Neurol 14: 445–449

5. Reder A T, Antel J P et al (1984) Ann Neurol 16: 242–249

© 1989 Elsevier Science Publishers B.V. (Biomedical Division)
Recent advances in multiple sclerosis therapy.
R.E. Gonsette, P. Delmotte, editors.

MAGNETIC STIMULATION OF MOTOR PATHWAY IN MULTIPLE SCLEROSIS PATIENTS. A COMPARISON WITH MULTIMODAL EVOKED POTENTIALS

P. DE CASTRO, J. ARTIEDA, S. FLORENTIN, J.M. MARTINEZ LAGE
Department of Neurology. Clinica Universitaria. University of Navarra.

INTRODUCTION

The study of conduction in central nervous system pathways is an established clinical value in diagnosis and evolutive control of patients with multiple sclerosis, but until recently it has been confined to afferent systems. Actually central motor conduction may be determined using percutaneous magnetic stimulation of the motor cortex. We have studied the conduction of central motor pathways using cortical and cervical magnetic stimulation in multiple sclerosis patients and healthy subjects. In addition the percentage of central motor conduction abnormalities and trimodal evoked potentials abnormalities founded were compared.

METHODS

Twenty patients with a diagnosis of definite multiple sclerosis (clinically or laboratory supported, Poser 1983 (1)) and fifteen healthy volunteers (age matched) were studied. The general and clinical characteristics of both groups are specified in Table I.

TABLE I

GENERAL AND CLINICAL CHARACTERISTICS OF MULTIPLE SCLEROSIS PATIENTS AND CONTROLS

	N	Sex	Height	Age	Kurtzke.S.	Piramidal.S.
C	15	8/7	161 ±8,94	41,36±15,3		(ext. Sup.)
MS	20	11/9	161,7±8,5	38,2 ±12,7	0 - 8	9/18

In each patient trimodal evoked potentials, and central motor conduction time for both upper extremities were analized.

The central motor conduction time was calculated bilaterally by using magnetic stimulation at the cortical level (vertex) and at the cervical level (C7). The evoked motor response was recorded on both abductor digiti minimi muscles (ADM). The procedure was carried out by using a magnetic field generated by a clockwise and anticlockwise current. Minimal latencies obtained were analyzed. All the recordings were made at absolute muscular rest. The central conduction time was calculated substracting the latencies of motor evoked potentials obtained after C7 stimulation and the latencies of motor evoked potentials after cortical stimulation.

The evoked potentials -visual (reversal pattern) brain-stem auditory (60 dB HL), and somatosensory (median and posterior tibial stimulation)- were carried out according to the American Academy EEG criteria (1986).

RESULTS

The MEP latencies obtained by cortical and cervical stimulation, the central motor conduction time and the assymetries between both sides were analized. The values that were more than three standard deviations from normal, were considered abnormal.

The motor evoked potential (MEP) latencies and the central motor conduction times, were significatively longer in the group of multiple sclerosis patients than in the control group. The statistical study and the values obtained are shown in Table II.

In many cases, the assymetries (between left and right side) in the latencies of motor evoked potentials obtained by cortical stimulation, were statistically more significant in the group of multiple sclerosis patients (Table III).

The incidence of abnormalities found using magnetic stimulation (75%) were greater than those obtained using trimodality evoked potentials (70%). The incidence of abnormalities increased to 85% when the four techniques (visual, auditory, somatosensory, motor evoked potentials) were used.

TABLE II

LATENCIES OF EVOKED MOTOR RESPONSES (MEP) BY CORTICAL AND CERVICAL
STIMULATION IN MULTIPLE SCLEROSIS PATIENTS AND CONTROLS

	Cortical St. Latencies (ms)		C7 St. Latencies (ms)		Central Conduction (ms)	
	RADM	LADM	RADM	LADM	R	L
CONTROLS	19,8	19,78	12,21	12,23	7,6	7,54
	± 1,28	± 1,33	± 0,78	± 0,80	± 1,03	± 1,01
	(18,1-23)	(17,7-22,9)	(11,1-13,7)	(11,2-13,7)	(5,4-9,3)	(5,8-9,2)
SM	27,9	29,11	13,41	13,42	14,80	16,08
	± 9,17	± 10,45	± 1,11	± 1,18	± 9,2	± 10,53
	(21-59,4)	(21,4-59,4)	(12,1-17)	(11,9-17)	(8,9-45,2)	(8,3-45,2)
	F= 23,02		F= 23,05		F= 18,53	
	P< 0,001		P< 0,001		P< 0,01	

RADM: Right abductor digiti minimi
LADM: Left abductor digiti minimi

TABLE III

MEP LATENCIES EVOKED BY CORTICAL AND CERVICAL MAGNETIC
STIMULATION IN MULTIPLE SCLEROSIS PATIENTS AND CONTROLS.
RIGHT LEFT ASIMETRIES IN RESPONSE

	Cortical St. (ms)	C7 Stimulation (ms)	Central Cond. (ms)
CONTROL	0.30 ± 0.40 (0-1.1)	0.39 ± 0.37 (0-1.1)	0.19 ± 0.31
MS	2.75 ± 3.02 (0-9.2) F= 9.66 P< 0.01	0.39 ± 0.37 (0-1.2) n.s.	2.5 ± 0.38 F= 6.95 P< 0.05

CONCLUSIONS

The central motor conduction time is prolonged in
patients with multiple sclerosis; there are assymetries
between left and right side in these patients. The magnetic
stimulation has the highest sensitivity in detecting
demielinating lesions of piramidal motor pathways. The
range of abnormalities detected in the motor pathways is
greater than the abnormalities in afferent sensitive
pathways using multimodality evoked potentials.

Our results point out the importance of this technique in
the diagnosis and evolutive control of M.S. patients and
should be included in M.S. protocols.

REFERENCES

1. Poser ChM, Donald MD, Paty MD, and col. (1983) New
   Diagnostic Criteria for Multiple Sclerosis: Guidelines
   for Reserarch Protocols. Annals of Neurology, pp
   227-231.

© 1989 Elsevier Science Publishers B.V. (Biomedical Division)
Recent advances in multiple sclerosis therapy.
R.E. Gonsette, P. Delmotte, editors.

MULTIPLE SCLEROSIS (MS) ETIOLOGY : THE PANCREATIC HYPOTHESIS

YVES DE SMET[1,2], JEAN MARIE BRUCHER[2]

1. Hôpital Régional du Nord, b.p.103, L-9002 Ettelbruck (GD of Luxembourg)
2. Laboratory of Neuropathology, ANPG 5260, UCL, B-1200 Brussels (Belgium)

MS etiology remains unknown and its pathogenesis a mystery. Two major complementary hypothesis have permanent supporters : a persistent slow viral infection
and/or a genetic alteration of the immune system. So, MS may be considered as
a four-stage viral-immunological disease[1,2,3], including : a) a genetically-
determined susceptibility in the immune system, but not associated with the
major histocompatibility system; b) an environmental initiatory event between
ages 5 and 15 producing a symptomless systemic illness (virus? vaccine?); c)
an unspecific vasculopathic alteration of the blood-brain barrier (BBB) permeability (hormonal? immune-mediated? trauma?); d) a myelinoclastic plaque-forming
mechanism. So, an unspecific viral disease in the late childhood, adolescence
or early adult life induces the formation of homologous circulating "antimyelin"
antigens and the secretion of gamma interferon, which respectively leads to
the activation or reactivation of antimyelin basic protein (MBP) circulating
T lymphocytes (through a crossed immunisation). The undetermined BBB alteration
permits the transfer in the CNS of (yet unknown!) anti-MBP lymphocytes. The
consequent autoimmune reaction induces demyelination and MS. But evidences for
an infective agent are lacking and much doubts remain concerning the pathogenetic significance of the reported alterations of the immune system. Moreover,
the primary acute MS lesion is a perivascular humoral inflammation, but not
a demyelinating lesion showing immune cells infiltrates[4]. The acute predemyeli-
nating MS lesion consists of a venular and perivenular fibrinous edema, but
the usually modest nature of this venulitis counts against a virulent bacterial
or viral attack; likewise, this non-necrotising inflammatory vasculitis is too
slight and too chronic for a floride autoimmune reaction; nevertheless, the
inflammatory agent inducing such a fibrinous exudate may be of a physical or
chemical nature[4]. On the other hand, the functionnal handicap during the first
attacks of MS seem secondary to the edema only; likewise, the rapid regression
of the symptoms after high doses corticotherapy seems the result of the inter-
ruption of the inflammatory transsudation's phenomena at the level of the recent
lesion. Swank also reported about fibrin-mediated subcutaneous hemorrhages in
MS[5]. Finally, the course of experimental allergic encephalomyelitis (EAE) may
be modified with prazosin, a drug known to affect only vascular tone[7].

So, other upholders emphasize marginal etiopathogenies, such as inflammatory process[5], trauma, diet[6], stress, toxins[8] or fat embolism[9,10]. Moreover, in presenting the evidences for subacute fat embolism in MS, James[9] did not argue that all relapses proceed from further embolism; but the proven damage to the BBB in lesions may allow many circulating toxic or infective agents access to brain tissue. On the other hand, pancreatic encephalopathy presents many resemblances to MS[12] : disseminated, patchy, often perivenular loss of myelin, occasional perivascular hemorrhages, moderate gliosis and no axonal destruction. In fact[13], inflammatory pancreatitis may be acute, relapsing or chronic; the causes of pancreatitis are very protean, including viruses, diet, stress or trauma, like MS; drugs against pancreatitis like proteinase inhibitors may modify the clinical and/or pathological course of EAE and MS[11,14]; the pancreas secretes lipoproteolytic enzymes which also are myelinolytic; a variety of factors (toxins, sepsis, inflammatory disorders, ischaemia, trauma) are believed to activate proenzymes within the pancreas. Activated proteolytic enzymes digest pancreatic tissue but also activate other enzymes and cause proteolysis, edema, interstitial hemorrhage and vascular damage; the liberation of activated enzymes produces enzymatic toxemia. In addition, activation and release of vasoactive substances produce vasodilatation, increased vascular permeability and edema. So, we suggest a Poser-like[1] four-stage process as etiopathogeny of MS, which take into account the viral-immunological cellular hypothesis, but as a secondary result of a genetically-mediated unspecific subclinical pancreatopathy, induced by unspecific environmental factors (trauma, stress, diet, virus, vaccine) and inducing through circulating enzymes, first an inflammatory humoral vasculitis (with BBB permeability alteration and perivascular edema), then an enzymatic demyelinating mechanism leading to an accessory autoimmune reaction. Such an hypothesis explains James' suggestion of MS as a BBB disease[15], first supported by Gonsette et al[16].

(13.HARRISON's Principles 9th ed McGraw-Hill 1980.)

REFERENCES

1.POSER CM ActaNeuropathol 1986;71:1-10. 2.POSER CM JNeurolSci 1987;79:83-90.
3.POSER CM JNeurolSci 1988;84:117-119. 4.ADAMS CWM JNeurolSci 1985;69:261-283.
5.SWANK RL Neurology 1958;8:497-499. 6.SWANK RL AmJMedSci 1950;220:421-430.
7.GOLDMUNTZ EA et al BrainResearch 1986;397:16-26.
8.WOLFGRAM R NeurochemicalResearch 1979;4:1-14. 9.JAMES PB Lancet 1982;ii:380-86.
10.HULMAN G Lancet 1988;ii:1366-67. 11.SIBLEY RE et al Neurology 1978;28:102-105.
12.BRUCHER JM et al In:Gonsette RE, Delmotte P (eds) Immunological and clinical aspects of MS. MTP Press Limited, 1984, p 362.
14.DAVISON X, CUZNER Y (eds) The suppression of EAE and MS. Academic Press, 1980.
15.JAMES PB Lancet 1989;i:46. 16.GONSETTE RE et al ActaNeurolBelg 1966;66:247-62.

© 1989 Elsevier Science Publishers B.V. (Biomedical Division)
Recent advances in multiple sclerosis therapy.
R.E. Gonsette, P. Delmotte, editors.

DEXAMETHASONE VERSUS SYNTHETIC ACTH IN THE TREATMENT OF ACUTE BOUTS IN MULTIPLE SCLEROSIS

GÜNTHER ESSINGER, KLAUS LAUER, WOLFGANG FIRNHABER

Department of Neurology, Academic Teaching Hospital,
Heidelberger Landstrasse 379, D-6100 Darmstadt (F.R.G.)

INTRODUCTION

Whereas numerous investigations demonstrated a short-term therapeutic effect of ACTH or steroids on symptomatology, CSF findings, CT or MRI findings in MS, only few studies compared both drugs with each other (1,2), but the results were inconclusive. Since we had changed our standard regimen in acute bouts from ACTH (1 mg/day over 28 days) to dexamethasone (initially 16 mg/day, declining over 6 weeks) in 1980, we were able to make a comparison by means of a retrospective evaluation of hospital files.

METHODS

150 treatment courses of dexamethasone in 137 patients with definite or probable MS were compared with 40 courses of tetracosactid (Synacthen^{TM}) in 32 patients. Both groups agreed well with respect to sex ratio, type of time course (75% intermittent), age, age at onset, duration(6vs.5.5 yrs.), prior relapse rate, duration of bout under study, percentage of azathioprine-treated patients (21 vs. 28%), and symptomatic treatment. DSS, ambulation index, and a 4-grade functional index for 6 systems were assessed immediately before therapy and 3-10 weeks later. In 111 patients (82 after dexamethasone over 2.5 years at average ; 29 after ACTH over 4.0 years at average), the subsequent annual relapse rate was analyzed. All comparisons were made by chi^2-contingency table analysis.

RESULTS

The pretreatment scores were lower in the ACTH group for sensory ($P < 0.01$) and vegetative ($P < 0.05$) functions, whereas no significant variations existed for the other systems. As shown in Tbl.1, the improvement in relation to basic level was more marked in the dexamethasone group for DSS, ambulation index, motor and sensory score, whereas only a borderline value was reached for vegatative functions. No difference in efficacy was found for visual, brainstem and coordination scores. The relapse rate after therapy decreased from 0.75 to 0.72 in the dexamethasone, and from 0.71 to 0.64 in the ACTH group.

DISCUSSION

The present data are in agreement with a recent double-blind
study in 30 patients (2). In contrast to Massacesi et al., however, we could not find a clear difference of the subsequent
relapse rate, which fact underscores the superior effect of
dexamethasone. Possible reasons for this more favourable effect
might be a high rate of penetration into the CNS (3), a longer
biological half-life (1), a pronounced antioedematous effect
(4) and/or an inhibitory effect on demyelination (5). In each
case, the more beneficial effect also on sensory symptoms argues in favour of a stronger antiinflammatory activity of
dexamethasone in addition to the antispastic effect which
might have influenced DSS and ambulation index.

Tbl. 1: Mean change between score before and after treatment

	Dexamethasone	ACTH	P
DSS	1.40	0.70	< 0.001
Ambulation index	1.16	0.25	< 0.001
Vision	0.78	0.60	n.s.
Brainstem function	0.75	0.54	n.s.
Motor function	0.74	0.15	< 0.001
Sensory function	0.78	0.39	< 0.001
Coordination	0.53	0.32	n.s.
Bladder/bowel	0.81	0.14	< 0.1

REFERENCES:

1. Troiano R,et al.(1987) Arch Neurol 4:803-807
2. Milanese C,et al.(1989) Eur Neurol 29:10-14
3. Balis FM,et al.(1987) J Clin Oncol 5:202-207
4. Reid AC,et al.(1983) Ann Neurol 13: 28-31
5. Triarhou LC,Herndon RM (1986) Arch Neurol 43: 121-125

FAILURE TO DETECT CYTOKINES IN SPINAL FLUIDS OF PATIENTS WITH
OPTIC NEURITIS AND MULTIPLE SCLEROSIS.

J. FREDERIKSEN[1], K. BENDTZEN[2], H.B.W. LARSSON[3], O. HENRIKSEN[3].
Dept. of Neurology[1], Gentofte Hospital, Dept. of Immunology[2],
Rigshospitalet, and Magnetic Resonance Dept. [3], University of
Copenhagen, Denmark.

In recent years magnetic resonance imaging (MRI) has led to
an increased knowledge of the pathophysiology of multiple scle-
roris (MS) and optic neuritis (ON), but still the immunological
correlates of the lesions seen on MRI are largely unknown. Interleukin (IL) 1 α/β are potent peptide hormones which are thought
to be involved in MS. Also, tumor necrosis factor (TNF) may
play an important role in inflammatory processes leading to MS.
The production by T-lymphocytes of patients with MS of interferon gamma (INF-γ) has previously been reported to be elevated.
The presence of these cytokines in spinal fluids of patients
with acute ON was investigated.

MATERIALS
Fifteen untreated patients (9 women, 6 men) aged 12-46 (median 28)
years with acute optic neuritis were equally divided into 3 groups:
Patients with isolated ON, patients with MS at onset of ON and
patients with subsequent evolution of MS. All patients, except
3 with isolated ON showed cerebral lesions on MRI. A control
material was available for each analysis.

METHODS
Lumbar puncture was performed within 1 to 30 (median 12) days
from onset of acute ON. At least 300 μ l CSF was immediately
frozen at -80° to be analyzed as follows: IL 1 α/β was measured
by a biological assay, El-4 (at 0.1 and 1.0 volume percent),
with a detection limit of 0.1 U/ml. IL 1 α/β inhibitors were
measured by a classical thymocyte costimulating assay, TNF by
a bioassay and IFN-γ was measured biochemically.

RESULTS
There were no measureable content of neither IL 1 α/β nor
IL 1 α/β inhibitors, which were measured by a very sensitive

assay at different concentrations of CSF. Also TNF and IFN-γ
were not present in measurable concentrations, even in patients
with big periventricular lesions as judged by MRI.

CONCLUSION

Judged from the results of examining CSF from selected patients
with acute optic neuritis (ON) the above mentioned cytokines
play to major role at clinical manifestation of acute ON, but
whether their role precide the attack of ON is unknown.

© 1989 Elsevier Science Publishers B.V. (Biomedical Division)
Recent advances in multiple sclerosis therapy.
R.E. Gonsette, P. Delmotte, editors.

NEOPTERIN IN SERUM AND CSF IN PATIENTS WITH MULTIPLE SCLEROSIS
AND/OR OPTIC NEURITIS.

J. FREDERIKSEN[1], P.R. HANSEN[2], H. LARSSON[3].
Department of Neurology[1], Gentofte Hospital, University of Co-
penhagen, Statens Seruminstitut[2] and MR-department[3], Hvidovre
Hospital, University of Copenhagen, Denmark.

Magnetic resonance imaging MRI has revealed a wide range of
abnormalities in the brain of patients with multiple sclerosis
(MS), to a certain extent depending upon the disease stage.
The wide spectrum of number, sizes and extents of lesions rises
the need for immunological parameters, which may be valuable to
follow the disease activity. Neopterin is a devirate in the synthetic pathway of biopterin, which acts as a co-factor in neuro-
transmitter synthesis. Neopterin is easily diffuseable and is
involved in a wide range of immunological processes. We investigated the concentration of neopterin in 3 well-selected
groups of patients.

MATERIAL
Concomitant serum and CSF was derived from 6 patients with
chronic progressive MS, 6 patients with stable MS (though recently a minor excercabation) and 6 patients with isolated acute
optic neuritis (ON). MRI was abnormal in all but 5 patients;
those had isolated ON. Patients (10 women, 8 men) aged 12-57
(median 34) years, were all untreated at the time of examination.
Six healthy persons aged 18-67 (median 38) years served as controls.

METHOD
Serum and CSF were frozen immediately at -80 degrees celcius,
and neopterin (nmol/l) was measured by RIA-analysis, the kit
being Neopterin-RIAcid (Hennig Berlin GMBH).

RESULTS
Median values and ranges of neopterin in serum were 3.4(2.7-6.3)
in progressive (p) MS; 4.3(2.3-5.0) in stable (s) MS, 4.9(2.3-9.0)
in isolated acute ON and 5.9(2.2-9.8) in healthy controls. The

328

concentration of neopterin in CSF was less than 3 nmol/l in all
examined persons except for 3 patients with values of 7.4(pMS),
6.2(sMS) and 12.6(sMS), respectively. The corresponding concentration of neopterin in serum were 3.4, 2.6 and 5.0, respectively.

CONCLUSION
We report the results of a pilot study of concentration of
neopterin in serum and CSF in subgroups of patients with MS.
With reservation of the small number of patients (and controls)
in each group, neopterin in serum seems to be lowered in MS
(especially progressive MS) as compared to controls. The results
in CSF gave no evidence of abnormalities in MS.

© 1989 Elsevier Science Publishers B.V. (Biomedical Division)
Recent advances in multiple sclerosis therapy.
R.E. Gonsette, P. Delmotte, editors.

MAGNETIC RESONANCE IMAGING IS A PREDICTOR FOR LATER DEVELOPMENT
OF MULTIPLE SCLEROSIS IN ACUTE MONOSYMPTOMATIC OPTIC NEURITIS.

J. FREDERIKSEN[1], H.B.W. LARSSON[2], O. HENRIKSEN[1].
Department of Neurology[1], Gentofte Hospital, University of Co-
penhagen and MR-Department[2], Hvidovre Hospital, University of
Copenhagen, Denmark.

Judged from the literature the risk of developing multiple
sclerosis (MS) following a first attack of monosymptomatic optic
neuritis (mON) ranges from 8-85%, primarily depending on length
of follow up. We undertook a prospective study of patients with
acute ON to increase the pathophysiological knowledge of monosymptomatic ON and to obtain a better understanding of the relationship between ON and MS.

MATERIAL
During 28 months, 83 consecutive patients with acute (defined
as duration of visual symptoms less than a fortnight) ON were
extensively screened for known ethiologies of ON. Sixteen had
clinically definite MS (CDMS), 7 patients could not participate
for various reasons. Serial magnetic resonance imagings (MRIs)
and neurological examinations were performed in the remaining
60 untreated patients (42 women, 18 men aged 12-53 (median 31)
years) with mON, in 7 bilaterally simultaneously. The initial
MRI was performed within 3-49 (median 16) days from onset of
symptoms. Twenty healthy control persons matched for age and
sex had normal MRIs.

METHODS
MR-scanning was performed at 1.5 T with 2 sequences (slice
thickness 4 mm, voxel size 1.2 x 1.2 x 4 mm^3): double spin echo
(TR = 1.8 s, TE = 30 and 90 ms, 12 slices axially) and inversion
recovery (TR = 2.45 s, TI = 400 ms, TE = 30 ms, 5 slices sagit-
tally).

RESULTS
Among patients presenting with mON, MRI revealed clinically
silent lesions in the CNS in 39/60 (=65%) of patients. The ap-

pearence, locations and extents of lesions were consistent with
demyelination. 12 of 60 (20%) patients developed CDMS during a
follow up of 1-28 (median 11) months, and they all had lesions
on MRI at onset. The clinical relapse was experienced within
1-9 (median 3) months from onset of mON.

CONCLUSION
Those patients with monosymptomatic acute ON showing lesions
on MRI at onset run a much higher risk of later developing
clinically definite MS. The results of MRI was the sole predictive factor, and the degree of visual loss did not influence
the risk of subsequently development of MS.

© 1989 Elsevier Science Publishers B.V. (Biomedical Division)
Recent advances in multiple sclerosis therapy.
R.E. Gonsette, P. Delmotte, editors.

SERIAL VEPs. A PROSPECTIVE STUDY OF 62 PATIENTS WITH ACUTE UNI-
LATERAL OPTIC NEURITIS.

J.FREDERIKSEN[1], H.B.W.LARSSON[2], and B.STIGSBY[3].
Department of Neurology[1] and Clinical Neurophysiology[3], Gentofte
hospital, University of Copenhagen and Magnetic Resonance Department[2], Hvidovre Hospital, University of Copenhagen, Denmark.

No clear consensus as to the clinical value of visual evoked
potential (VEP) changes in multiple sclerosis (MS) has emerged,
but it is a wide-spread opinion that VEP is always abnormal in
eyes affected by acute optic neuritis (ON) and is seldom normalized
at follow up. This study aimed to investigate VEPs in patients with
acute ON (either idiopathic or as an attack of MS) in the very
acute stage of ON and at follow up.

MATERIAL

Sixtytwo consecutive patients (41 women, 21 men) aged 12-57
(median 32) years were diagnosed with ON (duration less than 14
days) based on clinical criteria. Patients with known ethiologies
of ON apart from MS were excluded. Patients were followed prospectively thus VEP was performed immediately at referral and
2,4,13 and 26 weeks afterwards.

METHOD

Pattern reversal VEP was elicited by black-white checkerboard
pattern of 22.6° visual subtense (each square = 1.4°) presented
monocularly (stimulation frequency 1.5 Hz, 100 sweeps). The VEP
changes amplitude of the major positive peak and the shape of the
potential. Normal limits (mean +3SD) were derived from 61 healthy
subjects matched for age and sex.

RESULTS

Refer-ral	During follow up	Day 180	VEP in eyes with acute ON onset		VEP in contra-lateral eyes onset	
			−MS	+MS	−MS	+MS
A	A	A	22	11	13	5
A	N	A	1	0	1	1
A	A	N	11	3	2	1
N	A	A	5	0	7	1
N	A	N	3	0	4	1
N	N	N	6	0	21	5

A = abnormal, N = normal.

Focusing on the results in patients without MS at onset of acute ON (n=48) we emphasize that normal VEP ($\leq$ mean +3SD) at onset may occur, which might be explained by a very short interval between onset of ON and VEP in this study and referral of patients with only minor symptoms to this research project. In cases with a mild ON, the diagnosis was confirmed by findings of cerebral plaques on MRI. Complete normalization of VEP frequently occured. Abnormal VEP (sometimes only temporarily) was observed in 27/48 (56%) of the clinically unaffected eyes.

CONCLUSION

Serial VEPs is a valuable tool to monitor visual pathway conduction accurately, and the results indicate a big dynamic range of the VEP.

© 1989 Elsevier Science Publishers B.V. (Biomedical Division)
Recent advances in multiple sclerosis therapy.
R.E. Gonsette, P. Delmotte, editors.

MAGNETIC RESONANCE IMAGING AND ANALYSES OF CSF IN PATIENTS WITH ACUTE MONOSYMPTOMATIC OPTIC NEURITIS.

J. FREDERIKSEN[1], H.B.W. LARSSON[2], E. KJÆRSGAARD[3], J. OLESEN[1], O. HENRIKSEN[2].

Department of Neurology[1] and Internal Medicine[3], Gentofte Hospital, University of Copenhagen, and Department of Magnetic Resonance[2], Hvidovre Hospital, University of Copenhagen, Denmark.

Optic neuritis (ON) may often be the first clinical manifestation of multiple sclerosis (MS) and this sign offers a special opportunity to study the very early stages of MS.

MATERIALS AND METHODS

As a part of a prospective study of patients with acute ON, 68 patients were consecutively referred. Eleven had clinically definite MS, another 10 refused a lumbar puncture and seven could not participate for various reasons. In the remaining 40 untreated patients (28 female, 12 men) aged 12-53 years with monosymptomatic ON, we have studied the interrelationships of parameters measured in CSF (white cell count, IgG-index and presence of oligoclonal bands (OBs) and their relationship with MR aspects of the disease process. Lumbar puncture and MRI were performed within median 24 (1-48) and 16 (3-49) days from onset of acute ON, respectively. OBs were obtained by agarose gel-electrophoresis with immune fixation. MRI was performed at 1.5 T with double spin echo and inversion recovery sequences. All methods were evaluated in healthy controls and thereby normal limits were obtained.

RESULTS

Abnormalities in the CSF was found in a total of 62% of the patients, thus in 50% raised white cell count, in 35% raised IgG-index and OBs were present in 14% of the patients. MRI showed lesions in the cerebrum, cerebellum and brain stem in 62% of the patients, thus being more sensitive than each analysis of CSF. MRI, IgG-index and OBs are complementary to each other in revealing subclinical abnormalities in monosymptomatic acute ON.

334

CONCLUSION

The relationship between MRI of the brain and immunological studies of the CSF is, though not clearcut, helpful in better under-standing of the pathogenesis and dynamics of multiple sclerosis.

© 1989 Elsevier Science Publishers B.V. (Biomedical Division)
Recent advances in multiple sclerosis therapy.
R.E. Gonsette, P. Delmotte editors.

MRI, VEP, SEP AND BIOTESIOMETRY SUGGEST MONOSYMPTOMATIC ACUTE
OPTIC NEURITIS TO BE A FIRST MANIFESTATION OF MULTIPLE SCLEROSIS.

J. FREDERIKSEN[1], H.B.W. LARSSON[2], B. STIGSBY[3], J. OLESEN[1], O. HEN-
RIKSEN[2].
Department of Neurology[1], and Clinical Neurophysiology[3], Gentofte
Hospital, University of Copenhagen and MR-Department[2], Hvidovre
Hospital, University of Copenhagen, Denmark.

A cohort of fifty consecutive patients with acute monosymptomatic optic neuritis (mON) from a defined uptake area joined a
prospective study to compare the sensitivity of magnetic resonance imaging (MRI), electrophysiological methods (VEP and SEP,
(n. medianus and n.tibialis)) and quantitative vibration thres-
holds measured by biotesiometry to detect silent lesions in
the CNS outside of the affected optic nerve(s) during the acute
phase of mON.

MATERIAL AND METHODS
Fifty untreated patients (34 women, 16 men) aged 12-53 (median 31)
years with acute mON (7 patients bilateral simultaneously, 43 unilaterally) were immediately referred to our clinic to participate in this research project. VEP elicited by black-white pattern
shift was performed the same day, whereas SEP and biotesiometry
were performed within the following week. All but 2 patients
(both with contraindication to MRI) underwent MRI of the cerebrum,
cerebellum and brainstem 3-49 (median 16) days after onset of
symptoms. An adequate control material was established for each
method.

RESULTS
VEP recorded from the eyes with acute ON were abnormal initially
in all but 8 eyes, however, after one week the VEP of additio-
nally 5 eyes became abnormal. MRI proved to be the most sensitive
method (63% abnormal) as compared to VEP (42%) in the clinically
unaffected eye, SEP (17%) and biotesiometry (33%). The combination of all above mentioned methods except for MRI (and VEP in
eyes with acute ON) revealed abnormalities in 63% of patients.

Further combined with MRI, 79% of patients had abnormal findings suggesting additional - clinically silent - lesions in CNS.

CONCLUSION

MRI and neurophysiological examinations are complementary to each other and provide evidence that monosymptomatic acute ON is usually not a disease entity distinct from MS. The development of clinically definite MS in 7 of 50 patients during maximally 20 months of follow up support this view.

© 1989 Elsevier Science Publishers B.V. (Biomedical Division)
Recent advances in multiple sclerosis therapy.
R.E. Gonsette, P. Delmotte, editors.

INCREASED LEVELS OF IL-2 AND sIL-2R IN MS SERUM.

PAOLO GALLO, MARIA G. PICCINNO, VICENZA ARGENTIERO, SILVANA PAGNI, BRUNO

GIOMETTO, FELICE BOZZA, and BRUNO TAVOLATO

Institute of Neurology, University of Padua, 35128 Padova, Italy.

INTRODUCTION

Interleukin 2 (IL-2) plays an essential role in triggering proliferation of activated, antigen-reactive, T-cells, a response mediated by interaction of the factor with a high affinity membrane receptor (IL-2R). The soluble form of IL-2R (sIL-2R), usually detected at low levels in the serum of normal persons, can be found at higher levels in conditions associated with lymphocyte activation, and it is supposed to play a role in the down regulation of the immune system (included the IL-2/gamma interferon (γ IFN) regulatory circuit).

In order to define the relation between disease activity and lymphocyte activation "in vivo", we studied the serum levels of IL-2 and sIL-2R in 50 Multiple Sclerosis (MS) patients.

MATERIAL AND METHODS

Sera from 50 patients with clinically definite or laboratory-supported definite MS, and from 30 normal subjects were included in the study.

Two commercial ELISA systems were used (Intertest-2, Genzyme Co., and Cell-free, T-cell Sciences), according to the manufacturer's instructions.

RESULTS

Increased sIL-2-R levels (exceeding the range observed in control subjects) were found in 22 out of 50 MS patients (44%). The mean value was significantly higher in MS patients (mean $\pm$ SD = 428 $\pm$128) compared to the control group (mean $\pm$ SD = 185 $\pm$ 56, p $<$ 0.001) (Fig. 1a).

In testing sera with IL-2 ELISA, increased OD405 reading values were also

338

found in MS patients (Fig. 1b). The mean value was significantly higher in MS patients (mean ± SD = 187 ± 82) compared to the control group (mean ± SD = 100±36, p < 0.001). When compared against a standard IL-2 curve (made by using human recombinant IL-2), the IL-2 levels in units/ml were 37.6±23.8 in MS sera compared to 2.3±1.4 control sera. (Table 1).

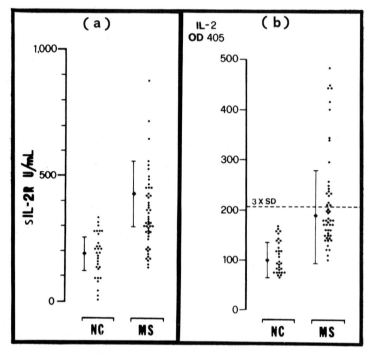

Fig. 1 (see text for explanations)

	Multiple Sclerosis (50)	Normal subjects (30)
IL-2 U/ml :	37.6±23.8	2.3±1.4
sIL-2R U/ml :	428±128	185±56

Table 1: Serum levels of IL-2 and sIL-2R in patients with Multiple Sclerosis and normal controls (number of subjects into brackets).

DISCUSSION

Increased sIL-2-R levels have been demonstrated in the sera of patients with autoimmune diseases and certain B- or T-cell malignancies, thus suggesting a role for sIL-2-R in the down-regulation of the immune system (including decreased natural cytotoxic activity and low γ IFN production) often seen in such patients.

We found significantly elevated titers od sIL-2-R in sera of MS patients compared to ormal control subjects. This increase is noteworthy because it further stresses a systemic T-cell activation in MS, and suggests that sIL-2-R may be involved in a systemic immune imbalance. Since sIL-2-R bind IL-2 efficiently, they may block the binding of IL-2 to cell surface receptors and therefore they may be involved in a down-regulation of at least some T-cell subsets. Such an event could conceivably explain the defects in the IL-2/ γ IFN regulatory circuit that have been described in MS patients and attributed to inhibitory factors such as prostagliandin E.

Our data leave no doubt that systemic T cell activation occurs in MS patients and support the hypothesis that an immunologic disorder exists in such patients. A time-course analysis to establish the relation bvetween IL-2 and sIL-2-R on one hand, and disease activity and progression on the other, is in progress.

ACKNOWLEDGEMENTS

This work was supported by grants from Associazione Italiana Sclerosi Multipla and from Regione Veneto.

© 1989 Elsevier Science Publishers B.V. (Biomedical Division)
Recent advances in multiple sclerosis therapy.
R.E. Gonsette, P. Delmotte, editors.

IMMUNOGLOBULIN FREE LIGHT CHAINS IN MULTIPLE SCLEROSIS CEREBROSPINAL FLUID

PAOLO GALLO*, AKE SIDEN**, and BRUNO TAVOLATO*

*Institute of Neurology, University of Padova, 35128 Padova, Italy, and

**Department of Neurology, Huddinge University Hospital, S-14186 Huddinge,

Sweden.

INTRODUCTION

Agarose gel isoelectric focusing (AIEF) and nitrocellulose (NC) immunoblotting were used for detection of immunoglobulin free light chains (FLC). The occurrence of CSF FLC was investigated in MS, other inflammatory neurological diseases (OID), other non-inflammatory neurological diseases (OND) and controls. The patient material included subjects with as well as without IgG oligoclonal bands (OB) in the CSF.

MATERIAL AND METHODS

Paired CSF and serum samples were obtained from 50 MS patients, 18 subjects with OID and 17 with OND as well as 15 control cases. Basic CSF investigations, including AIEF for detection of IgG OB, were performed. CSF FLC were visualized by AIEF, NC blotting and avidin-biotin amplified double-antibody peroxidase staining of IgG Fc-fragments and bound as well as free kappa and lambda chains. FLC positive samples were also examined by alpha and u chain staining.
Sodium dodecyl sulphate polyacrylamide gel electrophoresis (SDS-PAGE) and NC immunoblotting were applied to analyze if FLC occured in mono- and/or dimeric form.

RESULTS

The data are summarized in Table 1 and Figure 1 gives an example of the AIEF immunoblotting findings.

All sera as well as the CSF of controls and subjects with OND were negative for FLC. Among the MS patients, CSF FLC were detected in 44 cases; three of these subjects were negative for IgG OB in the CSF.

Table 1.

Diagnosis, No. of cases in brackets		No. of cases with:		
		IgG OB	FLC	IgG OB and FLC
MS	(50)	46	44	41
OID:				
Herpes simplex encephalitis	(6)	6	6	6
Neurosyphilis	(6)	6	6	6
Aseptic meningitis	(2)	0	1	0
Subacute sclerosing panencephalitis	(2)	2	2	2
Post chickenpox cerebellitis	(2)	1	2	1
OND:				
Dementia of Alzheimer type	(8)	0	0	0
Amyotrophic lateral sclerosis	(4)	0	0	0
Parkinsonism	(4)	0	0	0
Meningioma	(1)	1	0	0
Controls	(15)	0	0	0

Five out of the six MS patients without FLC in the CSF were positive for IgG OB. In OID, FLC were present in the CSF of 17 out of the 18 patients. Two of the FLC positive cases did not exhibit IgG OB in the CSF. The FLC negative subjects had no CSF IgG OB. The FLC components detected in MS and OID show clear restricted heterogeneities at AIEF where they were focused into distinct bands. FLC in the individual CSF samples were of kappa as well as lambda identity or either kappa or lambda type; samples exhibiting kappa as well as lambda free light chains were most frequent.

At SDS-PAGE of specimens being positive for FLC, dimers as well as monomers of such components were identified.

DISCUSSION

CSF FLC were detected in about 90% of patients with MS or OID and such findings were present also in subjects being negative for IgG OB in the CSF. There were no data favouring degradation of immunoglobulin molecules as the mechanism causing occurrence of FLC. Other mechanisms, e.g. a strong antigenic stimulation or a B-cell deregulation, seem to be more probable. AIEF with NC immunoblotting for FLC staining can be a valuable complementary tool for detection of intrathecal immunological phenomena.

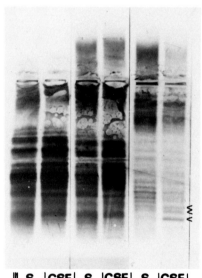

Ⅲ S ICSFI S ICSFI S ICSFI
1   2   3

Fig. 1: Paired serum (S) and CSF from a MS patient having not IgG OB. 1-2-3 indicate anti-IgG, anti kappa and anti-lambda immunofixations respectively. A clear pattern of lambda FLC was detected (arrow-heads).

ACKNOWLEDGEMENTS

This study was supported by grants from the Italian Society for Multiple Sclerosis, Regione Veneto, the Karolinska Institute, the Swedish Medical Research Council and the Swedish Multiple Sclerosis Society.

CLINICAL CONTROLLED RANDOMIZED TRIAL OF AZATHIOPRINE IN MULTIPLE SCLEROSIS.

A. GHEZZI, M. DI FALCO, C. LOCATELLI, M. ZAFFARONI, D. CAPUTO, S. MARFORIO,
C.L. CAZZULLO

Centro Studi Sclerosi Multipla, Ospedale di Gallarate, Via Pastori, 4
21013 Gallarate - Italy

INTRODUCTION

Among immunosuppressants, azathioprine (AZA) is one of the most widely used drug in the treatment of multiple sclerosis (MS). Several mainly uncontrolled studies have been published in the past, with conflicting results (1). In 1988 a randomized controlled trial of 354 MS patients has been concluded (2), showing a slightly lower number of relapses and a slightly lower deterioration in Kurtzke scores in AZA treated patients, but not at significant levels. A trend in favour of AZA + metilprednisolone for limiting disease progression was found by Ellison et al. (3) in a randomized trial of 98 chronic progressive patients. In a controlled study of 39 MS patients we did not find significant differences between AZA treated patients and controls (4).
Here we present the results of a controlled randomized trial of 185 MS patients.

MATERIAL AND METHODS

185 definite consenting MS patients took part in the study: 74 patients presented a relapsing course, 111 patients a relapsing progressive course. Patients with disease duration lower than 1 year, Kurtzke disability status higher than 7, concomitant diseases controindicating immunosuppression were excluded from the study; patients were randomized to receive AZA 2.5 mg/Kg daily or not. Relapses during the study were treated with corticosteroids. The follow up lasted 18 months. 24 AZA treated patients and 26 controls did not conclude the study, 13 AZA treated patients because of side effects (anaemia:3, gastric intolerance:5, hepatopathy:4, cutaneous rash 1)one patient after surgical operation. The others did not come back for further observations. Clinical status assessed by Kurtzke Func

Table 1: characteristics of the patients who concluded the study (range).

	AZA TREATED (32)	CONTROLS (22)
RELAPSING (54)		
Females/males	23/9	16/6
Age of onset (Ys)	26 (15–42)	26 (18–42)
Disease duration (Ys)	5 (1–14)	5 (1–20)
Relapse rate prestudy	1.2 (0.2–4)	1.1 (0.2–3)
Disability prestudy	2.1 (1–5)	2.2 (1–5)
RELAPSING PROGRESSIVE (81)	(37)	(44)
Females/males	22/15	27/17
Age of onset (Ys)	29 (12–44)	31 (16–47)
Disease duration (Ys)	6.5 (1–36)	8.5 (2–22)
Relapse rate prestudy	0.6 (0.1–3.3)	0.4 (0.1–2.5)
Disability prestudy	3.8 (1–6.5)	3.7 (1–7)

Table 2: Clinical evolution, assessed with Kurtzke Disability Status Scale (in brackets functional system scores), in relation to treatment and course.

RELAPSING (54)	IMPROVED	STABLE	WORSENED	x^2 test
AZA TREATED (32)	5 (7)	18 (15)	9 (10)	p > 0.10
CONTROLS (22)	0 (1)	14 (11)	8 (10)	
RELAPSING–PROGR. (81)				
AZA TREATED (37)	2 (2)	17 (13)	18 (22)	p > 0.10
CONTROLS (44)	3 (3)	22 (16)	19 (25)	

Table 3: Number of relapses in relation to treatment and course.

RELAPSING (54)	MEAN (SD) NUMBER OF RELAPSES	t-test
AZA TREATED (54)	0.87 (1.07)	p = 0.73
CONTROLS (22)	1.00 (1.44)	
RELAPSING–PROGR. (81)		
AZA TREATED (37)	0.70 (1.10)	p = 0.78
CONTROLS (44)	0.63 (1.08)	

tional System and Expanded Disability Status Scales by blind neurologists and re lapses before and at the end of the study were recorded for each patient. The cha racteristics of the patients who concluded the study are reported in table 1.

RESULTS AND COMMENT

Patients were classified as "improved", "stable", "worsened" in relation to the difference between final and initial Kurtzke scores: results did not show signifi cant differences between AZA treated and control patients. The number of relapses during the study are reported in table 3: results were not significant at t–test. Data were analyzed in relation to initial disability (EDSS $\leq$ 3/ > 3) disease du ration $\leq$ 5/ > 5 ys), sex, age of onset ($\leq$ 25/ > 25): no statistically signifi-cant result was observed for each correlation. In 13 patients AZA therapy was not continued because of side effects.

To conclude: clinical evolution and number of relapses did not differ signifi-cantly after a follow up of 18 months in relation to the treatment with azathio-prine. Clinical outcome was not influenced by clinical course, initial disability disease duration, sex, age of onset.

REFERENCES

1) Noseworthy JH, Seland TP, Ebers GC (1984) Therapeutic trials in multiple sclerosis. Can J Neurol Sci 11:355–362
2) British and Dutch Multiple Sclerosis Azathioprine Trial Group (1988) Double masked trial of azathioprine in multiple sclerosis. The Lancet,July,179–183
3) Ellison GW, Myers LW, Mickey MR et al. (1988) Clinical experience with aza-thioprine: the pros. Neurology 38:20–23
4) Ghezzi A, Zaffaroni M, Caputo D et al. (1988) Immunosuppression with azathio-prine in multiple sclerosis. In: Cazzullo CL, Caputo D, Ghezzi A, Zaffaroni M (eds) Virology and immunology in multiple sclerosis. Springer–Verlag, Berlin

© 1989 Elsevier Science Publishers B.V. (Biomedical Division)
Recent advances in multiple sclerosis therapy.
R.E. Gonsette, P. Delmotte, editors.

SERUM SEX HORMONE AND GONADOTROPINE CONCENTRATIONS IN MENSTRUATING WOMEN WITH MULTIPLE SCLEROSIS.

LOTTE GRINSTED, M.D.[1], HENNING DJURSING, M.D.[1], ANNE HELTBERG, M.D.[2], CLAUS HAGEN, M.D.[3].

[1] Department of Obstetrics and Gynecology, University Hospital of Copenhagen, DK-2650 Hvidovre, Denmark.

[2] Department of Neurology, Amtssygehuset Roskilde, DK-4000 Roskilde, and MS-Hospital, DK-4690 Haslev, Denmark.

[3] Department of Endocrinology, University Hospital of Copenhagen, DK-2730 Herlev, Denmark.

Serum concentrations of prolactin, gonadotropines, sex hormone binding globulin (SHBG) and free and bound estrogen- and androgen levels were measured in 14 regularly menstruating patients with clinically definite multiple sclerosis (MS). None had experienced fertility problems.

14 regularly menstruating normal women served as controls.

Both groups were sampled during the early follicular phase of the cycle.

Serum levels of prolactin were significantly ($P<0.05$) higher in the MS group compared to controls, and 2 patients displayed prolactin levels above the normal range. Gonadotropine levels were significantly ($P<0.05$) higher in MS patients compared to controls, and 6 MS patients had LH levels above the normal range while 5 had raised FSH levels. In addition, MS patients had significantly higher serum levels of testosterone ($P<0.01$) and androstenedion ($P<0.001$) and significantly lower serum levels of estrone sulphate ($P<0.001$) compared to controls

11 MS patients had estrone sulphate levels below normal range whereas other hormonal parameters were within the normal range for most of the patients. MS patients with disability status score of 6-7 had significantly ($P<0.01$) higher testosterone concentration compared with patients having disability status score of 2-4 (1.4 ± 0.1 nmol/l versus 1.0 ± 0.1 nmol/l). Other hormonal parameters were not related to age, degree of disability or MS activity.

None of the patients revealed clinical symptoms of hyperandrogenism, hypoestrogenism or hyperprolactinemia.

In a group of female patients with MS we found normal menstrual cycles despite raised serum concentrations of prolactin, LH, FSH, total and free testosterone and delta 4-androstenedion. The raised gonadotropines do not seem related to inadequate ovarian steroid production. A gradual increase in FSH levels appears to be an effect of reproductive aging.

Premature aging phenomenons within the CNS may be a possibility in MS.

In addition, the hormone concentrations found in patients with MS may in part be explained by a decreased ovarian estrogen response to gonadotropines leading to raised gonadotropine secretion and thereby augmented ovarian androgen secretion. - Or the raised androgen levels could, at least in part, be due to a peripheral abnormality which, however, does not change the secretion of estrogens and dehydroepiandrosterone sulphate (DHEAS).

Whether this increase in androgen secretion is of adrenal or ovarian origin is speculative, but it may, at least in part, be of ovarian origin as DHEAS secreted from the adrenals was within the normal range.

Alternatively MS may possess a central hormonal effect or dysfunction of the regulation of gonadotropine as well as prolactin secretion. Dopamine is a central inhibitor of prolactin and gonadotropine secretion. Therefore a lowered central dopaminergic tone may be a possibility in these patients.

In conclusion, MS leads to altered hormone secretion within the pituitary-gonadal axis. The altered plasma steroid levels in the MS patients had only minor, if any, clinical manifestations as the patients had regular menstrual cycles and no infertility problems.

The results may suggest that women with MS have an abnormal central regulation of pituitary prolactin and gonadotropines as well as peripheral resistance to these hormones.

The possible neuromodulators involved need further studies.

Recent advances in multiple sclerosis therapy.
R.E. Gonsette, P. Delmotte, editors.

METHOD FOR THE EVALUATION OF SMALL INTESTINE ACTIVITY IN MS

ANDRAS GUSEO

Department of Neurology, Central Hospital of County Fejer,
Szekesfehervar (Hungary)

INTRODUCTION

Lazy activity of small intestine in MS is a common symptom. The
measurement of small intestine motility gives the possibility to
follow external and internal influences resulting in activation
or inhibition of intestine function.

We demonstrate a new non invasive, computer assisted method to
demonstrate small intestine motility based on sound registration.

MATERIAL AND METHOD

Small intestine motility was registered by sounds caused by
clusters of peristaltic contractions. A piezoelectric microphone
/HM-622, sensitivity 15-1000 Hz/ was situated over the abdominal
region 4 cm lateraly and 3 cm distaly from navel in a quiet horison-
tal position. Sounds were registered by 3-NEK-116 electrocardio-
graph suitable for phonocardiography too.

Electric signals were transfered to IBM compatible XT PC, digi-
talized and analysed for frequency,amplitude hsitogram and power
spectrum.

Two minute registrations were made in the following time intervals: 0 minute /start/, 8 minute /base-line/, 20, 35, 50, 65, and
80 minutes.

The method have been used to evaluate the effect of various
frequency bands /2, 12, 50 Hz as well as placebo/ of pulsing
electromagnetic field therapy on small intestine motility compared
to cholinergic and anticholinergic drugs.

Ten healthy individuals served as controll and 5 MS patients
have been investigated.

RESULTS

After lieing down the very intensive high frequency motility
slows down continuously. The rapid fall is in the first 5-6 minutes
further diminishing is very slow and dont exceed more than 10-20%.

After placebo treatment a tendency of slowing down of motility
was observed. In contrary to the placebo treatment all frequency

bands of PEMF resulted in enhancement of frequency as well as
power spectrum immediately /12 Hz/ or protracted /50 Hz/. At
highest level the frequency reached +378% increase. The bigest
reaction were observed after 30 minutes of 2 and 12 Hz PEMF
treatment.

The increase in the power spectrum ment that the individual
sounds were more stronger.

In MS there was an overall reduction in frequency and power
spectrum as well as in reaction to PEMF treatment in the investigated patients.

DISCUSSION

Our non invasive method of measuring small intestine motility
is comparable to EMG registrations used for the detection of
small intestine muscle activity in animals.It is sensitive, follows
truly all movements causing sounds during the passage of intestinal
content in the investigated region. The occurrence of sound depends
on actual intestinal content, but it is the same during one investigation, therefore the tendency of action of external forces or
medication can be measured.There was an individual variation in
susceptibility to magnetic field as well as in healthy and MS
patients too.

SUMMARY

Non invasive computer asisted new method have been developed to
analyse small intestine activity based on sound registration
caused by clusters of intestine peristaltic movements.

Lazy activity of small intestine motility have been detected
in MS and compared to healthy individuals.

Various reactions to pulsing electromagnetic field treatment
have been detected in healthy individuals and in persons with MS.

© 1989 Elsevier Science Publishers B.V. (Biomedical Division)
Recent advances in multiple sclerosis therapy.
R.E. Gonsette, P. Delmotte, editors.

THE EFFECT OF LONG-LASTING AZATHIOPRINE TREATMENT ON CSF HUMORAL
PARAMETERS IN MS

ANDRAS GUSEO
Department of Neurology, Central Hospital of County Fejer,
Szekesfehervar (Hungary)

INTRODUCTION

Increased cerebrospinal fluid immunoglobulin G and de novo IgG
synthesis within the central nervous system are hallmarks of MS
throughout its course. In several studies Azathioprine /AZA/ has
been claimed to influence disease progression favorably, and
correcting abnormal effector B-cell function in MS without altering
T-cell regulation[1].

The aim of the study was to follow the changes in CSF humoral
immunological parameters in MS treated for years by AZA. The following questions should be answered:
Has any effect the AZA treatment on
1/ CSF IgG level?
2/ intrathecal IgG synthesis?
3/ disease progression?

MATERIAL AND METHODS

Six patients have been followed for 5-9 years after starting
AZA therapy and one patient after Cyclophosphamide therapy.
Two patients died after 4 and 6 years of treatment not due to
complications of the immunosuppressive treatment. In four patients
the treatment has been continued. Patients were hospitalized 2-4
times yearly, serum and CSF IgG level, agarose electrophoresis
stained by silver impregnation, IgG production per day /Tourtellotte
Kurtzke DSS and progression index have been evaluated.

RESULTS

The effect of long lasting AZA on CSF IgG level:
a/ there is no acute change in CSF IgG level after introduction
   of AZA therapy
b/ low IgG level at the beginning remained low after years
c/ high IgG level at beginning may elevate successively or it
   may remain on the same level

d/ intermittent steroid therapy lowers the IgG level only
   temporaly

e/AZA does not decrease the IgG level even after years of
   administration.

f/ the effect of Cyclophosphamide in one case was similar to
   those of AZA

The effect of long-lasting AZA on CSF IgG production per day:

a/ the IgG production per day runs parallel with the actual IgG
   level

b/ AZA therapy has no effect on IgG production per day

c/ AZA therapy can not stop the continuous IgG elevation

d/ AZA therapy does not decrease IgG production per day after
   years of administration.

The progression index decreased almost continuously in all treated patients despite of the two lethal cases.

CONCLUSIONS

   Long lasting AZA does not stop the disease progression in every
case.

AZA has neither acute nor late action on CSF IgG level or de novo
CNS IgG production per day.

   AZA does not prevent new exacerbations, therefore intermittent
steroid therapy is necessary.

   Early and late side effects can occour, therefore it's use
should be considered.

   AZA decreases the progression index in most of the cases.

REFERENCE

1. Oger J J-F, Antel JP, KUO HH, Arnason BGW /1982/ Influence
    of Azathioprine /Imuran/ on in vitro immune function in
    multiple sclerosis. Ann Neurol 11: 177-181

© 1989 Elsevier Science Publishers B.V. (Biomedical Division)
Recent advances in multiple sclerosis therapy.
R.E. Gonsette, P. Delmotte, editors.

353

VEP-changes reflect extent of disease in chronic multiple sclerosis

----

Paul E. Hänny MD and Felix A.J. Müller MD
Dept. of Neurology, University Hospital of
Zürich, Switzerland

INTRODUCTION

VEP-delay in multiple sclerosis results of slow conduction velocity within the visual pathways. This slowing often follows optic neuritis [1] and might improve or sometimes return to normal even years after the initial symptoms [2,3]. Additional factors such as local edema [4], substances with nerve blocking effects and adaptation mechanisms in demyelinated neural tissue [5] will contribute to VEP-changes. Earlier studies gave only scant evidence of a consistant correlation between VEP and loss of visual function [6], course and extent of the disease, nor of any coexisting impairement within other neurologic systems [7,8]. Our goal is to disclose a tight relation between the summated VEP-latency and the amount of hyperintense MRI-changes, particularly for the periventricular regions [9]. It would suggest that the retrogeniculate parts of the visual pathway become more important to explain the slowing of VEP during the later course of the disease.

MATERIAL AND METHODS

170 patients with with probable or definite MS:

Classification (Poser[10]):
1) definite: N = 100   category A = 76
                           category B = 24
2) probable: N = 70   (Duration < 6 mth; first bouts;
                           remitting symptoms; only one focus)

Correlations between VEP-latencies, MRI-abnormalities and clinical data could be established in 93 patients (52 with definite diagnosis Poser group A or B, 41 with probable diagnosis). Further grouping was done between a simple chronic, remittent-progressive and a strictly remittent course. A comparison between clinical, functional systems (FS) and the VEP's was evaluated in 125 patients.

VEP: checkerboard stimulation; P100;
        sum from both eyes = **sumRL**

MRI: periventricular white matter =
        pv = thickness * circumference

        thickness of belt: 0= none
                                 1= focal hyperintensities,
                                 2= thin periventricular line
                                 3= thick line and knobs >2mm
                                 4= thick coat

        circumference involved: 0= none   1= 0-20%
                                 2= 20-40%   3= 40-60%
                                 4= 60-80%   5= 80-100%

Correlations between sum of the VEP-Latencies of both sides
(LOG sumRL) and periventricular abnormalities in MRI (pv)
****

		duration:			
		all	< 3y	> 3y	> 10y

LOG sumRL

pv	\				
all courses:					
all (probable and	r	0.50	0.43	0.48	0.56
definite diagnosis)	N	93	46	47	19
	p <	0.0000	0.003	0.0007	0.013
Poser Cat. A and B	r	0.52	0.2	0.62	0.76
	N	52	16	36	15
	p <	0.0001	n.s.	0.0001	0.001
Poser Cat. A	r	0.58	0.01	0.73	0.83
	N	40	12	28	12
	p <	0.0001	n.s.	0.0000	0.0009
strictly remittent course:					
all (probable and	r	0.42	0.24	*	*
definite diagnosis)	N	48	33		
	p <	0.003	n.s.		
Poser Cat. A and B	r	0.39	0.33	0.48	0.78
	N	23	8	15	7
	p <	n.s.	n.s.	n.s.	n.s.
Poser Cat. A	r	0.31	-0.4	0.47	0.74
	N	19	5	14	6
	p <	n.s.	n.s.	n.s.	n.s.
remittent-progressive course:					
all (probable and	r	0.62	0.40	0.70	0.84
definite diagnosis)	N	29	9	20	8
	p <	0.0003	n.s.	0.0005	0.0093
Poser Cat. A and B	r	0.59	0.14	0.69	0.86
	N	26	8	18	7
	p <	0.0015	n.s.	0.0026	0.0132
Poser Cat. A	r	0.70	0.07	0.84	0.95
	N	21	7	14	6
	p <	0.0005	n.s.	0.0002	0.0044
FS visual equal 0 or 1:					
all (probable and	r	0.55	0.41	0.57	0.82
definite diagnosis)	N	73	38	35	13
	p <	0.0000	0.006	0.0004	0.0007
Poser Cat. A and B	r	0.54	0.04	0.69	0.85
	N	39	14	26	11
	p <	0.0003	n.s.	0.0001	0.001
Poser Cat. A	r	0.56	-0.01	0.72	0.86
	N	32	11	21	9
	p <	0.0012	n.s.	0.0002	0.0032

*only definite cases (Poser Cat. A and B)

Correlations between sum of VEP-latencies and visual FS (Rank
correlation coefficients)
****

		duration: all	< 3y	> 3y	> 10y
		sumRL			
FS visual					
all patients	r	0.54	0.47	0.54	0.28
(probable and	N	125	62	63	25
definite diagnosis)	p <	0.0000	0.0004	0.0000	n.s.

periventricular score equal 0 or 1:

all patients	r	0.49	0.26	0.73	0.97
(probable and	N	36	25	11	7
definite diagnosis)	p <	0.004	n.s.	0.021	0.017

RESULTS

1) The VEP latency-sum correlates to the extent of periventricular hyperintensities in MRI in patients with MS.

2) Increasing duration of illness and certainty of diagnosis
improves the correlation substantially. The linkage is
slightly better for the definite than for the probable forms
and it is strongest for the chronic-progressive courses.

3) Acute and strictly remittant forms of short duration do
not show any higher VEP/MRI-correlation.

4) Patients without visual impairment have better correlations than the average of all cases.

5) The correlation between visual impairment and VEP-
latencies is stronger for cases with short disease duration
than for the chronic courses. It is also much better, when
periventricular hyperintensities are absent.

CONCLUSIONS:

1) Slowing of visual conduction time (VEP) might happen at
pre- and/or retrogeniculate location.

2) A substantial amount of VEP-changes have retrogeniculate
origin, especially in patients with chronic forms of
disease.

3) Retrogeniculate lesions often are clinically silent but
slow visual conduction time.

4) VEP will provide a useful tool in monitoring the course
of the disease.

356

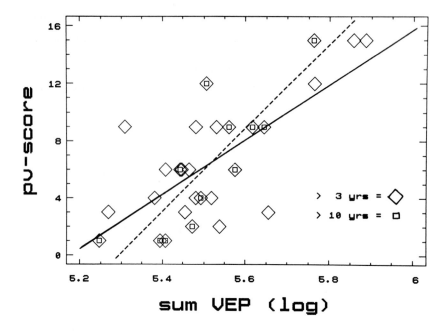

sum VEP (log)

REFERENCES:

1 Chappa KH, Parker SW, Shahani BT: Pathoneurophysiology of multiple sclerosis. In: Koetsier JC (ed): Handbook of clinical neurology. Elsevier, 1985, New York. Revised series Vol 3 (47), pp 131-145.
2 Matthews WB, Small M: Prolonged follow up of abnormal visual evoked potentials in multiple sclerosis: Evidence for delayed recovery. J Neurol Neurosurg Psychat 1983; 639-642.
3 Hely MA, McManis PG, Walsh JC and McLeod JG: Visual evoked responses and ophthalmological examination in optic neuritis. A follow up study. J Neurol Sci 1986; 75:275-283.
4 Dalakas M, Wright RG, Prineas JW: Nature of the reversible white matter lesion in multiple sclerosis. Effects of acute inflammation on myelinated tissue studied in the rabbit eye. Brain 1980; 103:515-524.
5 Raminssky M: Pathophysiology of demyelination. Ann N Y Acad Sci 1984; 436:68-80.
6 Aminoff MJ, Davis SL, Panitch HS: Serial evoked potential studies in patients with multiple sclerosis. Clinical relevance. Arch Neurol 1984; 1197-1202.
7 Nuwer MR, Packwood JW, Myers LW, Ellison GW: Evoked potentials predict the clinical changes in a multiple sclerosis drug study. Neurology 1987; 37:1754-1761.
8 de Weerd AW: Variability of central conduction in the course of multiple sclerosis. Serial recordings of evoked potentials in the evaluation of therapy. Clin Neurol Neurosurg 1987; 89-1:9-15.
9 Müller FAJ, Haenny PE, Wichmann W et al: CSF-immunoglobulins correspond to MRI- and VEP-abnormalities in multiple sclerosis. Arch Neurol 1989; 46:367-371.
10 Poser CM, Paty DW, Scheinberg L et al: New diagnostic criteria for multiple sclerosis: Guidelines for research protocols. Ann Neurol 1983; 13:227-231.

© 1989 Elsevier Science Publishers B.V. (Biomedical Division)
Recent advances in multiple sclerosis therapy.
R.E. Gonsette, P. Delmotte, editors.

THE CHANGING PREVALENCE OF MULTIPLE SCLEROSIS IN NORTHERN IRELAND WITH REFERENCE TO BENIGN MULTIPLE SCLEROSIS

DR S A HAWKINS AND DR F KEE

Department of Medicine, Institute of Clinical Science, The Queen's University, Grosvenor Road, Belfast BT12 6BJ, Northern Ireland.

INTRODUCTION

Previous estimates of the prevalence by Allison & Millar were based on the population of the whole Province. The prevalence studies in 1951, 51/100,000 (population 1,370,709) and 1961, 81/100,000 (population 1,484,775) are some of the largest studies ever completed. The present study was designed to endeavour to achieve optimal case ascertainment in a population of optimal size for the purpose i.e. approx 100,000. The Coleraine, Ballymoney and Moyle Unit of Management of the Northern Health Board occupies 555 square miles in the north east corner of Ireland. It was chosen for the survey because it is a well defined area geographically, being bounded on two sides by sea, and for the last 7 years has been served by the neurologist (S.A.H.). The estimated population is 86,500.

The definition of benign MS is not standard. Estimates of the percentage of 'benign' MS have varied from 5% to 40% in various studies.

METHODS

Cases resident in the area were ascertained through a postal survey of all Family General Medical Practitioners (G.Ps), through the listings of the MS Society, the records of the Regional Neurology Service in Belfast and by reviewing all hospital discharges of multiple sclerosis in Northern Ireland within the Hospital Activity Analysis (H.A.A.) dataset since its inception in 1968 to the present date. All cases were called for review and examination at the local hospital or if disability prevented this, were visited in their own home. Basic demographic data was collected and each patient had his/her disease catergorised according to both the taxonomy of Allison and Millar and that of Poser et al. Physical disability was assessed in each case using the Kurtzke Rating Scales.

We have chosen to designate patients who have Kurtzke disability status 3 or less, 10 years or more after the first symptom as 'benign' MS.

RESULTS

The response rate from GPs was 98% (n=49). 50 patients were known to the local MS Society and a further 26 were identified from the H.A.A. search, but in neither instance were cases identified from these sources who were not already known to their GPs. Altogether 119 cases resident in the area were ascertained. Five patients declined to participate, and were thus not examined. These five patients had their records reviewed and in all respects fulfilled the diagnostic criteria for MS., giving a crude prevalence rate of 138/100,000. Of these 5 cases, 3 had been seen personally by (S.A.H.) but did not attend for review, and hence were not given a DSS rating.

This leaves a residue of 114 cases, 65% were born within the study area and were still resident there, 91% were born in Northern Ireland. Of the 90 cases which were 'probable' according to Allison and Millar, 84 could be described as 'clinically definite' according to the criteria of Poser. (These categories are roughly comparable for relapsing remitting MS only). The prevalence rate for 'probable' cases on Allison and Millar criteria was 101/100,000.

The age of onset for females was 12-56 (mean 31.6) and for males 16-55 (mean 36.0) These figures are comparable to previous studies in Northern Ireland and elsewhere.

Using Millar's prevalence figures of 1961 for the population of Coleraine, Ballymoney and Moyle, the expected number would be 71. It should be noted that there is a striking excess in the number of cases in the older age groups.

TABLE 1

ACTUAL AND EXPECTED CASES OF MS IN COLERAINE/BALLYMENA/MOYLE
(calculated using age- and sex-specific prevalence rates for N Ireland 1961)

Age group	Male		Female		Total
	<54 years	>54 years	<54 years	>54 years	M + F (all ages)
Actual	21	21	48	24	114
Expected	26.85	6.86	29.03	8.28	71
$(A-E)^2/E$	1.27	29.15	12.39	29.87	27.27
Significance level	NS	P<.0001	P<.02	P<.001	P<.001

28 of 114 or (25%) of all cases and 25 of 87 (28%) of 'probable' cases (Allison and Millar criteria) had benign MS, i.e. Kurtzke Disability Status of 3 or less, 10 years after the first symptoms of MS.

CONCLUSIONS
1. The crude prevalence rate was 138/100,000 for a population of 86,500.
2. We have evidence of an excess of patients in older age groups.
3. 25% had 'benign MS'- Kurtzke D.S.S. 3 or less 10 years from first symptoms.

REFERENCES

1. Millar JHD, Allison RS.(1954) Prevalence and familial incidence of disseminated sclerosis. Ulster Med J 23 (Suppl)

2. Millar JHD. (1971) Multiple Sclerosis: A disease acquired in childhood. Springfield, Illinois: Charles C Thomas

3. Poser CM, Paty DW, Scheinberg L, McDonald WI, et al. (1983) New diagnostic criteria for multiple sclerosis: Guidelines for Research Protocols. Ann Neurol 13:227-231

© 1989 Elsevier Science Publishers B.V. (Biomedical Division)
Recent advances in multiple sclerosis therapy.
R.E. Gonsette, P. Delmotte, editors.

A POPULATION-BASED SURVEY OF THE PREVALENCE OF ANTIBODIES TO BORRELIA BURGDORFERI IN MULTIPLE SCLEROSIS PATIENTS IN A DISTRICT OF NORTHERN IRELAND.

S A HAWKINS, D KIDD, E T M SMYTH, W A ELLIS, W R HENRY, N T HEASLEY.
The Queen's University, Belfast, Northern Ireland.
The Royal Victoria Hospital, Belfast, Northern Ireland.
The Veterinary Research Laboratory, Belfast, Northern Ireland.

INTRODUCTION

In the last five years Lyme Disease has been described and characterised in New England, the causative agent, Borrelia burgdorferi (BB) has been found, and effective treatment has been instituted (1) (2). Since BB encephalomyelopathy can occasionally mimic Multiple Sclerosis (M.S.) the possibility has been raised that some patients with progressive neurological disease have been mis-diagnosed. Within the last two years we have performed a prevalence study of MS in a defined population. Patients ascertained in that study were used. To date, there have been few population-based serological studies of the prevalence of Borrelia burgdorferi in control groups or in multiple sclerosis patients.

In an independent study in our laboratories, the sera from 406 farmers from different parts of Northern Ireland have been obtained to study farmer's lung. 14.3% of these sera were found to have significant titres of antibodies to Borrelia burgdorferi.

Two cases of clinical Lyme disease have been found in our province. We felt it was important to investigate the overlap between Lyme disease and MS in Northern Ireland.

METHODS

A population of 119 MS patients has been identified in a population of 86,500 in Northern Ireland. This is a community comprising small towns and farms.

Controls were taken from family members who were otherwise healthy and had no history of multiple sclerosis.

Borrelia burgdorferi antibodies were detected by means of the Zeus indirect fluorescent antibody (IFA) technique (Zeus Scientific Inc. USA). Step 1: human sera are reacted with Borrelia burgdorferi (strain B31) immobilised on ten-well antigen slides and incubated at room temperature for 30 min. They are then washed with a stream of phosphate buffer solution. Step 2: is to bind fluorescein-labelled anti-human gamma globulin to the cell-wall antigens causing the Borrelia to fluoresce. Serial dilutions of serum were tested. A serum dilution of 1:256 has been established as a significant cut-off point, during standardisation of the kit.(3)

360

RESULTS

91 MS patients were tested (77% of those known in the community). The disease duration ranged from 2 - 42 years, 36% male and 64% female. 81 family members acted as controls.

10% of patients and 11% of controls had titres of > 256. The noted positive patients were reviewed for features particularly suggestive of Borreliosis. No such features were found.

CONCLUSIONS

We conclude that our results reflect the prevalence of positive serology in the community. We have detected no specific association with multiple sclerosis symptoms in our community.

REFERENCES

1.   Benach JL, Bosler EM, Hanrahan JP, Coleman JL, Habicht GS, Bast TF, Cameron DJ, Ziegler JL, Barbour AG, Burgdorfer W, Edelman R & Kaslow RA. (1983) Spirochetes isolated from the blood of two patients with Lyme Disease. New Eng J Med 308:740-742

2.   Steere AC, Malawista SE, Bartenhagen NH, Spieler PN, Newman JH, Rahn DW, Hutchinson GJ, Green J, Snydman DR & Taylor E (1984)   The Clinical Spectrum and Treatment of Lyme Disease. Yale J Biol Med 57:453-461

3.   Mertz LE, Wobig GH, Duffy J & Katzman JA (1985)   Ticks, Spirochetes and new diagnostic tests for Lyme disease. Mayo Clin Proc 60:402-406.

© 1989 Elsevier Science Publishers B.V. (Biomedical Division)
Recent advances in multiple sclerosis therapy.
R.E. Gonsette, P. Delmotte, editors.

ANALYSIS OF LONG-TERM CULTURED MONONUCLEAR CELLS IN MS: WITH SPECIAL REFERENCE TO REVERSE TRANSCRIPTASE.

PER HÖLLSBERG[1], ANNE MØLLER-LARSEN[1], FINN SKOU PEDERSEN[2], JUST JUSTESEN[2], HANS-JACOB HANSEN[3], SVEN HAAHR[1].

[1] Institute of Medical Microbiology, [2] Institute of Molecular Biology, [3] Department of Neurology, Municipal Hospital of Aarhus.
University of Aarhus, DK-8000 Aarhus, Denmark.

INTRODUCTION.
In searching for a retrovirus in MS we have chosen methods that allow detection of all different types of retroviruses, albeit with some differences in sensitivity, as opposed to the very sensitive, but narrow assays, like PCR amplification.

MATERIAL AND METHODS.
Peripheral blood mononuclear cell (PBMNC) cultures were established from 33 MS patients, 9 with other neurological diseases (OND), an 24 normal controls (C). Cultures were stimulated with interleukin-2 (IL-2) (10 units/ml) and IL-2 + PHA (0.01 units/ml), respectively. Supernatants were analysed with a reverse transcriptase (RT) assay - using poly (rA), oligo (dT), and Mn^{++} as template, primer, and divalent cation, respectively - after 1,3,6,9,12, and 15 weeks of culture. Cells were analysed with a 2'-5'oligoadenylate synthetase assay. Cultures and Giemsa stained cytocentrifuge preparations were regularly examined in an inverted microscope (400 x magnification) for the presence of multinucleated macrophages and aberrations in cell morphology. Moreover, CSF cell cultures were analysed for the presence of RT activity in the culture supernatants.

RESULTS.
PBMNC cultures from MS patients did not grow for an extended period, and were dependent on exogenous IL-2. Table 1 shows the mean life and range for these cultures.

Table 1.
Mean life span and range for cultured peripheral blood mononuclear cells.
Cells were cultured in IL-2 containing medium in presence or absence of PHA. ± SEM.

	N	Life span (days) PHA		Range (days) PHA	
		-	+	-	+
MS	33	104±11	99±11	38-273	40-228
OND	9	111±17	89±18	38-237	40-222
C	24	93±11	90± 8	23-193	40-219

By regular microscopic examinations no aberrations in cell morphology, such as multinucleated macrophages and/or changes in nuclear appearence in Giemsa staining, could be revealed. Furthermore, RT activity from the supernatants were not significantly above the background level. Table 2A and 2B show the relative values for IL-2 (A) and IL-2 + PHA (B) cultures, respectively. Likewise, no RT activity could be detected in the CSF cell culteres (Table 3). Moreover, these cultures had a limited life span (between 8 and 13 weeks), and were dependent on exogenous IL-2.
All cultures were analysed for the presence of 2'-5' OAS (fig. 1). Their were no significant differences between the 3 groups.

Table 2.
Reverse transcriptase activity in the supernatants from cultured peripheral blood mononuclear cells.
For details, see text. ±SEM.

A.			Weeks		
	1	3	6	12	15
MS	107±17	113±13	100±14	161±33	117±39
C	77±11	123±23	127±26	124±28	187±64
OND	79±33	70±11	79±16	112±38	161±57

B.					
	1	3	6	12	15
MS	103±10	127±20	104±13	155±26	129±22
C	99±10	111±13	101±18	111±19	109±48
OND	99±33	89±16	60± 9	101±25	113±60

Table 3.
Reverse transcriptase activity in supernatants from cultured cerebrospinal fluid cells from patients with multiple sclerosis.
Mean values are presented and expressed as percentage of the background level (relative RT). Variable numbers of supernatants were harvested (N) between week 2 and 12, but all cultures were examined after 6 weeks of culture.

Pt. no.	N	Rel.RT
A	3	141
B	4	130
C	2	129
D	3	99
E	1	138
F	2	166
G	6	134
H	1	126
I	5	110
J	1	113
K	4	115

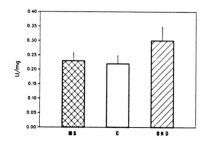

Fig. 1. Activity of 2'-5' oligoadenylate synthetase in peripheral blood mononuclear cells. Mean values are presented and expressed as units of enzyme per mg protein. SEM are indicated on the top of the bars. From MS, OND, and normal controls (C) 67, 17, and 39 samples were analysed respectively.

DISCUSSION

These results did not reveal any signs of a retrovirus in MS. If one assumes that MS patients are infected with such a virus, then our failure to detect it could be due to several possibilities: 1) No expression of the viral genes under the employed conditions 2) Extremely few productively infected cells. The sensitivity of our RT assay corresponds to approx. one virusproducing cell in 10^4 cells. 3) Culturing the cells may result in negative selection. 4) Differing preferences for template, primer or divalent cation. For some virus groups sensitivity can be increased by use of poly (rC)-oligo (dT).Despite the negative results, we find it highly relevant to continue the search for a retrovirus in MS. In particular, analysis of different cell types may be relevant.

© 1989 Elsevier Science Publishers B.V. (Biomedical Division)
Recent advances in multiple sclerosis therapy.
R.E. Gonsette, P. Delmotte, editors.

LYMPHOCYTE SUBTYPING IN CEREBROSPINAL FLUID OF PATIENTS WITH MULTIPLE SCLEROSIS, USING THE ALPHA-NAPHTHYL-ACETATE-ESTERASE STAINING METHOD.

J. HUYBRECHTS, P. VANDERDONCKT, J. DE REUCK

NEUROPATHOLOGY LABORATORY, DEPARTMENT OF NEUROLOGY, UNIVERSITY HOSPITAL, GHENT, BELGIUM.

INTRODUCTION

Alpha-naphthyl-acetate esterase (ANAE) staining is easy to perform and much cheaper than the use of monoclonal antibodies. Also the staining procedure is less versatile in cerebrospinal fluid cytology (1).

The present study investigates the significance of the different types of ANAE positive cells in CSF of 11 patients with an active form of multiple sclerosis, of 14 patients suspected of MS but paraclinically unproven and of 14 normal controls. None of the patients was treated with corticosteroids or immunosuppressive drugs.

MATERIAL & METHODS

ANAE staining was performed on CSF cells obtained by lumbar puncture in 39 patients. This population was divided into 3 groups :

I. Definite diagnosis of MS (N=11)
   a. oligoclonal pattern in CSF (N=7)
   b. no oligoclonal pattern in CSF (N=4)

II. Tentative diagnosis of MS (N=14)

III. Control group (N=14)

In each slide, a minimum of 30 lymphocytes were evaluated. These cells were qualified as :
- L_N : ANAE negative
- L_D : ANAE positive - dotted pattern
- L_G : ANAE positive - granular (or diffuse) pattern.

The last two groups have been shown to correspond to mature T-lymphocytes. The dotted cells are thought to be equivalent to T-helper cells, whereas the granular cells are considered to be T-suppressor/cytotoxic cells.

RESULTS

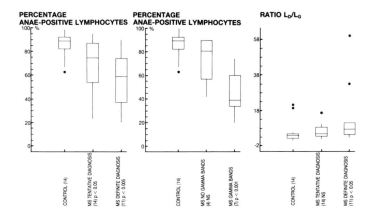

We observed a decrease in percentage of ANAE positive cells in the groups I and II versus the control group. Statistical significant difference was seen in groups

I   versus control (p<0.005)
I_a versus control (p<0.001)
II   versus control (p<0.05)
I_a versus II (p<0.05)

Comparing the subsets of ANAE positive lymphocytes, we observed an increase of the ratio L_D/L_G in MS patients (group I) versus controls (p<0.05).

In the group of proven multiple sclerosis patients a significant increase in L_N cells and decrease in L_G are observed, compared to the control group. These changes are even more pronounced in these CSF fluids with oligoclonal bands on agargel electrophoresis.
In the group of the suspected multiple sclerosis patients the results are intermediate between the proven multiple sclerosis patients and the control groups.

CONCLUSION

This study confirms that in active multiple sclerosis there is a decrease of the percentage of T-lymphocytes in cerebrospinal fluid (1). There is also a significant correlation between the diminuation of the T-lymphocytes and the occurrence of gamma-bands on agargel-electrophoresis. In addition the decrease of the L_G lymphocytes, observed in the multiple sclerosis patients, probably corresponds to a loss of T-suppressor/cytotoxic cells. (2,3,4,5).

REFERENCES

1. De Reuck J., Vanderdonckt P. (1988) Acta Neurol Scand 78 : 190.

2. Lisak RP, Levinson AT, Zweiman B, Abdou NI. (1975) Clin Exp Immunol 22 : 30.

3. Manconi PE, Marrosu MG, Cianchette C, Ennas MG, Mangoni A, Zaccheo D. (1980) Acta Neurol Scand 62 : 165.

4. Reinherz EC, Weiner HL, Hauser SL, Cohen JA, Distase JA, Schlossmann SF. (1980) Engl J Med 303 : 125.

5. Cazzullo CL, Caputo D, Ghezzi A, Zaffaroni M. (1987) Eur Neurol 27 : 5.

© 1989 Elsevier Science Publishers B.V. (Biomedical Division)
Recent advances in multiple sclerosis therapy.
R.E. Gonsette, P. Delmotte, editors.

ANALYSIS OF BLOOD IN MS PATIENTS FOLLOWING A PUFA RICH DIET

R. JONES, E. GROVE, G. FITZGERALD and A. FORTI
Biophysics Group, Radiotherapy & Oncology Unit, Horfield Road, Bristol BS2 8ED
(United Kingdom)

INTRODUCTION

Analysis of blood, blood cells (1,2) and CSF (3) show that levels of linoleic acid (LA) are lower in patients with multiple sclerosis (MS) than in healthy controls. Studies employing dietary supplementation with LA indicate a reduction in severity and length of relapses (4). In the present study a diet designed to increase the intake of polyunsaturated fatty acids with reduction in saturated fat intake has been tested (5). Previous studies have shown that red cell surface charge (electrophoretic mobility, EPM) is correlated with choline phosphoglyceride levels of LA (6) both of which are low in MS patients not on diet or supplements. In addition to neurological assessment, red cell EMP and other blood biochemical parameters have been measured in patients following the diet for up to 5 years.

PATIENTS AND METHODS

	Male (8)	Female (32)
Age at entry (yrs)	32 - 55	32 - 66
Time from diagnosis (yrs)	2 - 13	1 - 17
Kurtzke EDSS at entry	5.0 - 6.5	3.0 - 7.0

Dietary Advice and Analysis

Nutrient intakes based on 7 day weighed intakes were calculated 6 monthly and a diet score (DS) derived.

Blood Preparation

Erythrocytes were separated from venous blood anti-coagulated with sodium citrate, fixed in 1% glutaraldehyde in phosphate buffered saline (PBS) and EPM was measured "blind" as described in Ref. 7.

RESULTS

Table 1 shows values for red cell EPM, diet score (DS) and linoleic acid intake (LA) for the 5 years of the study.

TABLE 1   Mean Values (±SD)

	PRE DIET	YR1	YR2	YR3	YR5
	n=40	n=40	n=20	n=19	n=11
EPM	46.5 (8.5)	52.7[*](8.5)	48.9 (10.3)	37.7 (6.5)	39.7 (8.0)
Control EPM	50.7 (7.4)	51.5 (6.8)			
DS	40.6 (14.3)	60.6[†](11.6)	59.2[†](16.3)	56.8[†](11.9)	50.8[†](16)
LA	12.9 (6.3)	21.7[†](9.3)	19.5[†](8.1)	18.0[*](6.4)	13.0 (6.3)

[*] p>0.05   [†] p>0.01

DISCUSSION

There is a significant increase in all values at year 1 compared to the pre-diet values. These improvements are maintained for the second year but start to decrease by year 3 and return to pre-diet values by year 5. The change in patient numbers did not influence the statistical validity of the finding when the mean for all patients was compared to the paired means for each of the groups remaining at 3 and 5 years (Jones et al in preparation).

Although improvements in diet can be recognised as early as 3 months after counselling, improvements in red cells were not seen for 6 to 9 months, suggesting that changes are due to alterations at the stem cell stage. Whether such changes in cell membrane construction can be equated with improved myelin formation or an alteration in immune properties has yet to be established.

ACKNOWLEDGEMENTS

Supported by ARMS (Action for Research into Multiple Sclerosis).

REFERENCES

1. Gul, S. et al (1970) J.Neurol.Neurosurg.Psychiat. 33:506-10

2. Cherayil, G. (1984) J.Neurol.Sci. 63:1-10

3. Neu, I.S. (1983) Acta.Neurol.Scand. 67:151-163

4. Dworkin, R.H. et al (1984) Neurology 34:1441-5

5. Fitzgerald, G., Harbige, L.S., Forti, A. and Crawford, M.A. (1987) Human Nutrition:Applied Nutrition 41A:297-310

6. Harbige, L.S. et al (1986) Prog.Lipid Res. 25:243-248

7. Jones, R. Preece, A.W., Luckman, N.P. and Forrester, J.A. (1983) Phys.Med.Biol. 28:1145-1151

© 1989 Elsevier Science Publishers B.V. (Biomedical Division)
Recent advances in multiple sclerosis therapy.
R.E. Gonsette, P. Delmotte, editors.

PSYCHOLOGICAL REHABILITATION IN PATIENTS WITH MULTIPLE SCLEROSIS

M.G.LANDONI,C.P.G.OGGIONNI,M.G.SINATRA,D.CAPUTO,C.L.CAZZULLO

Centro Universitario Sclerosi Multipla, Fondazione Don Gnocchi,Via
Capecelatro 66, 20148, Milano (Italy)

Multiple Sclerosis, being an inabilitant chronic disease with an
unforeseeable evolution, produces serious qualitative and
quantitative changes in the life and relationships of patients and
involves problems concerning the mind-body relationship.
Theoretically patients with MS could accept the impairment of
their autonomy and elaborate a kind of "mourning" of some
abilities: this renouncement may allow an investment on the
surviving autonomy and healthy functions in order to organize more
successful defensive systems.
Nevertheless more often we observe in these patients a
psychological discomfort, wich occurs before the manifestation of
psychiatrical symptoms, due to the difficulties in integrating the
pulsional load invested on reality with the new objective
limitations due to the disease.
Thus the patients have to face simultaneously the problem of the
loss of their autonomy and the inability to elaborate the new
needs of the modified reality and therefore they manifest the
feeling of loss of their role and disbalance in relationship.
Quite often these patients convey the frustration and depressive
effect consequent to the loss of self-esteem. Depression is
frequent and it manifest itself, in the gravest cases, as a
primary affective disorder (PAD). Some Authors, like C.L.Cazzullo
and others, point out that the PAD is more frequent in MS then in
general population, as expression of the common immunogenetic
pattern of depression due to the awareness of the disease.
Furthermore in these patients often occur emotional disturbances
as emotional lability, dysforia, dissyntonia, fatuity,
effusiveness and loss of criticism. These symptoms are correlated
for the most part with the cognitive impairment and with the
worsening of the patient's psychiatrical functions and
relationships.
If we consider the body schema as a fundamental support to the
mind-body relationship and we believe that this schema is a
somatic Ego expression, thus we can easily understand how much the
modifications produced by such invalidating disease may affect the
psychological balance of patients.
In fact we make use of the body to enter into relation with others
and on this we base our affective-emotional external perception.
Thus they may find an adaptation if they successfully elaborate
the mutation of body schema and the conseguent limitations.
In patients with MS the modifications of body-schema are
associated with a decrease of autonomy and the new needs of
gratification are complicated by difficulties to organize adequate
psychological defenses.
For all these reasons it is important to take charge of the
psychological problems of patients with MS. The main goals of
psychological rehabilitation should be both to cure the
psychiatrical discomfort and to stimulate the recovery of
individual autonomy.
Rehabilitation should be started at the onset of disease in order
to avoid that when they are aware of diagnosis of MS, patients
organize their discomfort and develop a psychiatrical disturbance

and an impairment of the functional autonomy.
We individuate four areas of rehabilitative treatment:
- Individual psychoterapy of support
- Group psychotherapy: so that the group becomes the mean to
  exchange experiences and to hold anguish.
- Support to the family: this is useful in order to avoid
  distortion in comunication and behaviour between familials and
  patient.
- Social intervent: these are raccommended mainly in patients
  with long duration disease.

References

1)   MANARA F., CARTA I. e CAZZULLO C.L. (1980)
      Riabilitazione Psicosociale nei Malati Neurologici.
      Il Pensiero Scientifico Editore.

2)   Schilder P. (1973)
      Immagine di Sé e Schema Corporeo.
      Franco Angeli Editore

3)   LANDONI M.G. (1987)
      "Una Psicoterapia per Pazienti con Sclerosi Multipla"
      in: C.L. Cazzullo, A. Ghezzi, M. Zaffaroni e D. Caputo
      Sclerosi Multipla.   Masson Ed. pp.223 - 232

© 1989 Elsevier Science Publishers B.V. (Biomedical Division)
Recent advances in multiple sclerosis therapy.
R.E. Gonsette, P. Delmotte, editors.

USE OF SPECIFIC HTLV-1 PEPTIDES IN SEARCH FOR ANTIBODY
REACTIVITY IN MULTIPLE SCLEROSIS

JAN LYCKE[1], OLUF ANDERSEN[1] and BO SVENNERHOLM[2].
[1] Department of Neurology, [2] Department of Virology, University of Gothenburg,
Sahlgren Hospital, S-413 45 Gothenburg (Sweden)

INTRODUCTION
   The complete nucleotide sequence of HTLV-1 has been reported (1). By solid
phase peptide synthesis using an Applied Biosystem peptide synthesizer (Model
430A L.A. CA) thirty-five overlapping peptides spanning the complete envelope
glycoprotein -gp 46- of HTLV-1 were produced.These peptides with length of twenty
to twenty-eight amino acids were encoded by the nucleotide sequence of the HTLV-
1 genome encompassing base pairs 5202 through 6668. All synthetic peptides have
been tested in ELISA against panels of Western blot confirmed HTLV-1 positive
sera and cerebrospinal fluids. Four distinctly separated regions representing
different continuous epitopes of the HTLV-1 envelope protein were defined. They
reacted with 70-100 % of HTLV-1 confirmed positive sera from European and US
patients, while 41-78 % of HTLV-1 positive sera from Japan gave positive reactions.
No false positive reactions in ELISA were demonstrable when tested with panels of
200 true negative sera as well as 30 HIV-1 and 8 HIV-2 positive sera. In order to
examine a possible involvement of HTLV-1 in the pathogenesis of MS the four
specific immunoreactive HTLV-1 peptides as well as disrupted adult T-cell
leukemia virus (ATLV) were used as antigens.

MATERIAL AND METHODS
Patients
   Paired serum and CSF specimens were obtained from 41 patients with definite MS
based on the criteria of Poser et al.(2) including 39 with relapsing-remitting course
and 2 with chronic progressive course, and from 15 patients with other neurologic
diseases (OND), 9 non-neurologic control patients submitted to transurethral
prostatectomy (TURP) and CSF from 10 healthy normal controls. All MS patients
except one demonstrated oligoclonal IgG bands and all except two had elevated IgG
index ($\geq$ 0.7). None of the MS patients had been treated with immunosuppressive
drugs. Out of 125 paired MS samples of serum and CSF 59 were obtained from 9
patients submitted to repeated sampling during five to sixteen months. Thirty-one
pairs were collected during exacerbations.

Assays of HTLV-1
   ELISA of synthetic HTLV-1 peptides. Four immuno-reactive HTLV-1 peptides
designed A, B, C and H were coated onto 96 well microtiter plates. IgG reactivity of
sera and CSF was tested in an indirect ELISA according to standard procedures.
The presence of antibodies reactive with HTLV-1 peptides in sera and CSF
specimens were determined by relating the absorbance to cut off values which were
adjusted to an increased sensitivity. In peptide ELISA, background optical density

(OD) values of negative control sera and CSF are low, indicated by arithmetic means for all four specific HTLV-1 peptides of 0.034 OD in sera and 0.033 OD in CSF of non-neurologic controls and of 0.035 OD in CSF of healthy normal controls. Cut off values of 3 SD above an absorbance mean for control sera and CSF were used where 3SD corresponded to 0.011-0.036 OD in sera and 0.013-0.033 OD in CSF, respectively, for all four HTLV-1 peptides.

In "standard" peptide ELISA cut off values of 0.1 OD above background absorbance were used. Specimens with absorbance values greater than or equal to cut off values in repeated tests were considered as positive.

Particle agglutination test of HTLV-1. All samples of sera and CSF were also assayed by a commercial passive agglutination test (Serodia-ATLA, Fujirebio Inc.) The antigen used derives from detergent treated and partially purified adult T-cell leukemia virus (ATLV) and the assay is reported to be reactive with envelope but primarily core antibodies (3).

RESULTS

In previous assays of synthetic HTLV-1 peptides a high degree of specificity and sensitivity were achieved. Using the same criteria for positive reactions in ELISA in the present study no antibody reactivity was demonstrable in sera or CSF from MS patients, OND-patients or controls (Table 1).

In order to increase sensitivity in peptide ELISA the criteria for positive reactions were adjusted to the absorbance mean of sera and CSF from the control population. Cut off values were determined to 3SD above these values (Table 2).

Reactivity with either of the specific HTLV-1 peptides were demonstrable in 15 MS CSF specimens (12 %) collected from 11 patients (37 %) and in sera and CSF specimens from 2 patients in the OND population (13 %), one with a cerebral arteriovenous malformation (AVM) and one with normal pressure hydrocephalus (NPH). 3 out of 15 positive MS CSF samples were obtained during exacerbation which indicates that the clinical activity did not influence the results. As a confirmatory test Western blot (NEA-8005, Du Pont) analysis was carried out on all positive serum and CSF samples but no antibodies that were reactive with HTLV-1 proteins were detectable.

TABLE 1
"STANDARD" SYNTHETIC HTLV-1 PEPTIDE ELISA
Reactivity of peptides with confirmed HTLV-1 positive sera from Japan, USA and Europe and sera and CSF from adult T-cell leukemia (ATL), tropical spastic paraparesis (TSP), multiple sclerosis, other neurologic patients (OND), non-neurologic control patients submitted to transurethral prostatectomy (TURP) and CSF from healthy normal controls (Positivity ≥ 0.1 OD above background absorbance mean for negative controls).

Study population	n	Peptide			
		A	B	C	H
HTLV-1 Japan	32	16	13	25	22
HTLV-Europe-USA	10	9	7	10	N.D.
ATL SERA	3	3	3	3	N.D.
CSF	1	1	1	1	1
TSP SERA	4	4	4	4	4
CSF	4	4	4	4	4
MS SERA	125	0	0	0	0
CSF	125	0	0	0	0
OND SERA	15	0	0	0	0
CSF	15	0	0	0	0
TURP SERA	9	0	0	0	0
CSF	9	0	0	0	0
HEALTHY CONTROLS	210	0	0	0	0

n = number of samples
N.D. not done

TABLE 2
HTLV-1 PEPTIDE ELISA AND HTLV-1 PARTICLE AGGLUTINATION TEST
Reactivity of HTLV-1 peptides in ELISA and of disrupted partially purified adult
T-cell leukemia virus (ATLV) in particle agglutination test with samples of sera and
CSF from patients with multiple sclerosis, other neurologic diseases (OND), non-
neurologic controls (TURP) and CSF from normal healthy controls (Positivity $\geq$ 3
SD, corresponding to 0.011-0.036 OD, above the absorbance mean for control sera
and CSF for HTLV-1 peptides).

Study population	n	Peptide				Part. aggl. test
		A	B	C	H	
MS SERA	125	0	0	0	0	0
CSF	125	7	9	10	8	0
OND SERA	15	1	0	0	0	0
CSF	15	1	2	0	1	0
TURP SERA	9	0	0	0	0	0
CSF	9	0	0	0	0	0
Healthy CSF controls	10	0	0	0	0	0

n = number of samples

CONCLUSIONS
- Four synthetic HTLV-1 envelope peptides A,B,C and H that were immunoreactive with 70-100 % of HTLV-1 confirmed positive sera from Europe and USA did not react with paired samples of sera and CSF from 41 MS patients and 15 patients with other neurologic diseases (OND) when tested in ELISA with "standard" criteria for positive reactions.

-Using disrupted and partially purified Adult T-cell leukemia virus as antigen in a particle agglutination test, primarily sensitive for the core proteins of HTLV-1, no antibody-reactivity was observed in sera and CSF samples from the same MS and OND-populations.

-Adjusting the cut off values for increased sensitivity 15 MS CSF samples, 1 OND sera and 2 OND CSF samples were considered positive. However, when all positive samples were tested in a confirmatory Western blot test no antibodies were demonstrable.

-Serial CSF and serum samples were obtained in 9 MS patients with relapsing-remitting course but no indication of HTLV-1 antibodies was found.

REFERENCES
1. Seiki et al.,Proc.Nat.Acad.Sci. USA. 1983. 80:3618-3622.
2. Poser et al.,Ann. Neurol.,1983. 13:2278-231.
3. Ikeda M et al., Gann 1984, 75:845-848.

© 1989 Elsevier Science Publishers B.V. (Biomedical Division)
Recent advances in multiple sclerosis therapy.
R.E. Gonsette, P. Delmotte, editors.

DETECTION OF BRAINSTEM INVOLVEMENT IN MULTIPLE SCLEROSIS: SUPERIORITY OF MRI
VERSUS EVOKED POTENTIALS.

VITTORIO MARTINELLI, GIANCARLO COMI, MASSIMO FILIPPI, MARIA GRAZIA NATALI SORA,
GIUSEPPE MAGNANI, TIZIANA LOCATELLI, ANNA VISCIANI, GIUSEPPE SCOTTI, NICOLA CANAL.

Centro Sclerosi Multipla, Scientific Institute S.Raffaele, University of Milan,
via Olgettina 48, 20132 Milan, Italy.

INTRODUCTION

Several studies have widely confirmed that Nuclear Magnetic Resonance Imaging
(MRI) is superior to multymodality Evoked Potentials (EPs) in detecting brain
lesions in patients with Multiple Sclerosis (MS). However as far as the brainstem
is concerned in a previos study (1) we found that the combined use of Somatosensory Evoked Potentials (SEPs) and Brainstem Auditory Evoked Potentials (BAEPs)
was superior to 1.5 T MRI conventional spin-echo T2 weighted sequence in revealing
MS plaques. The recent application of the Gradient Refocusing Technique, which
suppresses the influence of CSF and vascular motion artifact on MRI sensitivity
resulted in an improvement in image quality. We applied this MRI technique,
combined with BAEPs and median SEPs in the evaluation of the braistem in 30 MS
patients with clinical signs of involvement of this structure in order to re-
evaluate the sensitivity of the two techniques.

PATIENTS AND METHODS

We studied 30 MS patients (21 female and 9 male). According to Mc Donald and
Halliday's criteria (2) they were classified as definite (18), probable (7) or
suspected (5) cases. Mean age was 36.5 years (range 16-67 years). All the patients
had clinical neurological signs of brainstem involvement.

BAEPs and mSEPs were performed bilaterally as previously described (1).
MRI studies were obtained with a 1.5 Tesla magnet in 2 spin echo sequences (TR 2.1
sec., TE 35/120 msec.). Both axial and sagittal slice thickness was 5 mm. Gradient
motion refocusing technique utilizes modifications of gradient waveforms to
eliminate phase shift due to motion that occurs between the 90° pulse and data
collection.

RESULTS

Brainstem MRI lesions were observed in 22 patients (73%): 15/18 definite,
6/7 probable and 1/5 suspected cases. Single brainstem lesions were demonstrated

in 13/22 patients (59%). 5 patients had MRI lesions located in the medulla oblongata, 17 in the pons and 6 in the midbrain. Cerebellar lesions were shown in 9 patients; only one of these patients had a normal brainstem MRI. Supratentorial multiple white matter abnormal areas were found in 24 patients; 2 of these patients had no braistem or cerebellar lesions. Only 1 patient with a single brainstem lesion had normal supratentorial brain MRI.

Median SEPs were abnormal in 9 cases (3 patients were not considered because the P11 or N13 components were absent bilaterally). The median SEP abnormalities were unilateral in 7 patients and bilateral in 2. The P14 and N18 components were absent, respectevely in 2 and in 7 evaluations. The P11-P14 interpeak latency was increased in 3 patients while the P11-N18 interpeak latency was abnormal in only one patient.

BAEPs were abnormal in 9 patients; the abnormalities were unilateral in 2 cases and bilateral in 7. Seven patients had abnormal I-III and III-V IPLs, while two patients had only an increased III-V interpeak latency.

BAEPs and/or mSEPs were abnormal in 12 patients (40%). Comparing the sensitivity between MRI and neurophysiological techniques in detecting brainstem lesions, we can observe a significant superiority of MRI (Table I).

TABLE I

CORRELATION BETWEEN BRAINSTEM MRI AND EPs

	ABNORMAL EPs	NORMAL EPs
ABNORMAL MRI	11*	11*
NORMAL MRI	1	7*

* In 1 patient the mSEPs were not evaluable bilaterally
(absent P11 or N13 components)

DISCUSSION

Our study shows that a thin-slice MRI investigation with the motion artifact suppression technique is far more sensitive than EPs in demonstrating demyelinating brainstem lesions. In fact only one patient with normal brainstem MRI (but with disseminated lesions in the periventricular regions and in the hemispheric white matter) had abnormal BAEPs. On the contrary 11 of the 22 patients with abnormal brainstem MRI had normal neurophysiological tests.

Our patients had a variety of clinical symptoms or signs of brainstem involvement, which in some cases cannot be surely attributable to an isolated focal neurological lesion of the brainstem (i.e. horizontal, upbeat or downbeat nystagmus, vertigo). This is why it is difficult to find a good correlation between clinical features and neurophysiological or MRI abnormalities. On the other hand we found a better correspondance between the clinical picture and the site of MRI lesions in the case of cranial nerve palsies associated or not with long tract signs (6 of the 8 patients with these clinical features had a MRI lesion correctly located).

In our cases MRI lesions were more frequently located in the pons than in the medulla or in the midbrain.

Our results suggest that the use of EPs is obsolete for the demonstration of brainstem lesions in MS patients. However, due to the complementary information of MRI and EPs, both examinations should be used in longitudinal studies in order to demonstrated the appearance of new brainstem plaques.

REFERENCES

1. Comi G, Martinelli V et al: Comparison of sensitivity of Magnetic Resonance Imaging and Evoked Potentials in the detection of brainstem involvement in MS. In Trends in European MS research. Confavreux C, Aimard G, Devic M (eds);(1988) Elsevier Science Publishers: 307-310.

2. McDonald WI, Halliday AM: Diagnosis and classification of MS. (1977) Br. Med. Bull. 33: 4-9.

© 1989 Elsevier Science Publishers B.V. (Biomedical Division)
Recent advances in multiple sclerosis therapy.
R.E. Gonsette, P. Delmotte, editors.

CONCENTRATION-RELATED EFFECTS OF RETINOIC ACID ON LYMPHOPROLIFERATIVE RESPONSE IN EAE

MASSACESI L., SARLO F., CASTIGLI E., VERGELLI M., OLIVOTTO J., RAIMONDI L.*, MEDICA A.* and AMADUCCI L.

Department of Neurology and *Department of Pharmacology, University of Florence, Italy.

Experimental Autoimmune Encephalomyelitis (EAE) is a model of immune mediated disease involving the central nervous system (CNS). We previously described the suppressive activity of the Vitamin A derivative Retinoic Acid (RA) on EAE (1). This non-antimitotic non-cytotoxic agent is extensively studied for its antineoplastic and cell differentiation inducing activity. Moreover, being highly liposoluble, RA easily passes the brain blood barrier (BBB), and seems to suppress delayed type hyperreactivity-mediated immune reaction (2).

We investigated the presence of concentration related effects of RA on lymphocyte proliferative response to Concanavaline A (ConA), assumed as a marker of T cell activation. The study was performed in vitro, adding scalar concentrations of RA to spleen cells harvested from EAE rats. Furthermore, ex vivo activity of RA was evaluated by culturing spleen cells collected from RA-treated EAE rats at different times after the last administration. Spleen cell proliferative response to ConA was correlated to seric levels of RA.

Several _in vitro_ experiments showed a tight relationship between RA concentration and suppression of ConA-induced lymphocyte proliferation, expressed by concentration-response curves which do not differ significantly between them. Such curves have a sigmoidal shape suggesting a non-cytotoxic, possibly receptor-mediated mechanism of action. We observed an optimal inhibiting concentration between 10^{-6} M and 10^{-5} M, and an ID50 of about 10^{-9} M. Similar values were observed for the binding of RA to its intracellular receptor (3).

Proliferative responses to myelin and MBP were similarly influenced by the concentration of RA, even if in a less evident manner.

_Ex_ _vivo_ studies showed a significantly decreased response to

ConA by spleen cells collected from RA-treated EAE rats, in which RA serum concentrations of 5×10^{-6} M or more were determined at killing time by reverse phase HPLC. Such concentrations are comparable to those obtained in the human therapy of some neoplastic diseases (4).

Our data seem to indicate a concentration-related effect of RA in vivo. Maximal suppression of ConA-induced proliferation corresponded to the serum peak of the drug, between 1 and 2 hours after the last administration. In the next hours such suppressive activity decreased as RA serum concentration diminished. This is shown by the marked recovery of proliferative response to ConA. A reversible effect of RA in vivo, due to merely functional lymphocyte suppression, could account for such recovery.

Further indirect evidence of non-antimitotic, non-cytotoxic activity of the drug was obtained adding RA (at a final concentration of 10^{-6} M) to EAE rat lymphocyte cultures, at different culture times. Proliferative response to ConA was markedly reduced adding RA within the first eight hours. If added later, the drug was progressively less effective, until no suppression was observed, in respect to the background, after 40 hours. On the contrary a cytotoxic mechanism of action would have caused suppression of lymphocyte proliferation irrespective of what time RA was added to the cultures. Moreover, since ConA-induced synthesis of DNA begins after about 36 hours (5), these data may suggest that the immunosuppressive activity of RA is not due to inhibition of DNA synthesys, but is carried out, in reversible manner, on the earlier events of lymphocyte activation.

REFERENCES

1. Massacesi L., Abbamondi A.L., Giorgi C., Sarlo F., Lolli F. and Amaducci L. (1987) J. Neurol. Sci., 80:55.
2. Uhr J.W., Weissman G. and Thomas L. (1963), Proc. Exp. Biol. Med., 112:287.
3. Petkovich M., Brand N.J., Krust A. and Chambon P. (1987), Nature, 330:444.
4. Sporn M.B., Roberts A.B., Goodman D.S. (1984) The Retinoids, Academic Press, New York.
5. Ashman R.F. (1984) in Paul W.E., Fundamental Immunology, Raven Press, New York.

© 1989 Elsevier Science Publishers B.V. (Biomedical Division)
Recent advances in multiple sclerosis therapy.
R.E. Gonsette, P. Delmotte, editors.

THE PATTERN OF HANDICAPS IN MULTIPLE SCLEROSIS IN EUROPE

J.M. MINDERHOUD (GRONINGEN), G. GRONNING (BERGEN), R. MIDGARD (MOLDEN), O. FERNANDEZ (MALAGA), S. POSER (GOTTINGEN), K. LAUER (DARMSTADT), W. FIRNHABER (DARMSTADT), G. PALFFY (PECS).

Data from Multiple Sclerosis (MS) patients in centers in Europe were used to describe the patterns of handicaps as can be seen during the course of the disease.

In total the scores on the Expanded Disability Status Scale (EDSS, Kurtzke) and on the Incapacity Status Scale of 1096 patients were used. Handicaps were clustered being "motor", related to "communication", to "bowel, bladder or sexual functions" or regard fatigability (see table 1).

TABLE 1:

CLUSTERS OF HANDICAPS

A.	Motor performance	B.	Communication
1.	stair climbing	8.	vision
2.	ambulation	9.	speech/hearing
3.	transfer	10.	mood and thought
4.	bathing	11.	mentation
5.	dressing		
6.	grooming		
7.	feeding		

C.	Bowel, bladder and sexual functions	D.	Fatigability
12.	bowel functions		
13.	bladder functions		
14.	sexual functions		

It proved that in cases with a low EDSS signs and symptoms were especially related to "communication functions" (vision, speech and hearing, mood and thought and mentation), to bladder disturbances and to fatigability, although the handicaps were low. In case with a higher disability showed more motor handicaps. These were related to arm functions (bathing, dressing, grooming and ambulation and transfer)(fig. 1). Although the pattern of handicaps in patients with a secondary progressive course differed from the pattern of patients with a primary progressive course in cases with a low disability, the patterns of these groups of patients were identical in cases with a high disability (EDSS)(fig. 2).

Slight differences were found between the data form the different participating centers, but in general the pattern through Europe proved to be stable. The results also indicate that Multiple Sclerosis, notwithstanding a variety of signs and symptoms, is one disease.

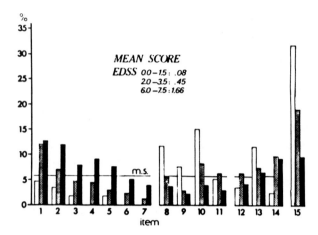

Fig. 1: Relative severity of handicaps in patients with ESS 0.0-1.5, 2.0-3.5 or 6.0-
7.5. Numbers see table 1.

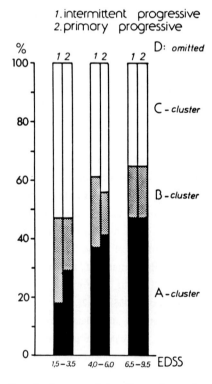

Fig. 2: Relative severity of clusters of handicaps in patients with an intermittent/
progressive course in groups with EDSS 1.5-3.5, 4.0-6.0 and 6.5-9.5. For cluster see
table 1.

© 1989 Elsevier Science Publishers B.V. (Biomedical Division)
Recent advances in multiple sclerosis therapy.
R.E. Gonsette, P. Delmotte, editors.

LEFT-HANDEDNESS AND MULTIPLE SCLEROSIS

THIBAULT MOREAU, ALAIN VIGHETTO, GILBERT AIMARD,
CHRISTIAN CONFAVREUX
Clinique de Neurologie, Hôpital Neurologique,
59, boulevard Pinel, 69003 LYON, FRANCE

Geschwind and Behan (2) postulated that left-handedness and auto-immunity could be associated as testosterone influence simultaneously neuronal development in the left hemisphere and immune maturation. We tested this hypothesis in Multiple Sclerosis (MS) by studying 85 patients with definite (47/85),
probable (22/85) and possible (16/85) MS (Poser classification) (1-4). These patients were compared to 87 normal controls with similar age and sex distribution. A laterality quotient, derived from the Oldfield questionnaire (3) was used. Three categories were defined : strict right-handers (quotient=+100); predominant right-handers (0<quotient<+100); predominant and strict left-handers (-100≤quotient<0). Strict right-handers were more prevalent while predominant right-handers and left-handers were less prevalent among MS patients by comparison with controls. This distribution difference was significant according to the Chi-2 test (X2=10.1; p<0.05). The same trends were observed for each sex and diagnostic classification category of MS patients. Mean laterality quotient was also calculated. It was 90.1 ± 18.6 for MS patients and 72.4 ± 44,3 for controls. The difference was significant (Student test : t=3.42 ; p<0.05). The same tendency was found for males and females.

By contrast with the Geschwind and Behan hypothesis, we did not find the expected over-representation of left-handers in our MS population. Interestingly, these authors reached the same results when studying 118 MS patients. The same was true for Schur (5) in 88 systemic lupus erythematosus patients. If MS is an auto-immune disease, the theory linking auto-immunity and sinistrality is, at least, not generalizable.

382

REFERENCES

1. CONFAVREUX C., AIMARD G., DEVIC M., (1980)
Brain, 8O, 103 : 281-300.

2. GESCHWIND N., BEHAN P. (1982)
Proc. Natl. Acad. Sci USA, 79 : 5 O97-5 100.

3. OLDFIELD R.C. (1971)
Neuropsychologie, 9 : 97-113.

4. POSER CM., PATY DW., SCHNEINBERG L. (1983)
Ann. Neurol. 83, 13 : 227-231.

5. SCHUR P.H. (1986)
Arthritis Rheum 29 : 419-420.

© 1989 Elsevier Science Publishers B.V. (Biomedical Division)
Recent advances in multiple sclerosis therapy.
R.E. Gonsette, P. Delmotte, editors.

LONG-TERM TREATMENT WITH AZATHIOPRINE IN 80 PATIENTS WITH MUL-
TIPLE SCLEROSIS: A RETROSPECTIVE UNCONTROLLED STUDY

KAMIL MÜLLER, KLAUS LAUER, WOLFGANG FIRNHABER
Department of Neurology, Academic Teaching Hospital,Heidel-
berger Landstrasse 379, D-6100 Darmstadt (F.R.G.)

INTRODUCTION

Therapeutical trials of azathioprine in MS revealed conflicting results.In particular, a strong discrepancy between uncontrolled (1,2) and controlled (3,4) studies was evident. As
a contribution to discussion, our experience in patients with
definite or probable MS treated for 2 years or more, shall be
reported.

METHODS

Alltogether, 84 treatment courses with azathioprine (100 mg/
day) in 80 patients (60 intermittent,20 chronic progressive)
were evaluated. Mean duration was 5.5 and mean period of treatment 4.2 years in the intermittent, and 6.3 and 5.9 years, respectively, in the progressive cases. Annual relapse rate,(excluding the first bout marking onset of MS), DSS, and the abilities to walk and to work were compared between pretreatment
and treatment period in our cases, and with published data on
the natural course during comparable periods after onset(5-11).

RESULTS

The mean annual relapse rate declined from 1.12 to 0.52 in the
intermittent cases; it increased again to 0.94 in those 14 patients who finished therapy. The DSS remained fairly stable during treatment (Fig.1),whereas a continuous increase comparable
to the natural course, was observed in progressive cases.No intermittent patient became unable to walk or unable to work during 7 years' treatment, whereas 20% were unable to walk and
63% unable to work in the chronic progressive group after 5 years
therapy, as is to be expected from the natural course.One case
of fatal ovarial carcinoma occurred after 2.5 years of treatment,
corresponding to a rate for female cancers of 0.017.This contrasts
with 0.0018 for the West German female population age 24-44 (odds
ratio 9.6; P <0.05).

384

DISCUSSION

Our findings in the intermittent cases are in agreement with
earlier reports (1,2). Since no fall of the relapse rate was
found in the natural course of MS when the first bout was omitted
(5), our data indicate a favourable effect of azathioprine on the
relapse rate. The fact that the DSS remained constant and the
gap to the natural course became wider in the intermittent,but
closer in the progressive cases, argues in favour of a stabilizing effect also on disability in the former group. This is
confirmed by the absence of severe disability to walk and to work
in intermittent cases after 5-7 years'treatment, whereas chronic
progressive cases developed similarly as reported in the natural
course (6-11). In spite of statistical significance, the small
numerical basis of our cancer data suggests a careful interpretation.

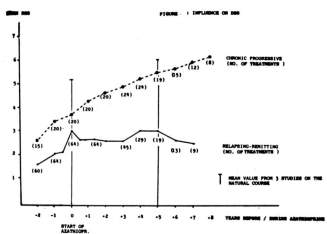

Fig. 1

REFERENCES:
1. Frick E,et al.(1977) Münchn Med Wschr 119:1111-1114
2. Sabouraud O,et al.(1984) Rev.Neurol.140: 125-130
3. Mertin J,et al. (1982) Lancet 2: 351-354
4. Brit.Dutch MS Azathiop.Trial Group (1988) Lancet 2: 179-183
5. Lhermitte F,et al.(1973) J Neurol 205: 47-59
6. Veterans Admin.Study Group (1964)Arch Neurol 11: 583-592
7. Kurtzke JF,et al.(1977) J Chron Dis 30: 819-830
8. Cendrowski W (1986) Arch Suisse Neurol Psychiatr 137:5-13
9. Müller R (1949) Acta Med Scand 133 (Suppl.222) : 1 - 214
10.Müller HR (1961) Deutsch MEd Wschr 86: 1800-1808
11.Lauer K,Firnhaber W (1987) Acta Neurol Scand 76: 12-17

ASTROCYTES OF OPTIC NERVE : MORPHOLOGICAL, IMMUNOCYTOCHEMIICAL AND FUNCTIONAL
PROPERTIES IN LONG-TERM TISSUE CULTURES

FRANCOIS X. OMLIN*, MARIA KIRALY** AND MAURICETTE MAILLARD**
Institutes of Histology*, Embryology* and Physiology**, Faculty of Medicine,
University of Lausanne, Rue du Bugnon, CH - 1005 Lausanne (Switzerland)

INTRODUCTION

The optic nerve offers ideal prerequisites for developmental, functional,
pathological and experimental studies of glia cells; this is documented in a
large body of investigations (1-6). In fact, in situ optic nerves which are free
of neuronal cell bodies, represent in terms of their development, histology and
function a simple but prestigious part of the central nervous system (CNS).

Previously, we elaborated a long-term tissue culture using small pieces of
newborn rat optic nerve, called minisegments, which allow to investigate simultaneously developmental and functional aspects of CNS glia and precursor cells
(7, 8). We have shown that precursor cells differentiate in vitro into functional myelin-forming oligodendrocytes, which appear at day 3 and are present up
to 210 days in vitro, expressing proteins specific for this type of macroglia;
These findings suggest that oligodendrocytes are to a certain degree, neuron-
independent.

In the present in vitro study we attempt to elucidate whether morphological
and immunocytochemical criteria of the other type of glia, the astrocyte,
correlate or not with its functional properties. This is of interest since
interactions between oligodendrocytes and astrocytes could play a key role in
normal development, as well as in aging, degeneration and regeneration of the
CNS.

MATERIAL AND METHODS

Tissue preparation for cultivation: The basic procedure of this tissue culture
system is previously described (7, 8). Briefly, optic nerves (ON) of newborn
Wistar rats were dissected and the meninges removed . In each culture experiment the nerves of 30-50 animals were then cut into small pieces (5-7 per
nerve), called minisegments; over 40 independent dissection experiments and
series of cultures have been carried out. For the present study, minisegments
were kept during 12d up to 7 months as floating explants in a Dulbecco-Vogt
modified Eagle's medium supplemented by 10% FCS (9). At 2-14d intervals,
minisegments were removed from the flask for morphological, immunocytochemical
and electrophysiological investigations.

Single cell recordings and horse radish peroxidase (HRP) labeling: Mini-segments cultured for 40-60d were mounted in a conventional recording chamber which was superfused with prewarmed Krebs solution. Intracellular recordings of 71 single astrocytes were carried out by the use of glass microelectrodes filled with 2M potassium acetate. HRP was then injected into some of these cells by passing depolarizing current pulses of 0.5 nA intensity (10).

Morphological and immunocytochemical methods: For light- and electron micros-copic investigations of minisegments a fixative solution containing 1.5% para-formaldehyde and 0.5% glutaraldehyde in 0.1M phosphate buffer at a pH of 7.6 was used. Postfixation was carried out in 1% osmium tetroxide followed by dehy-dration in ethanol and embedding in Epon. Monoclonal- and polyclonal antibodies recognizing glial fibrillary acidic protein (GFAP) and Vimentin served as immunocytochemical markers of astrocytes. Most of the immunostaining was performed on plastic (1 ym thick) or cryostat (8-13 ym thick) sections obtained from those minisegments, which were used before for intracellular recordings. Both, PAP and immunofluorescence techniques were applied.

RESULTS AND CONCLUDING REMARKS

The most striking difference concerning the cellular organization of an optic nerve minisegment obtained from a newborn rat and cultured during 5d (Fig. 1b) compared to an in situ optic nerve of a 5d old rat (Fig. 1a), is the formation of a compact, well organized *glial tissue* (Fig. 1b and c). This glial tissue is composed of scattered myelinating oligodendrocytes, differentiated astrocytes, phagocytes and progenitor cells. After about 2-3 weeks in culture up to 7 months the cellular organization within the minisegment remains stable. At the peri-pheral part of the explant the following cells are localized: most myelinating oligodendrocytes, some astrocytes and neuron-like cells (the latter appear after 4-5 weeks) (8) and a complex network of loosely communicating cell processes. The compact center is mainly formed by astrocytes and astrocytic processes (Fig. 1c), which frequently are connected to each other with intercellular junctions.

Already at day 3-4 in vitro oligodendrocytes form myelin and the activity of myelination increases up to about 7 months. During this main period of myelin formation in vitro, the functional capabilities of 71 astrocytes have been investigated by the use of microelectrodes. The mean resting membrane potential of these cells was -75 mV (Fig. 2). This value corresponds to that of in situ astrocytes. Following recording, some of the cells were labeled with HRP, which allowed to identify the type of cell using morphological and electron microscopical characteristics (Fig. 3a-c). The fine structure revealed was

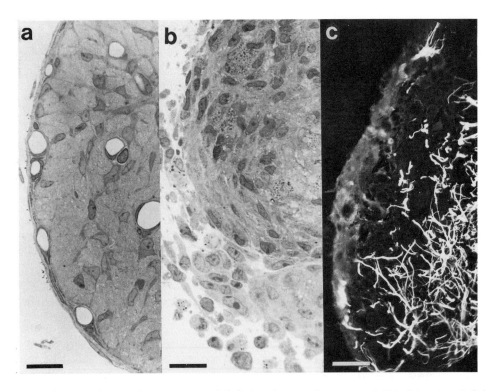

Fig. 1a-c. Light micrographs of (a) in situ optic nerve of 5d-old rat and (b) optic nerve minisegment of newborn rat cultured during 5d. The formation of a glial tissue in vitro is present in both b and c; the latter (50d in vitro) shows astrocytes immunostained with glial fibrillary acidic protein (GFAP) antibodies. Bars: 20 µm.

identical to that of in vivo astrocytes; HRP labeled cells showed long and tiny processes containing bundles of intermediate filaments (Fig. 3c). On serial sections the three dimensional shape of these astrocytes could be determined, some cells showed an extension up to 150 µm.

We suggest that several factors may influence the formation of this *functional glia tissue in vitro*: (i) **Tissue selection and preparation**: The optic nerve of the newborn rat is an anatomically well defined structure, which allows other parts (e.g. brain, mesenchym etc) to be eliminated during dissection, in order to avoid contamination with cells of an other origin (other than the optic

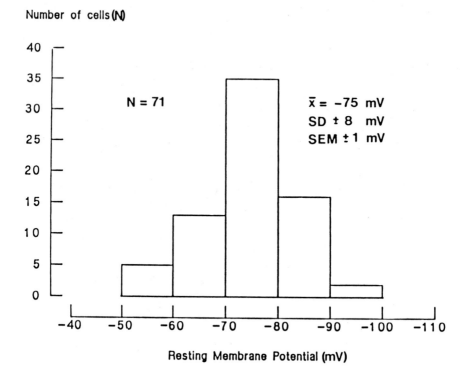

Fig. 2. Histogram showing the distribution of membrane potentials (mV) recorded from 71 single astrocytes, which have been cultured in minisegments during 40-60d.

nerve). About 50-60% of its cells are undifferentiated progenitors; differentiated myelin-forming oligodendrocytes are absent. (ii) **Lack of dissociation and three dimensional organization of cultured cells:** From the beginning of the tissue culture up to the time-point of experimentation (and final tissue fixation) the three-dimensional organization of these cells was respected and the cells maintained it during months in culture forming intercellular junctions. (iii) **Size of minisegments:** Not only the intercellular junctions but also the size of the minisegments (200-250 μm) may allow a well equilibrated exchange of the medium and this permits the cells a very long survival time. (iv) **Fast elimination of cellular debris:** Within the first 2-3d in culture almost all axonal and cell debris within a minisegment is liberated into the

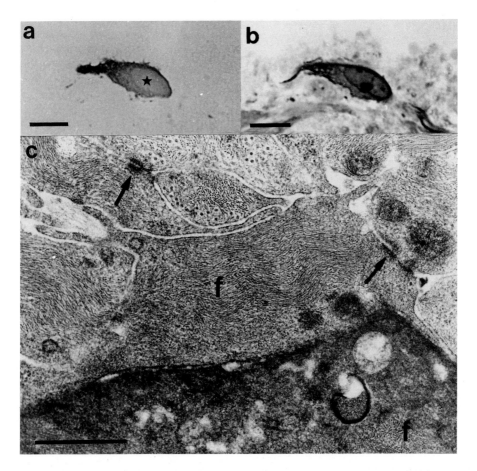

Fig. 3a-c. Light- and electron micrographs of a horse radish peroxidase (HRP*) labeled astrocytes before (a) and after (b) counterstaining. The labeled cell shows both tiny processes filled with bundles of gliafilaments (f) and inter-cellular junctions (arrows, in c). Bars : 10 ɥm in a and b, 0.5 ɥm in c.

medium or eliminated by the phagocytosing activity of cells.

This original optic nerve tissue culture provides a useful and complementary tool to identify and analyze mechanisms, involved in cell-to-cell interactions, which may play a crucial role in processes of degeneration, regeneration and aging.

ACKNOWLEDGEMENTS

Supported by the Swiss MS Society, NSF of Switzerland grants 3100-009237 and 3.258-0.85.

REFERENCES

1. Vaughn JE (1969) Z Zellforsch 94 : 293-324
2. Skoff RP, Price DL, Stocks A (1976) J Comp Neurol 169 : 291-312
3. Tennekoon GI, Cohen SR, Price DL, McKhann GM (1977) J Cell Biol 72: 604-616
4. Juurlink BHJ, Fedoroff S (1980) Dev Biol 78 : 215-221
5. Privat A, Valat J, Fulcrand J (1981) J Neuropath Exp Neurol 40 : 46-60
6. Raff MC (1989) Science 243 : 1450-1455
7. Omlin FX, Waldmeyer J (1986) Exp Brain Res 65 : 189-199
8. Omlin FX, Waldmeyer J (1989) Dev Biol 133 : (in press)
9. Honegger P, Richelson E (1976) Brain Res 109 : 334-354
10. Kiraly M, Maillard M, Omlin FX (1989) Experientia 45 : A19.

© 1989 Elsevier Science Publishers B.V. (Biomedical Division)
Recent advances in multiple sclerosis therapy.
R.E. Gonsette, P. Delmotte, editors.

IMMUNOSUPPRESSANT ACTION IN VITRO

SAMANTHA OWEN AND ALAN DAVISON
Dept of Neurochemistry, Institute of Neurology, London WC1N 3BG, UK

INTRODUCTION

We have proposed that multiple sclerosis (MS) originates within the central nervous system (CNS) (1). Activated lymphocytes bearing IL-2 receptors and producing IL-2 are found close to or within acute lesions and levels of IL-2 receptor positive lymphocytes and IgG in the CSF are elevated in comparison to blood. Glia expressing MHC class II antigens are also found throughout the normal appearing white matter permitting localised antigen presentation. Effective therapy in MS therefore requires immunosuppressants to penetrate into the CNS to prevent local T cell activation and ongoing immune activity within the CNS. One of the most effective but toxic immunosuppressants is cyclophosphamide which enters the brain. Azathioprine is of limited value probably due to its failure to enter the CNS. The potent immunosuppressive cyclosporin A (CsA) which inhibits transcription of mRNA for IL-2 receptors does not affect the level of IL-2 receptor positive lymphocytes in the CSF despite causing a decrease in the blood. Even at relatively high concentrations it fails to penetrate into the CNS and reach the sight of ongoing disease activity (2). Finally methylprednisolone (MPD) is an effective therapy in acute relapse. It penetrates the CNS, however its exact mode of action in MS is unclear. A reduction in oedema, temporary physiological effects on nerve conduction and immunosuppression are all possible mechanisms. The phytohaemmaglutinin (PHA) induced proliferation assay was used to test inhibition of T cell activation.

RESULTS

The inhibitory effect of MPD increased with concentration to a maximum of 500ng/ml where the proliferation was less than 15% of non-treated PHA blasts. FR900506 has much in common with CsA and is more potent (3). Proliferation is reduced by 70% at the lowest concentration of 5ng/ml. Finally mitoxantrone, a novel anthracenodione with antineoplasmic activity suppresses EAE in rats (4). It is a more potent inhibitor of T cell proliferation (Fig 1) and is 3 times more effective than MBP at 10ng/ml. It remains to be shown whether mitoxantrone+FR900506 can suppress immune activity within the CNS.

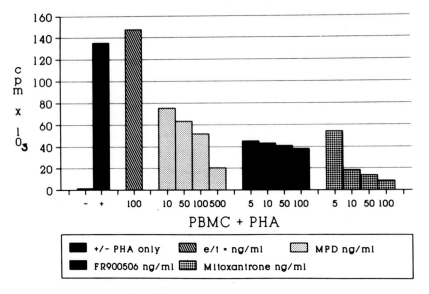

Fig.1. Peripheral blood mononuclear cells (PBMC) were plated out at 2×10^5 cells/well in 96 well plates in 0.1ml aliquots, PHA-P (1μg/ml) and a range of concentrations of the immunosuppressants were added in 0.1ml aliquots. After 72h proliferation was measured by incorporation of ^{3}H-thymidine over the last 8h. Results were mean counts per min (cpm) for triplicate cultures. Stock concentrations of the immunosuppressants were dissolved in 1ml of premixed solvent of 0.8 ml ethanol+0.2ml Tween 80. Further dilution was made in culture medium. The data shown are from a single healthy control sample, comparable results have been obtained from 5 MS patients and 2 other controls.

ACKNOWLEDGEMENTS

Supported by: MS Society; Lederle (Mitoxantrone) and Fujisawa (FR900506).

REFERENCES

1. Calder VL, Owen S, Watson C, Feldmann M, Davison AN (1989) Immunology Today, 10:99-103.

2. Calder VL, Bellamy AS, Owen S, Lewis C, Rudge P, Davison AN, Rudge P (1987) Clin. exp. Immunol. 70:570-577.

3. Sawada S, Suzuki G, Kawase Y, Takaku F (1987) J. Immunol. 139: 1797-1803.

4. Ridge SC, Sloboda AE, McReynolds RA, Levine S, Oronsky AL, Kerwar SS (1985) Clin. Immunol. Immunopath. 35:35-42.

© 1989 Elsevier Science Publishers B.V. (Biomedical Division)
Recent advances in multiple sclerosis therapy.
R.E. Gonsette, P. Delmotte, editors.

QUANTITATIVE EEG AND COGNITIVE PROFILE IN MULTIPLE SCLEROSIS

LUIGI PUGNETTI, *ACHILLE MOTTA, ANNAMARIA CATTANEO, PAOLO BISERNI,

DOMENICO CAPUTO, CARLO L. CAZZULLO, LAURA MENDOZZI

Centro Universitario Sclerosi Multipla "Don Gnocchi", via Capecelatro 66, 20148

Milano, and *Casa di Cura Biffi, via Amati 111, Monza, Italy.

INTRODUCTION

An important link in the neurophysiological study of MS is the absence of
reliable laboratory support to observed cognitive disturbances. Neuroradiologi_
cal images, in fact, do not easily lend themselves to such correlations, while
the new EEG mapping tecniques produce images that are meaningful in terms of
cortical functioning and therefore should be more confidently correlated with
other measures of brain function.

In a recent study on 14 drug-free MS patients, we have shown that patients
who are cognitively impaired have more delta and less alpha than non-impaired
patients, particularly over anterior brain regions (1).

The aim of this study was to extend and replicate these preliminary findings.

MATERIAL AND METHODS

Twenty-seven inpatients with definite MS and three with possible MS according
to McAlpine's criteria were studied (see ref. 1 for inclusion criteria).

Mean age was 30 $\pm$ 9, mean duration of illness was 80 $\pm$ 6 months, mean disabi_
lity score (Kurtzke) was 2.5 $\pm$ 1, female-to-male ratio was 1.1.

The EEG was recorded from 16 scalp electrodes while patients were resting
with eyes closed. Classical spectral parameters were obtained from Fast Fourier
Transformation of 3 minutes of artifact-free EEG, a/d sampled at 128 Hz. Spectral
values were then log-transformed and compared to those of 35 age-matched con_
trols. All patients underwent a complete neuropsychological assessment (NPA) con_
sisting of the Wechsler Adult Intelligence Scale (WAIS) and the Luria-Nebraska
Neuropsychological Battery (LNNB) within one week of the EEG recording. None was
taking psychotropics at the time of evaluations. The NPA scores were also compa_
red with those of age-matched controls. Statistical comparisons were made by
means of parametric univariate tests. To compare topographic EEG distributions
the tecnique of Statistical Probability Mapping (SPM) after Duffy (2) was used.

RESULTS

Quantitative EEG analysis (QEEG) showed that, as a group, MS patients had
significant increases of both absolute and relative EEG power in the delta
(1-4 Hz; $p = .05$) and theta (4-8 Hz; $p = .01$) frequency bands. Mean frequency
of the 1-32 Hz total band was also significantly reduced ($p = .05$). Alpha (8-13
Hz.) was not significantly decreased and slow beta (13-20 Hz.) power was not
significantly increased. The SPM topographic display showed that most involved
were both bi-frontal and the right posterior areas (Fig. 1).

Total MS group verbal, non-verbal and full IQ were significantly lower than
in normal controls ($p = .05$). On the LNNB, MS patients' mean T-scores were
significantly higher than in normals in left frontal and sensorymotor ($p = .04$),

394

right temporal (p = .04) and right parieto-occipital (p = .001). Fourty-eight
percent of the patients had at least two LNNB clinical scales above their
critical level. Using the above criterion for defining impaired patients (3) a
slower EEG (delta and slow alpha) over bitemporal and right posterior areas
(p = .05) was found in relation to the presence of a cognitive deficit. Impaired
patients showed significant elevations on the following LNNB localization scales
T-scores: right temporal (p = .009), right parieto-occipital (p = .01) and both
right and left frontal (p = .01).

Topographic Mapping

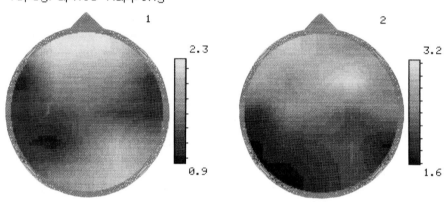

Fig. 1. Statistical Probability Maps. The two maps show the topographic
distribution of t-test differences between MS patients (n.=30) and matched
healthy controls (n.=35) for the relative Delta EEG power (left) and the
relative Theta power (right).

Quantitative EEG findings confirm our previous report dealing with a smaller
patients' group (1). We consider the good concordance between LNNB and QEEG
findings at a statistically descriptive level as a confirmation of each respec_
tive contribution, and as a tool for generating future hypotheses on the nature
of the cognitive dysfunction in MS.

REFERENCES
1. Pugnetti L., Mendozzi L., Cattaneo A.M., Biserni P., Hafele E., Caputo D.,
   Sinatra M.G., Cazzullo C.L. (1989) In: Proceedings of the International
   Multiple Sclerosis Conference. Monduzzi Editore, Bologna.

2. Duffy F.H., Burchfiel J.L., Lombroso C. (1979) Ann Neurol 5:309-321

3. Golden C.J., Hammeke T.A., Purish A.D. (1980) Manual for the Luria Nebraska
   Neuropsychological Battery. Los Angeles Psychological Service.

© 1989 Elsevier Science Publishers B.V. (Biomedical Division)
Recent advances in multiple sclerosis therapy.
R.E. Gonsette, P. Delmotte, editors.

BRAIN BANKING IN MULTIPLE SCLEROSIS; THE BRIDGE BETWEEN CLINIC AND ANIMAL MODELS

RIVKA RAVID AND DICK.F. SWAAB

The Netherlands Brain Bank, Meibergdreef 33, 1105 AZ Amsterdam ZO (The Netherlands).

Brain bank organizations for various neurological diseases serve at present more and more as an important link between the clinician and the basic scientist who needs brain tissue specimens; they support medical research that seeks means for diagnosis, causes. and develops treatments for devastating diseases.

Experimental allergic encephalomyelitis (EAE) can serve as a good example in order to illustrate how brain banking in multiple sclerosis (MS) can serve as a bridge between the clinic and the animal model. EAE resembles MS in many aspects; one of the more popular hypotheses about the pathogenesis of MS, but not necessarily the correct one, is that MS is an auto-immune-disease, similar to EAE. There is though at least one crucial difference; the immunological mechanism producing EAE, delayed hypersensitivity, can be suppressed by corticosteroids or immunosupressive drugs, which is unfortunately not the case for MS-patients.

In order to be able to explore the similarities and differences between EAE and MS, one needs to have access to post-mortem human brain tissue of MS patients as well as cerebro-spinal-fluid (CSF) samples of these patients. However, at present these facilities are not readily available in the Netherlands whereas there is an increasing demand from many research groups to be able to investigate brain tissue of MS-patients.

We are currently aiming at organizing a brain bank for MS tissues, similar to the readily functioning Alzheimer's Disease Brain Bank, that will collect, store and distribute brain tissue of donors, MS-patients and control subjects who have willed their brain for scientific research. This brain bank should be internationally oriented and distribute the collected brain specimens to various research groups and exchange techniques, knowledge and material with other brain banks.

All tissue used should come from well-documented clinical cases and be confirmed by neuropathological examination. In addition, a collection of ante- and post-mortem CSF samples will be initiated. The brain bank will be based upon research proposals submitted in advance, specifying a variety of requirements such as: total number of brains needed, kind of tissue (fixed or fresh) post-mortem delay, anatomical boundaries of the brain region and subsequently treatment requirements of the tissues.

This brain bank will have two unique features:

1. MS brain tissue will be obtained mainly by means of rapid autopsies with a very short post-mortem delay, between 2-4 hours.

2. Fresh brain tissue dissection procedure will be used; this is necessary for the immediate use of brain tissue and advantageous in increasing the range of morphological, neurochemical, immunocytochemical, metabolic and other procedures which can be applied on this tissue.

Vital support would come from the fascilities and knowledge already available in the Alzheimer's Disease Brain Bank, such as:

1. procedure for rapid autopsies;

2. neuropathological examination;

3. the use of the same controls;

4. contacts with nursing homes;

5. active membership in Eurage subgroups on tissue banking and diagnostic criteria, and international scientific cooperation. In this way better exchange of material, knowledge and information can be achieved.

The infrastrucure described in the present paper enabled the Netherlands Brain Bank to function efficiently; in the past three years this bank supplied 107 Alzheimer brains and 131 control brains to 37 different research groups in Europe and in the U.S.A.

For information:
Dr. R. Ravid
The Netherlands Brain Bank
Meibergdreef 33, 1105 AZ Amsterdam ZO
Telephone: 31-20-5665500
Fax: : 31-20-5664440

© 1989 Elsevier Science Publishers B.V. (Biomedical Division)
Recent advances in multiple sclerosis therapy.
R.E. Gonsette, P. Delmotte, editors.

SIGNIFICANCE OF MAGNETIC COIL POSITION IN PERIPHERAL MOTOR-EVOKED-
POTENTIAL RECORDING

MADS RAVNBORG, MORTEN BLINKENBERG, KRISTIAN DAHL*
Departments of Neurology and *Clinical Neurophysiology,
Rigshospitalet, Copenhagen, Denmark

INTRODUCTION

The latencies of compound motor action potentials (CMAPs) evoked
by magnetic stimulation of the cerebral cortex and the spinal roots
can be used for estimation of the central motor conduction velocity. Thus, the method may be of value for objective assessment of
motor functions in multiple sclerosis. However, before the method
can be used for clinical routine it must be standardized.

Stimulation with a magnetic coil, usually 10-14 cm in diameter,
makes definite localization of the depolarization difficult. We
made this study **to define the optimal position of the magnetic
coil** in relation to **a peripheral nerve**, searching for the most constant relationship to the electrically evoked CMAP. Having found
this coil position, we compared the **reproducibility of magnetically
evoked CMAPs** with those obtained by electric stimulation.

MATERIAL AND METHODS

10 healthy volunteers participated in the study. A Dantec magnetic stimulator was used (Dantec, Copenhagen). The outer diameter
of the stimulating coil is 14 cm. 7 lines were drawn on the coil
with 1 cm intervals from the center (L-0) to the outer rim (L-6).
The recordings were made with a Counterpoint (Dantec, Copenhagen).
An surface electrode was fixed over the **1st dorsal interosseus
muscle.** The neurovascular bundle in the medial bicipital groove
was localized by palpation, and the course of **the brachial segment
of the ulnar nerve** was marked on the skin. On this nerve line a
point, 14 cm above the medial epicondyle, was indicated and defined as the stimulation point. CMAPs evoked by supramaximal electrical cathode stimulations were recorded.

The magnetic coil was placed on the skin with the center line
(L-0) over and parallel to the line indicating the ulnar nerve
with the center of the coil at the stimulation point. CMAPs were
recorded from threshold to 100% SI at 10% intervals. This procedure was repeated as the coil was displaced parallelly in 1 cm

steps in lateral direction.

The full procedure was repeated with PVC plates of 1 cm, 2 cm
and 3 cm thickness interposed between coil and skin.
Using the optimal coil position, the intraindividual variations
of the CMAPs were analyzed in 2 persons.

RESULTS

Stimulation with the coil center positioned 3 cm laterally to
the nerve yielded the largest amplituted. With minimal variability
and latencies with the most constant relationship to electrically
evoked CMAPs. In this position the inter- and intraindividual
variations of the magnetic evoked latencies were smaller than
those of electric stimulation when coil-skin distance was $\leq$ 2 cm.

CONCLUSION

Magnetic stimulation of nervous tissue involves more variables
than the traditional electric stimulation, and our results
emphasize the importance of standardization of these variables.
If standardized, CMAP latencies evoked by magnetic stimulations
of peripheral nerves seem as reproducible as those obtained by
electric stimulation.

© 1989 Elsevier Science Publishers B.V. (Biomedical Division)
Recent advances in multiple sclerosis therapy.
R.E. Gonsette, P. Delmotte, editors.

EFFECT OF HORMONES ON EXPERIMENTAL ALLERGIC ENCEPHALOMYELITIS (EAE)
a preliminary study of a hormonal therapy for Multiple Sclerosis

W.J.TROOSTER, A.W.TEELKEN, J.PUISTER, J.G.LOOF, P.VERNIMMEN,
J.KAMPINGA* and J.M.MINDERHOUD.
Dept. of Neurology;*:Dept. of Histology, University Hospital,
Groningen, The Netherlands.

INTRODUCTION
In Multiple Sclerosis (MS) changes in the levels of some hormones are correlated to changes in the clinical manifestations of the disease. This is for instance apparent in the period during and following pregnancy. In addition other data indicate MS to be the result of a wrong function of the immune system (auto-immunity), while further it is known that hormones influence the action of the immune system. So a hormonal therapy in the treatment of MS may be considered. In this study the effect of application of the synthetic sex-hormone 17-alpha-ethynylestradiol is investigated in EAE, an animal model of MS.

METHODS
Acute EAE was induced in 10 female Lewis rats (170-190 gr.) by immunization with 50 ul of an emulsion,consisting of a homogenate of 1 gr. guinea pig spinal cord in 1 ml. saline, 1 ml. Complete Freund's Adjuvans and 10mg. Mycobacterium tuberculosum. This emulsion was injected intradermally in the left hind foot.
From five days before immunization 5 of the animals received daily orally 0.5 ml. of a suspension of 10 ug. 17-alpha-ethynylestradiol/ml. maize oil. Five control animals received only 0.5 ml. maize oil during the same period.
Investigated was the repression of clinical manifestations of EAE by this hormone. All animals were evaluated daily by a clinical rating scale (table 1).

TABLE 1
CLINICAL RATING SCALE FOR EAE

Grade 0: Well,no signs.
     1: Weakness of the hind limbs, weight loss, no definite neurological disease
     2: Paralysis of the tail
     3: Paralysis of the tail and spasticity of the hind limbs
     4: Paralysis of the tail, paresis of the hind limbs
     5: Paralysis of the tail, paralysis of the hind limbs

The leucocytes and T-lymphocytes in the peripheral blood of the control rats and of the rats treated with the hormone were compared. The leucocytes were counted with a Coulter Counter. Ratio's of (sub)sets of T-lymphocytes were determined by two-color immunofluorescence using a fluorescence-microscope. Especially the T4/T-ratio of lymphocytes was investigated. In addition a subset of T4-lymphocytes was studied containing the marker OX22. Presumably the OX22+ subset of T4+ cells consists of suppressor-inducer cells and the OX22- T4+cells represent a helper-inducer subset (1,3).
The spinal cord infiltrates were investigated in control rats and rats treated with the hormone.Histological paraffin sections of the thoracic spinal cord were cut at 15 um. and stained according to May-Grunwald.

RESULTS

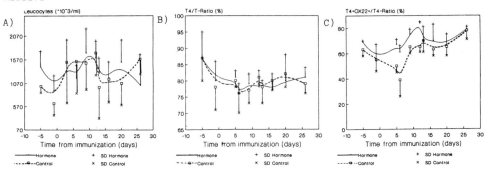

400

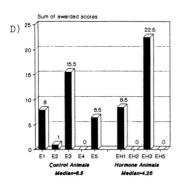

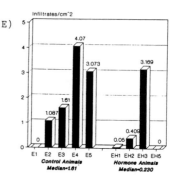

Fig.1. The effect of 17-alpha-ethynylestradiol on: A The number of leucocytes;
B The T4/T-ratio;C The T4+OX22+/T4-ratio;D The clinical manifestation of
EAE;E The infiltration into the spinal cord.

DISCUSSION
 In control rats and rats treated with 17-alpha-ethynylestradiol the amount of
leucocytes rised to a maximal value at +/- day 10 after the induction of EAE. From
this time the amount decreased back to normal (fig.1A).
 Both the course of the amount of leucocytes and the course of the T4/T-ratio did
not differ significantly for the control rats and the rats treated with the
hormone (fig.1B).
 A significant difference was achieved by the hormone in the T4+OX22+/T4-ratio. In
the control rats a temporary decrease of this ratio was found at +/- day 6
(fig.1C). This relative loss of suppressor-inducer function that was found in the
control rats was prevented by 17-alpha-ethynylestradiol. By this mechanism this
hormone probably counteracted a loss of suppression of the immune system.
 The human analogue of the OX22 marker is the CD45R marker (1). Interestingly in
the peripheral blood and CNS lesions of MS patients decreases of the
CD4+CD45R+/CD4-ratio have been found that may correlate negatively with the
disease activity (2,3,4). Therefore a study of 17-alpha-ethynylestradiol in MS
would be interesting.
 Some such study is warranted the more so as in rats treated with this sex-hormone
the clinical manifestations of EAE were repressed, compared to the control rats
(fig.1D). Moreover the amount of infiltrates in the thoracic spinal cord in rats
treated with hormone was lower than in control rats (fig.1E). Yet these last two
differences were not significant.
 In the literature (5) however a significant repression of the clinical
manifestations of EAE and significant less infiltrates in the spinal cord have
been reported in rats after similar application of 17-alpha-ethynylestradiol.
Probably this significance can be reached by using more animals and a more severe
EAE model.
 This investigation is a preliminary study within the scope of a series
experiments for the development of a therapy of MS, based on sex-hormones.

REFERENCES

1. Powrie F,Mason D (1988).Phenotypic and functional heterogeneity of CD4+
   T-cells. Immunol.Today 9(9):274-277.

2. Rose LM, Ginsberg AH, Rothstein TL et al. (1988). Fluctuations of CD4+ T-cell
   subsets in remitting-relapsing Multiple Sclerosis. Ann.Neurol. 24:192-199.

3. Morimoto C,Hafler DA,Weiner HL et al. (1987). Selective loss of the
   suppressor-inducer T-cell subset in progressive Multiple Sclerosis: Analysis with
   anti-2H4 monoclonal antibody. N.Eng.J.Med. 316(2):67-72.

4. Sobel RA,Hafler DA,Castro EE et al. (1988). The 2H4 (CD45R) antigen is
   selectively decreased in Multiple Sclerosis lesions. J.Immunol. 140(7):2210-2214.

5. Arnason BG, Richman DP (1969).Effect of oral contraceptives on experimental
   demyelinating disease. Arch.Neurol. 21:103-108.

© 1989 Elsevier Science Publishers B.V. (Biomedical Division)
Recent advances in multiple sclerosis therapy.
R.E. Gonsette, P. Delmotte, editors.

TO PATHOGENESIS OF MULTIPLE SCLEROSIS: LOSS OF GLIAL PROGENITOR CELLS SPECIFIC ANTIGEN IN MULTIPLE SCLEROSIS PLAQUES

KRYSTYNA WARECKA
Neurological Department, University of Lübeck, Fed. Rep. Germany

INTRODUCTION

It is not too much known about immuno-biochemical and morphological events preceding the formation of plaques in the CNS tissue in
case of multiple sclerosis (MS). Little is known how far the grade
and the timing of the arised pathological changes depends from the
genetic information and/or from secondary events, respectively
how strong is the reciprocal dependency and how far each component could be manipulated.

METHODS

This work presents data on a CNS-glia-specific glycoprotein,
which was isolated originally from normal human brain tissue by affinity chromatography and CON A Sepharose. This glycoprotein is water soluble, has a MW 45.000 and a relatively high content of NANA.
This glycoprotein is a strong antigen (methods see references 1-6).

RESULTS

This glia-specific glycoprotein could be found in lower mammals
in the range from Macaca Mulatta to the mouse, in human embryonic
and fetal brain as well as in a child brain, nevertheless in an
"abortive" or in a non mature, respectively fetal form. So, altogether these experiments illustrate, firstly, the phylogenetic development of this glycoprotein, secondly, it shows that the phyloge-
nesis reproduces the ontogenesis.
The concentration of the glia specific glycoprotein, which is a
sum of the two components i.e. of the fetal and adult form, increases during the period of myelination and remains quite constant thereafter. The "fetal form" of the glycoprotein remains
in the adult brain the whole life through. In the contrary, the
fetal brain contains some amount of "adult protein": the each-
other-relation is age dependent.

Previous immuno-cytochemical studies on E.M. clearly showed that
astrocytes rather than oligodendroglia were labeled with specific
antibodies directed against this glycoprotein. It was concluded
that the antigen represents an index of astrocytes maturation or
its degree of differentiation.

Investigations on multiple sclerosis brain tissue show that this
glial marker disappears in MS-plaques. On the junction between
brain tissue and plaques the amount of this glycoprotein decreases as well in the so-called normal tissue of MS-brain.
In the cultures of brain cells of new-born rats (immunocytochemical techniques) an expression of this glycoprotein could be shown
in precursors of glial cells. These precursor cells develop into
astrocytes type II or to oligodendrocytes as based on our experiments with A2B5.

CONCLUSIONS

The results of our experiments carried out with human brain tissue as well with new-born rat brain cells in cultures confirmed once more the in last years described facts, that astrocytes and oligodendrocytes are vivid cells with their own metabolism and with a high degree of plasticity, i.e. for instance, oligodendrocytes can transform into astrocytes under specific conditions and are susceptible to alterations of the environment. This means as well, that they could be manipulated resp. influenced. It was stated, that the fetal form of this glycoprotein , which possibly corresponds to precursor glial cells, remains for the whole life in adult human brain. Recent experiments are in agreement with these findings. So it could be assumed, that the absence of this glycoprotein could alter the course of normal development of astrocytes and/or oligodendrocytes to maintain myelin throughout the life span. Concerning multiple sclerosis it could be said, that this glycoprotein decreases in quantity consecutively to the following sequence: "normal" multiple sclerosis brain tissue; junction between this tissue and MS-plaque; and MS-plaque itself. In some MS- plaques no traces of the glycoprotein could be found.

OUTLOOK

It seems necessary to demonstrate, that a damage of precursor glial cells presenting this glycoprotein, prevents at least a local myelin synthesis or otherwise it has to be shown, by which way to manipulate the cultures of the progenitor glial cells in order to bring them to myelination

REFERENCES

1. Tripatzis I, Warecka K, Man-Chung Wong (1971) Nature (London) 230: 250-252

2. Warecka K, Möller HJ, Vogel HM, Tripatzis I (1972) J Neurochem 19: 719-725

3. Brunngraber EG, Susz JP, Warecka K (1974) J Neurochem 22: 181-182

4. Ghandour MS, Langley OK, Gombos G, Vincendon G, Warecka K (1982) Neuroscience 7: 231-237

5. Langley OK, Ghandour MS, Vincendon G, Gombos G, Warecka K (1982) J Neuroimmunol 2: 131-143

6. Bhat NR, Arimoto K, Warecka K, Brunngraber EG (1986) Dev. Brain Res 29: 31-36

© 1989 Elsevier Science Publishers B.V. (Biomedical Division)
Recent advances in multiple sclerosis therapy.
R.E. Gonsette, P. Delmotte, editors.

IN VITRO STUDIES OF DEMYELINATION

CAROLYN WATSON, SAMANTHA OWEN AND ALAN DAVISON
Department of Neurochemistry, Institute of Neurology, Queen Square,
London WC1N 3BG, UK

INTRODUCTION

Measurement of 2':3'-cyclic nucleotide 3' phosphodiesterase
(CNPase;EC 3.1.4.37) activity in cell free myelin preparations
provides the basis for a simple and reliable model for the study of
myelin lysis in vitro (1). In experimental allergic encephalomyelitis there is evidence that myelin basic protein (MBP) reactive T
cells can mediate demyelination, however, the precise mechanism of
demyelination is uncertain. The role of MBP primed lymph node
cells (MBP LNC) in initiating myelin degradation was studied.

MATERIALS AND METHODS

Cells. Balb/c mice were injected subcutaneously with 200μg MBP
emulsified in complete Freund's adjuvant. 7-10 days post-inoculat-
ion MBP LNC were prepared from the axillary and inguinal lymph
nodes. Adherent peritoneal exudate cells (ADH) were prepared as
described in (1).

Demyelination assay. MBP LNC with ADH (20:1 ratio LNC:ADH) were
set up in culture with either MBP (1μg/ml) or PHA (1μg/ml) then
each day, for up to 5 days, cells and supernatants (SNT) were
tested for their ability to degrade myelin in vitro following the
protocol in (1). Myelin degradation was expressed as % loss
CNPase (myelin incubated with cells/myelin incubated without cells
x 100).

BLT esterase assay. BLT esterase activity was measured (2) in
MBP LNC lysates and SNTs. 1 unit enzyme activity = absorbance of
1.0. All BLT esterase activity was expressed as units BLT
esterase/1×10^6 LNC.

RESULTS AND CONCLUSIONS

1. MBP LNC degrade myelin in vitro (Fig 1A). Insufficient ADH
were present to cause this effect on their own (1). 2. A soluble
factor(s) released by MBP LNC appears to be involved (Fig 1A).
3. There is no correlation between observed myelin degradation
and BLT esterase activity (Fig 1B).

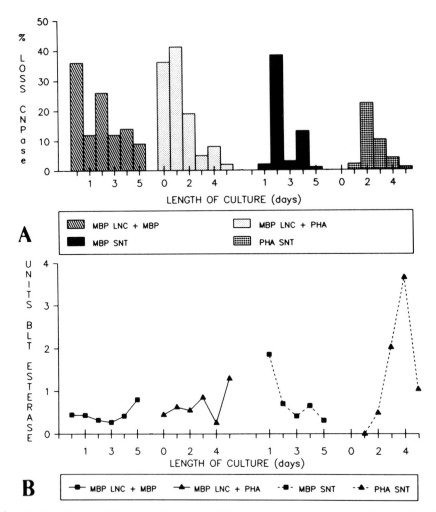

Fig 1A Loss of CNPase following 24h incubation of myelin with MBP LNC (2x10⁵ LNC/10μg myelin protein) or SNT from MBP LNC (75% SNT/ 10μg myelin protein) after 0-5 days culture with either MBP (1μg/ml) or PHA (1μg/ml).
Fig 1B BLT esterase activity detected in MBP LNC lysate or SNT at the start of the incubation with myelin.

ACKNOWLEDGEMENTS

This work was supported by the MS Society of Great Britain.

REFERENCES

1. Watson CM, Najbauer J, Owen SJ, Davison AN (1988) J. Neurochem. 50:1469-1477.

2. Coleman PL, Green DJ (1981) Methods Enzymol 80:408-414.

© 1989 Elsevier Science Publishers B.V. (Biomedical Division)
Recent advances in multiple sclerosis therapy.
R.E. Gonsette, P. Delmotte, editors.

In vitro functional blocking of Myelin Basic Protein-specific cytolytic human T lymphocyte clones by immunosuppressives and monoclonal antibodies

Wim E.J. Weber1,2, Marc M.P.P. Vandermeeren1, Jef C.M. Raus1 and Wim A. Buurman3

From the 1Dept. of Immunology, Dr.L.Willemsinstitute, Diepenbeek, Belgium, depts. of 2Neurology and 3General Surgery, Academic Hospital Maastricht, University Limburg, Maastricht, The Netherlands.

Cellullar immune responses against Myelin Basic Protein (MBP), a major protein constituent of the neuronal myelin sheath are held responsible for the occurrence of postinfectious and postvaccination encephalomyelitis. In animals, as SJL/J mice and Lewis rats, experimental auto-immune encephalomyelitis (EAE) has been proven to be transferable by MBP-specific helper-independent MHC Class II-restricted cytotoxic T lymphocyte clones. MBP-sensitized T lymphocytes have also been implicated in the pathogenesis of Multiple Sclerosis (MS).

From several MS patients, we recently isolated and generated as long-term cell lines, MBP-specific CD4+ cytolytic T lymphocyte clones expressing a number of MBP-specific T cell functions, including proliferation, cytolysis, and production of Interferon-g (IFN-g) (Weber and Buurman 1988). In the present study we report the effects of prednisolon, Cyclosporin A, and anti-T lymphocyte monoclonal antibodies on the functions of two auto-immune MBP-specific CTL clones derived from two different MS patients.

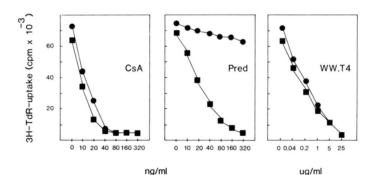

Fig. 1. Effects on MBP-specific proliferation by clone JVA16.4. Proliferation was measured in microcultures with (●) and without exogenously added IL2 (■). Each point is based on the mean of quadruplicate microwells (standard deviation was < 5%). Experiments with clone AH.F4 gave similar results (data not shown).

As can be seen from fig. 1, both CsA and Pred inhibited antigen-specific proliferation of the two auto-immune MBP-specific T cell clones tested in a 4 days-assay. Addition of exogeneous r-IL2 (100 U/ml) at the beginning of the culture could overcome the blocking effect of Pred, but had almost no effect on blocking by CsA and WW.T4.

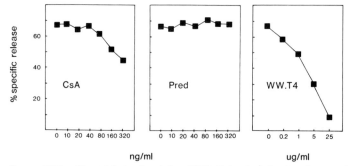

Fig. 2. Direct effects on MBP-specific cytolytic function of clone AH.F4. Each point is based on the mean of quadruplicate microwells (standard deviation was < 8%). Maximum release was always > 7 times spontaneous release. Cytolytic functions of clone JVA16.4 were affected in a similar mode.

The effect of the drugs and MAbs on the in vitro activation of MBP-specific CTL function was tested in a 7 day culture system. To this end, clone cells were incubated with MBP and irradiated autologous presenting cells (without exogeneously added IL2) for 7 days as described with the indicated amounts of drugs or MAbs. Cells were harvested and washed several times, counted by trypan blue dye exclusion test and used as effector cells in the cytolysis-assay. CsA decreased cytolytic effector functions by both T cell clones after 7 days of culture. At concentrations higher than 80 ng/ml almost no effector cells were generated in the 7 day culture period (Fig. 3). Pred did not affect the induction of CTL function in both MBP-specific T cell clones. WW.T4, in contrast, did decrease the induction of cytotoxic function in both T cell clones, as given in fig. 3.

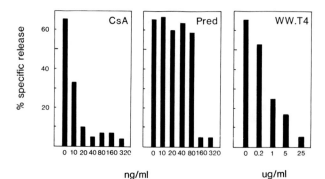

Fig. 3. Effects on generation of MBP-specific function in a 7-day culture period studied on clone JVA16.4. Each column is based on the mean of quadruplicate microwells (standard deviation was < 5%). Experiments on clone AH.F4 gave similar results.

Weber, W.E.J., and W.A. Buurman. 1988. Human Myelin Basic Protein-specific CD4+ cytolytic T lymphocyte clones isolated from Multiple Sclerosis patients. Hum. Immunol.22 : 94.
Weber, W.E.J., and W.A. Buurman. 1989. In vitro functional blocking of Myelin Basic Protein-specific cytolytic human T lymphocyte clones by immunosuppressives and monoclonal antibodies. J. Neuroimmunol. 22 : 1.

A METHOD FOR ESTIMATING THE LATENT PERIOD OF MULTIPLE SCLEROSIS

CHRISTINA WOLFSON, DAVID B. WOLFSON, JAN M ZIELINSKI
Department of Epidemiology and Biostatistics and Mathematics and
Statistics, McGill University, 1020 Pine Avenue West, Montreal,
Quebec H3A 1A2 CANADA

A widely accepted hypothesis is that Multiple Sclerosis is
the result of a childhood infection with a long period between
disease initiation and clinical onset of symptoms. Currently
very little is known about the interval between initiation and
onset (the latent period). The results of migrant studies have
led researchers to propose that there is a susceptibility period
somewhere between birth and adolescence (most commonly taken to
be age 15) within which disease initiation takes place. Ranges
of susceptibility considered are 0-5 years, 5-10 years, 10-15,
5-15, and 0-15 years. Migrant studies in MS have been the source
of many attempts to study the latent period of the disease.
Efforts have been invariably directed towards estimating the
mean, the median and the support of the distribution of the
latent period. The methods used have been ad hoc and have not
depended on any mathematical model describing the natural history
of MS (1-3), resulting in a wide range of estimates for the mean
latent period from five years (3) to over twenty years (4). In
the migrant studies, the time of disease initiation for an
individual is often taken arbitrarily to be the age at migration.
In this paper a more systematic approach to the investigation of
the latent period is proposed.

METHODS

The approach is to model the ages of onset of MS as the
times that customers exit from an infinite server queue (5, 6).
The input stream is taken to follow a nonhomogeneous Poisson
process. In this setting the estimation of the latent period
distribution is equivalent to the estimation of the service time
distribution. The service time (latent period) distribution was
estimated both parametrically (i.e. fit to known distributions)
as well as non-parametrically, for all susceptibility periods
considered.

RESULTS

The data consisted of approximate ages of onset of 528 patients under care at the Multiple Sclerosis Clinic of the Montreal Neurological Institute. The average age at onset was 30.34 years. In all cases where a susceptibility period of 10 years or more was considered, (i.e. 0-10 years, 5-15 years, and 0-15 years), the estimated latent period distributions were multi-modal and, as such, are unlikely candidates for the true distribution. The remaining candidate susceptibility periods are 0-5 years and 10-15 years, both of which result in reasonable unimodal latent period distributions. Both the chi-square and log-normal parametric estimators produce estimated modes for the onset intensity of around 20 years when the former susceptibility period is used. This contradicts values obtained in the literature which are most often between 25 and 35 years (7). On the other hand both the chi-square and log-normal estimators yield estimated modes for the onset intensity of about 30 years when the 10-15 year susceptibility is used, consistent with most age-specific incidence rate curves. The estimated mean and median for the latent period distribution corresponding to the 10-15 year susceptibility period are 18.08 years and 16 years respectively.

DISCUSSION

This work offers a new and more sophisticated approach to the study of the latent period of MS than has been previously attempted. Our research leads us to seriously consider that the most likely susceptibility period is between the ages of 10 and 15 years. This period has also been suggested by the results of migrant studies using a variety of approaches.

1. Kurtzke JF, Beebe GW, Norman JE (1985). Neurol. 35:672-676.
2. Atler M, Kahana E, Loewenson R (1978). Neurol. 28:1089-1093.
3. Fischman HR (1981). AJE. 114:244-252.
4. Schapira K, Poskanzer DC, Miller H (1963). Brain. 86:315-332.
5. Newell GF (1966). J Siam Appl Math. 14:86-88.
6. Clarkson DB, Wolfson DB (1983). Stat Neer. 37:21-28.
7. Acheson ED (1972). In: McAlpine D, Lumsden CE, Acheson ED, eds. Multiple Sclerosis: A reappraisal. Livingston, Edinburgh, pp. 42-80.

INDEX OF AUTHORS

410